362.1 SHE

D0320898

Providing Compassionate Healthcare

Despite the scope and sophistication of contemporary health care, there is increasing international concern about the perceived lack of compassion in its delivery. Citing evidence that when the basic needs of patients are attended to with kindness and understanding, recovery often takes place at a faster level, patients cope more effectively with the self-management of chronic disorders and can more easily overcome anxiety associated with various disorders, this book looks at how good care can be put back into the process of caring.

Beginning with an introduction to the historical values associated with the concept of compassion, the text goes on to provide a bio-psycho-social theoretical framework within which the concept might be further explained. The third part presents thought-provoking case studies and explores the implementation and impact of compassion in a range of healthcare settings. The fourth part investigates the role that organizations and their structures can play in promoting or hindering the provision of compassion. The book concludes by discussing how compassion may be taught and evaluated, and suggesting ways for increasing the attention paid to compassion in health care.

Developing a multi-disciplinary theory of compassionate care, and underpinned by empirical examples of good practice, this volume is a valuable resource for all those interesting in understanding and supporting compassion in health care, including advanced students, academics and practitioners within medicine, nursing, psychology, allied health, sociology and philosophy.

Sue Shea is a Psychologist and Researcher working with the University of Crete, Greece, and as an independent consultant with various UK institutions.

Robin Wynyard is Visiting Research Fellow in Education at the University of Derby, UK.

Christos Lionis is Professor of General Practice and Director of the Clinic of Social and Family Medicine, University of Crete, Greece.

Routledge Advances in Health and Social Policy

New titles

Health Care Reform and Globalisation
The US, China and Europe in comparative perspective
Edited by Peggy Watson

Power and Welfare
Understanding citizens' encounters with state welfare
Nanna Mik-Meyer and Kaspar Villadsen

International Perspectives on Elder Abuse
Amanda Phelan

Mental Health Services for Vulnerable Children and Young People
Supporting children who are, or have been, in foster care
Michael Tarren-Sweeney and Arlene Vetere

Providing Compassionate Healthcare
Challenges in policy and practice
Edited by Sue Shea, Robin Wynyard and Christos Lionis

Teen Pregnancy and Parenting
Rethinking the myths and misperceptions
Keri Weed, Jody S. Nicholson and Jaelyn R. Farris

Forthcoming titles

M-Health in Developing Countries
Design and implementation perspectives on using mobiles in healthcare
Arul Chib

Alcohol Policy in Europe
Delivering the WHO ideal?
Shane Butler, Karen Elmeland, Betsy Thom and James Nicholls

The Invisible Work of Nursing
Organising work and health service delivery in hospitals
Davina Allen

Innovation in Social Welfare and Human Services
Rolf Rønning and Marcus Knutagard

International Perspectives on Support for Trafficked Women
Developing a model for service provision
Delia Rambaldini-Gooding

Maternity Services and Policy in an International Context
Risk, citizenship and welfare regimes
Edited by Patricia Kennedy and Naonori Kodate

Social Development and Social Work Perspectives on Social Protection
Edited by Julie Drolet

Providing Compassionate Healthcare

Challenges in policy and practice

**Edited by Sue Shea,
Robin Wynyard and Christos Lionis**

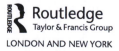
Routledge
Taylor & Francis Group

LONDON AND NEW YORK

First published 2014
by Routledge
2 Park Square, Milton Park, Abingdon, Oxon OX14 4RN

and by Routledge
711 Third Avenue, New York, NY 10017

*Routledge is an imprint of the Taylor & Francis Group, an informa
business*

British Library Cataloguing-in-Publication Data
A catalogue record for this book is available from the British
Library

Library of Congress Cataloging-in-Publication Data
Providing compassionate health care : challenges in policy and
practice / edited by Sue Shea, Robin Wynyard and Christos Lionis.
p. ; cm. — (Routledge advances in health and social policy)
Includes bibliographical references.
I. Shea, Sue, editor of compilation. II. Wynyard, Robin, editor of
compilation. III. Lionis, Christos, editor of compilation. IV. Series:
Routledge advances in health and social policy. [DNLM: 1. Attitude
of Health Personnel. 2. Empathy. 3. Organizational Culture. 4.
Professional-Patient Relations. W 21.5]
R697.A4
610.73'7069—dc23
2013050069

ISBN: 978-0-415-70496-0 (hbk)
ISBN: 978-1-315-89018-0 (ebk)

Typeset in Baskerville
by Swales & Willis Ltd, Exeter, Devon, UK

Contents

Figures

Tables

Contributors

Elizabeth Adamson is a Senior Lecturer within the School of Nursing, Midwifery and Social Care at Napier University Edinburgh, Scotland. She has 14 years of experience in education both within clinical practice and university. Her current role includes responsibility for student experience and she plays an active part in the Leadership in Compassionate Care Programme within the school which is a collaborative project involving the University and NHS Lothian that aims to embed compassionate care within practice and education.

Sanjay Basu is Assistant Professor of medicine and epidemiologist at the Prevention Research Centre at Stanford University, and was previously a Rhodes Scholar at Oxford University. He has worked with a number of organizations including Oxfam International and is a member of the New York Academy of Sciences. His work has featured in the *Wall Street Journal*, the *Boston Globe*, and the *New York Times*.

Ann Bradshaw is Senior Lecturer in pre-registration adult nursing in Oxford Brookes Faculty of Health and Life Sciences. She has a wide range of nursing experience as a staff nurse in medicine, surgery, district nursing, hospice care, oncology, palliative and end-of-life care and as a sister and clinical lecturer in the care of older people. Before she joined Oxford Brookes University she was Macmillan Clinical Fellow at the Royal College of Nursing. Ann's interests include nursing ethics and values of compassion, educational preparation for nursing competence, nursing ethics in the curriculum, the care of people with dementia, end-of-life care, nursing history, its interpretation and its relation to nursing policy, and the use of primary and secondary data.

Craig Brown retired in 2012 after 35 years in general practice on the south coast of England. He has always been interested in practising holistic medicine and in particular 'physician heal thyself' and the spiritual aspect of care. Over the last 13 years he has been involved in developing 'Values in healthcare, a spiritual approach', which is a training programme for healthcare practitioners. He was President of The

National Federation of Spiritual Healers from 1998–2001, Chairman of the British Holistic Medical Association from 2009–2012, and a trustee of the Janki Foundation from 2007.

George P. Chrousos is Professor and Chairman of the First Department of Pediatrics at the University of Athens School of Medicine, Athens, Greece, and former Chief of the Pediatric and Reproductive Endocrinology Branch of the National Institute of Child Health and Human Development (NICHD), National Institutes of Health (NIH), Bethesda, Maryland. He also holds the UNESCO Chair on Adolescent Health Care at the University of Athens and held the 2011 John Kluge Distinguished Chair in Technology and Society at the Library of Congress, Washington DC. He is internationally recognized for his research on the glucocorticoid signalling system of the cell, on the diseases of the hypothalamic-pituitary-adrenal axis, and on the physiological and molecular mechanisms of stress.

Alys Cole-King is a Consultant Liaison Psychiatrist (Betsi Cadwaladr University Health Board) and Co-Founder of the Connecting with People Programme. She works nationally with Royal Colleges, voluntary bodies, academics, patient leaders and sits on the All Party Parliamentary Group for Suicide and Self-harm Prevention. She is the Royal College of Psychiatrists' (RCPsych) spokesperson on suicide and self-harm and also sits on their Patient Safety Working Group. She has an interest in promoting compassion, patient safety and a public health approach to suicide prevention. She has collaborated with the media to promote a compassionate approach, led two World Suicide Prevention Day social media campaigns and the development of the RCPsych portfolio of compassionate self-help resources.

Susan Frampton is President of Planetree, a not-for-profit advocacy, consultation and membership organization that works with a growing international network of healthcare provider organizations across the continuum of care to implement Planetree's comprehensive patient-/person-centred model of care. She has authored numerous publications, and speaks internationally on culture change, patient-centred quality and safety, and the patient experience.

Paul Gilbert is Consultant Clinical Psychologist, at Derbyshire Health Care NHS Foundation Trust. He has a long-standing interest in compassionate care, and his research is internationally known. He developed the 'compassionate mind approach' as a way of integrating the scientific study of compassion and behaviour into healthcare. He has written several bestselling books, been extensively published, and has been awarded the OBE for his contribution in this field.

Joanna Goodrich is currently Research and Development Manager at the Point of Care Foundation and has a background in social science (anthropology/sociology). She has worked with the King's Fund' Point of Care programme since it was set up in 2007, as researcher and programme manager. She has worked for many years as a healthcare researcher in the voluntary and public sectors.

Valerie Iles has been developing clinical managers and leaders for 25 years. She has an in-depth understanding of management and leadership theory, a breadth of practical experience of the behaviours and dynamics of healthcare organizations and a wide-ranging interest in other fields of study. She uses these skills to enable healthcare professionals and teams to re-find enthusiasm for their roles, enhancing their ability to interact effectively with others and encouraging them to help their organizations act with care and compassion for patients. She is visiting Professor at Bucks New University, and honorary Senior Lecturer at the London School of Hygiene and Tropical Medicine and FRCGP.

Marina Karanikolos works with the Department of Public Health & Policy, London School of Hygiene & Tropical Medicine, and is seminar leader on Issues in Public Health. She joined the European Observatory on Health Systems and Policies and the ECOHOST in April 2010, after five years of work as public health information analyst for the NHS. Her work involves health systems performance assessment, and research on the impact of the Global Financial Crisis on population health.

Alexander Kentikelenis is a Research Associate in Sociology at Cambridge University; previously he was a Research Fellow at Harvard University. He has published on the social and health consequences of economic crises and austerity policies, and his work has featured in various media outlets, including the *New York Times*, Reuters, the Associated Press and Bloomberg.

Christos Lionis is qualified in both internal medicine and social medicine and is Professor of General Practice and Primary Care and Director of the Clinic of Social and Family Medicine, University of Crete, Greece. His fields of expertise comprise needs assessments, morbidity in general practice, diagnostic studies and probability, disease determinants, and health care services and quality in primary care. He has published over 200 papers in international journals. He has a strong interest in the concept of compassionate care and considers that against the back-drop of the current economic crisis in Greece and elsewhere, the benefits of compassion may prove even more essential. He operates a compassionate care elective, and is involved in various activities relating to compassionate care. He is also Co-Editor in Chief of the recently launched open access *Journal of Compassionate Health Care*.

Jill Maben is Director of the National Nursing Research Unit, King's College London. She is a registered nurse and recently experienced being part of the direct care nursing workforce again, working on an elderly care ward in an acute trust. Jill's expertise lies in research in the healthcare and nursing workforce, particularly the quality of the work environment and nurses' working lives and the effects of these on patient and staff outcomes and on the patient experience. Jill is particularly interested in links between staff well-being and patient experience, and recently completed a national research study in the UK examining staff and patient experience in two acute and two community trusts in England.

Adelais Markaki is Clinical Specialist in Public/Community Health Nursing and Instructor at the Primary Health Care Department of Social Medicine, Faculty of Medicine, University of Crete, Greece. She is a community health nurse and a medical anthropologist who strongly believes in bringing back the humanistic values to healthcare professions through interdisciplinary teaching and collaborative care. She is also involved in the teaching of compassionate care elective which is delivered to medical students at the University of Crete.

Martin McKee is Professor of European Public Health at the Department of Public Health & Policy, London School of Hygiene & Tropical Medicine. He qualified in medicine in Belfast, Northern Ireland, with subsequent training in internal medicine and public health. As Professor of European Public Health at the London School of Hygiene and Tropical Medicine he co-directs the European Centre on Health of Societies in Transition (ECOHOST), a WHO Collaborating Centre that comprises the largest team of researchers working on health and health policy in central and eastern Europe and the former Soviet Union. Professor McKee is also research director of the European Observatory on Health Systems and Policies.

Irene Papanicolas works with the Department of Social Policy, London School of Economics. In the past she has worked as a researcher at the Health Economics Research Centre at the University of Oxford and the Department of Economics at the London Business School. She has a PhD in Health Economics from the London School of Economics, and MSc degrees from the University of Oxford and University College London. Her current research interests are focused on performance measurement, international comparisons of health systems and performance based payment systems.

Stathis Papavasiliou is Associate Professor and head of the Department of Endocrinology, Diabetes, and Metabolic Diseases, University of Crete School of Medicine, Crete. His interests focus on clinical and basic research on diabetes mellitus, thyroid disease, reproductive endocrinology, growth hormone replacement in adults, chaos and hormone secretion. He believes that compassionate patient care represents the sum total of all medical decisions and actions that take into conscious account the distress and discomfort a patient experiences by the illness itself, compounded by the discomfort caused by diagnostic and thera-peutic actions.

Magdalena Schamberger is Artistic Director, CEO and Co-Founder of Hearts & Minds, the home of Clowndoctors and Elderflowers, based in Edinburgh, Scotland. She has over 25 years' experience in performing, directing and teaching physical theatre and theatre clowning around the world. In 2001 she launched the Hearts & Minds Elderflowers pro-gramme, using the performing arts to improve the quality of life for elderly people with advanced dementia in a health care environment.

Martin Seager is a Consultant Clinical Psychologist and an Adult Psychotherapist. He is a clinician, lecturer, campaigner, broadcaster and activist on mental health issues, and has worked in the NHS for nearly 30 years. He had a regular mental health slot on BBC Radio 5 Live from 2007–2009. He spent over a year working in the home-lessness field with St Mungos and also the *Big Issue*. He is currently working part-time with the South West Yorkshire Partnership NHS Foundation Trust and in private practice. He is also an honorary con-sultant psychologist with the Central London Samaritans and a mem-ber of the Mental Health Advisory Board of the College of Medicine. His work on psychological-mindedness has embraced the importance of trauma, neglect, broken attachments and failures of compassion during the developing years as a key factor in all serious mental health problems.

Sue Shea has a background in psychology and research into psychoso-cial aspects of chronic disorders, and works partly from the UK, and partly with the University of Crete. She has a strong interest in the concept of compassionate care, and since 2010 she has been involved in a number of initiatives in this field including organization of a sym-posium on compassion; development of a Continuing Professional Development course; assistance in the development and delivery of an elective on compassionate care for medical students at the University of Crete; various related publications; member of various compassion related discussion forums; and involvement in research and a number of activities in the field of compassionate care. She is also Co-Editor in Chief of the recently launched open access *Journal of Compassionate Health Care*.

Stephen Smith is a Senior Lecturer and Lead Nurse for the Leadership in Compassionate Care Programme at Edinburgh Napier University and NHS Lothian. Stephen has led the compassionate care programme since 2007 supporting developments which embed compassionate care within healthcare practice and education. Stephen has a background in palliative care nursing and has held a variety of roles in education, practice development, management and research.

David Stuckler is a Senior Research Leader at Oxford University; he also currently holds research posts at London School of Hygiene & Tropical Medicine and Chatham House. He has published over 100 peer-reviewed scientific articles in major journals on the subjects of economics and global health, and his work has featured on the cover of the *New York Times* and *The Economist*, as well as on BBC, NPR, and CNN, among others.

Robin Wynyard retired after several years working for British universities and universities abroad. He draws on his experience as a sociologist in understanding the concept of compassion. He continues to contribute to work in the field of compassion, and is currently visiting Research Fellow in Education at Derby University. He has published widely in academic journals and is co-editor of two books. His current research interests are in cultural transmission theory and its relationship to how popular culture deals with compassion.

Robin Youngson is an anaesthetist in New Zealand, internationally renowned for his leadership in strengthening compassion in healthcare. He is the co-founder of Hearts in Healthcare.com, a global social movement for health professionals, students, patient activists and all those passionate about rehumanizing healthcare. He is an honorary senior lecturer at Auckland University and is the author of the book *Time to Care – How to Love Your Patients and Your Job*.

Foreword

Robin Youngson

In the last two years our work on compassion in healthcare has taken us to many countries: to Ireland, the UK, the Netherlands, the USA, Canada, Australia, New Zealand and Hong Kong. In every country we find a prevailing sense of unease: a strong feeling that modern healthcare had become dehumanised, is lacking essential qualities of caring and compassion, and has forgotten its deeper purpose. Almost everyone we meet has a distressing story of the experience of being a patient in an uncaring system. But in the same breath they tell us of their profound gratitude for small acts of kindness, empathy, caring and compassion and how much these small acts helped them on the journey to healing and recovery.

The personal stories are mirrored by media reports of widespread and scandalous failings of compassionate care. Every country has its own version of the UK Francis Report (Francis 2013), a high-level inquiry into one or more healthcare institutions where there is a horrifying failure of the most basic human caring.

It's not only patients who are suffering. We see widespread reports of health professional disillusionment, depression and burnout; we witness first-hand the sadness, despair and cynicism of good-hearted health professionals who find their ideals compromised and crushed. In the USA, 60 per cent of physicians want to quit medicine.

While we find these deep concerns in every county we visit, what's fascinating are the competing theories used to explain this sorry state of healthcare.

In the UK, much is written about the management culture of the National Health Service (NHS). It's argued that a top-down approach to production, efficiency and financial accountability has created a fear-based culture, where rewards and penalties are based on meeting arbitrary targets rather than caring for patients. It's argued that this culture of fear is driving out compassion.

In the USA, the dehumanisation of patient care is largely blamed in the financial systems underpinning healthcare: the relentless cost-cutting by managed care organisations; the denial of coverage by insurance companies leaving many patients without care; and the greed of physicians who regard patients as 'profit-centers' where treatment is based on maximising revenue, not what is best for the patient. In the USA, the commonest cause of personal bankruptcy is unpaid healthcare bills.

In both countries, the high cost of litigation, adversarial relationships between patients and doctors and defensive medical practice are also cited as factors that drive out compassion.

But it's instructive to look as these claims from a New Zealand perspective. It's fun for me to explain to a USA audience that working as an anaesthesiologist I have yet to bill for a procedure in my entire career! I'm simply paid a salary. Moreover, my medical malpractice insurance premiums are less than $2,000 a year. In New Zealand it's against the law to sue a doctor; we have a national, no-fault compensation scheme for victims of medical error. And when I explain that our public hospitals don't have a billing department and that all treatment is free – there's frank disbelief!

And in comparison to the UK, here in New Zealand we have a benign management culture in healthcare. I was a member of the national Quality Improvement Committee that advised the government that setting multiple target would do harm to the health system. We did not want to emulate the culture of the NHS. In New Zealand we have a very small number of targets on largely sensible measures like waiting times and preventive health measures like immunisation and smoking cessation.

So as a clinician in New Zealand, my day-to-day clinical decisions are little influenced by financial considerations, rules on eligibility, or management targets. I have unprecedented clinical freedom. As an anaesthetist working in a public hospital, the only paperwork I complete is the clinical record.

And yet in New Zealand we are seeing similar patterns of dehumanised patient care, neglect of the basic human needs of patients, lack of caring and compassion, and epidemic levels of stress and burnout among health professionals. Something deeper about the culture of medicine (or society) is responsible for the lack of compassion – and financial drivers and management culture are merely contributing factors, not the fundamental cause.

In New Zealand, the rights of patients are defined in law. The Health and Disability Services Act 1998 defines ten rights for health and disability consumers, including the right to have needs assessed and met, the right to be given information, and the right to be treated with dignity and respect. If patients are dissatisfied with care, they can make a complaint to the independent Health and Disability Commission (www.hdc.org), which may result in mediation, a formal investigation, or prosecution of health professionals or provider organisations. All registered health professions have their standard of care judged against the legal code of patients' rights.

In the hope of establishing a precedent for the right of patients to be treated with compassion, we took a test case to the Health and Disability Commission. Our teenage daughter Chloe had spent three months in hospital in spinal traction, following a car crash. She had a broken neck and other serious injuries but fortunately made a full recovery. In our complaint we said we were satisfied with the standard of clinical care but that Chloe's basic human needs had been profoundly neglected. The hospital provided no disability or communication aids: Chloe couldn't read a book, watch TV or have any form of interest or entertainment, and she was disconnected from the outside world. She often went without food and was sometimes abandoned in severe, untreated pain.

The Health and Disability Commission investigated her case but, other than our letter of complaint, could find little evidence to support or refute our claims. The investigation was based almost entirely on the clinical record, which contained no account of the experience of the patient or the family. With the lack of evidence, the Commissioner was unable to find a breach of patient rights but wrote a four-page letter of education to the chief executive of the hospital trust, raising numerous concerns.

On the positive side, we met many compassionate and caring health professionals during the course of Chloe's long hospital stay. In the early days, when we felt so traumatised and frightened, we were profoundly grateful for small acts of kindness, like the transit care nurse who stopped Chloe's trolley at a join in the floor and lifted each wheel carefully over the join, so as to avoid painful jarring of her broken bones. The memory of that act still brings tears to my eyes many years later.

So knowing how much suffering was caused by the neglect of Chloe's basic human needs, and how profoundly we were grateful for small acts of kindness and compassion, we decided to take action.

In 2006, I co-founded the Compassion in Healthcare Trust and we mounted a public campaign to add a new right to the HDC Code of Rights: *the right to be treated with compassion*. The HDC Act and Code is revised every five years and the Commissioner calls for public submissions. Our proposed amendment was highly controversial.

The professional bodies were forced to declare their position in written submissions. The NZ College of Nurses strongly supported our proposal. The NZ Medical Association opposed it – patients had enough rights already, they argued.

Our controversial proposal raised many questions. What exactly is compassion? Is it different from empathy or pity? Can we measure compassion? If it becomes a legal right, how would we assess the performance of health professionals? Can you regulate for compassion? Should it be part of professional standards?

These are some of the questions explored so fully in this wonderful book.

In the chapters that follow, these questions are examined in the broader societal context. What is the influence of neo-liberalism, management theory, economic policy and austerity measures? How much are politicians, bankers and managers to blame for the sorry state of healthcare?

There is a tendency for clinicians to be critical of managers, complaining about the 'idiocy' of taking a complex organisation like a hospital and treating it like a machine: dividing it into different departments, screwing down the budgets, and holding managers accountable for managing the efficiency and targets of their bit of the system. Of course we all know that the different parts of a hospital are highly interdependent. A cost-saving in one manager's budget may have serious adverse consequences for patient care in another part of the system. An example is cost-cutting in patients' meals; the consequence is that many patients are left without the nourishment required to heal from injuries and illness. Research shows that many hospital patients have malnutrition, leading to increased complications, poor healing, delayed recovery and prolonged hospital stay – at a cost vastly greater than the savings in food budget.

There seems to be little understanding of complexity and interdependence – all parts of the hospital system affect one another and the only way to improve the cost-effectiveness of patient care is to coordinate all parts of the system and get all staff working together, aligned to common purpose. Fragmentation and competition – the hallmarks of modern management and economic theory – do great harm to complex organisations.

But is this a case of the pot calling the kettle black? Is the approach of doctors any better than the managers they deride? Modern medicine ignores the complexity of the human being and fragments care among many specialists: care of the heart, the lungs, the kidneys, the brain, the joints, the skin and the emotions is separated into different hospital departments even though they are all parts of an highly interdependent whole.

> One commentator called it N^2D^2 medicine: Name of Diagnosis = Name of Drug.

The typical elderly patient has six or ten diagnoses – managed independently by different specialists – and takes ten or more prescription drugs. Moreover, the evidence base for many of these treatments only looks at morbidity or mortality in the single organ system and neglects the unintended consequences in other body systems. For instance, lipid-lowering drugs reduce cardiac mortality but may increase mortality from all causes. A recent large study showed that patients with (untreated) raised total cholesterol in the range 5 to 8 had a 35 per cent lower overall mortality rate compared to patients with the recommended cholesterol level less than 5 (Bathum et al. 2013).

That compassionate whole-person care is critical to good patient outcomes is beyond debate. Numerous studies show that compassionate care results in more satisfied patients, greater trust, better concordance with advice and treatment, safer care, fewer complications, time saving, cost-savings, and happier and more resilient health professionals (Youngson 2012). For instance, a recent research showed that diabetic patients who rated their doctor as having high empathy had 42 per cent fewer hospital admission for diabetic crisis, compared with patient with low-empathy physicians (Del Canale et al. 2012).

So how do we promote compassionate, whole person care in healthcare systems that are under-resourced and suffering stress?

The authors of this book attempt to answer that question. In these pages you will find internationally renowned experts exploring the concepts of compassion, from historical models to the latest findings in neuroscience; then an exploration of the complex relationships between spiritual values, the well-being of health workers, the culture of healthcare organisations and the quality of care delivered to patients. Finally, the leaders in the field describe their pioneering efforts to rehumanise the system.

But as you explore the chapters in this book and hear accounts of how 'the system' is destroying compassion, remember that *we are the system*. Until we reflect individually on our own attitudes, assumptions and behaviours we'll not create a more compassionate system.

My greatest hope for culture change is a grassroots movement of concerned health professionals, students, patient activists and leaders – like the authors of this book and the people who will be drawn to read it. Social movements have the power to change the world much more quickly than political systems. Atul Gawande writes about 'Slow ideas' in *The New Yorker* magazine – how simple but effective changes in practice diffuse across the system (Gawande 2013). He gives as examples, developing nations' attempts to implement oral hydration therapies for childhood diarrhoea, and basic standards in midwifery care.

What was the surprising success factor identified by Gawande in implementing practices that can save the lives of millions of children and mothers? The barefoot trainers were 'nice', they 'smiled a lot', they felt like 'a friend come to help me, not to criticise my practice'. Each of us has the power to enact positive change in our efforts to rehumanise healthcare.

Compassionate care is revealed in the smallest of acts. It needs no permission and no resources other than our individual willingness to be present, to be kind, to listen, to show appreciation and gratitude, and to respond to suffering. When we bring these attributes to our daily practice, we influence others around us. Compassion is contagious.

Hearts in Healthcare (www.heartsinhealthcare.com) is the global social movement for human-centred healthcare.

References

Bathum, L., *et al.*, Association of lipoprotein levels with mortality in subjects aged 50 + without previous diabetes or cardiovascular disease: A population-based register study. *Scandinavian Journal of Primary Health Care*, 2013. 31(3): p. 172–80.

Del Canale, S., *et al.*, The relationship between physician empathy and disease complications: An empirical study of primary care physicians and their diabetic patients in Parma, Italy. *Academic Medicine: Journal of the Association of American Medical Colleges* 2012. 87(9): p. 1243–9.

Francis, R., *Mid Staffordshire NHS Foundation Trust Public Inquiry*, 2013. http://www.midstaffspublicinquiry.com/

Gawande, A.A., 'Slow ideas' in *The New Yorker*, 2013. http://www.newyorker.com/reporting/2013/07/29/130729fa_fact_gawande/

Youngson, R., *Time to Care: How to Love Your Patients and Your Job.* 2012, Raglan: Rebelheart Publishers.

Preface

Compassion

I'm a member of the public. I have chronic medical conditions and have been in Patient & Public Involvement for about 20 years. My particular interest in compassion in healthcare was generated by Sue Shea a couple of years ago and helped define more concisely my understanding that caring by healthcare professionals is a necessary component of good outcomes.

My chance link with Sue demonstrated that compassion has a part to play in chronic pain conditions on which my lay group and I are giving public perspectives at the moment. However, it has become apparent to me that the emotion, although assumed to be present is very often 'assumed' but rarely discussed. What I believe has always been a necessary constituent in healthcare and more so in this high-speed technological society is a thorough understanding of all aspects of compassion by all partners (including the patient) in care.

Compassion is wide ranging and applicable in very many life activities; healthcare may be an obvious example but nurses, doctors and the many other professionals, all overworked, will benefit from reminders of the benefits to be accrued in being compassionate.

I feel that I may be stating the obvious but by concentrating my thoughts, I quickly realise the power of compassion; you may perhaps be similar. Research will I'm sure demonstrate the need for increased knowledge in compassion and its power. I'm so grateful for Sue Shea's initial work on the topic which has the capacity to develop healthcare every bit as much as other major research. May her book gain wide circulation and recommendations adopted.

Ron Marsh
Hon Researcher, University of Aberdeen

Acknowledgements

The editors wish to express their great gratitude and thanks to the following:

- Grace McInnes, Managing Editor (Routledge), for her initial support and encouragement for this project;
- James Watson, Editorial Assistant (Routledge), for his help and attention to detail throughout;
- Irene Vasilaki (University of Crete) for her administrative support;
- Elsevier Ltd, for their permission to re-print 'The health impact of financial crisis: Omens of a Greek tragedy' (previously published in *The Lancet*);
- David Peters (Editor of the *Journal of Holistic Healthcare*) for permission to re-print 'Compassionate care: The theory and the reality';
- Colin Dickson, Lasswade Scotland, and Susan Burrell, Susan Burrell Photography, Dalkeith, Scotland for photographic material contained in Chapter 10;
- Joan Halifax for the diagram in Chapter 3;
- Janki Foundation for photographic material contained in Chapter 5;
- Ueli Grueninger, M.D. Executive Director, Swiss College of Primary Care Medicine and WONCA Europe, for permission to use the WONCA Tree diagram included in Chapter 8;
- Robin Youngson for inclusion of the 'compassion conversation' included in Chapter 15;
- David Zigmond and David Peters (Editor of the *Journal of Holistic Healthcare*) for permission to re-print the letters included at the end of the book.

Very importantly we express our great thanks to all of the service-users, carers, and members of the public who have shared with us their experiences for inclusion in this book.

Introduction

Sue Shea, Robin Wynyard and Christos Lionis

This book was inspired by the apparent need to restore humanity to healthcare, particularly within a period of austerity, affecting many countries. Furthermore it was intended to look at the broader picture at various levels of the healthcare system, as compassion across the health care teams themselves, and from an organizational level are essential factors. In 2011, the editors of this book organized a Symposium at Greenwich University on the topic of compassion in health care (Shea *et al.* 2011). The intention was to bring together key people from various backgrounds with an interest in moving forward with the science and art of compassion. The realization, following the symposium, was that people are united in moving forward on this topic, thus this experience has led us to conduct further work in bringing key people together with the common aim of enhancing compassion in health care

Compassion is a growing field requiring a multidisciplinary approach, thus we are privileged to have contributions from a range of different fields, covering medicine, nursing, psychotherapy, psychology, sociology, and organizational factors, to reflect the multidisciplinary nature of the book. Furthermore, a key feature of this book is the inclusion of service-user, carer, patient representatives and health care professionals' experience. These are interwoven throughout, drawing attention to positive as well as negative experiences with the aim of providing a valuable 'real-life' learning tool for our target readership.

Although there is an apparent interest globally with regards to the issue of compassionate care, in general the subject is still relatively new and developing with regards to the medical and nursing curricula. Thus, a further motivation for developing this book was to provide an academic aid to support health care students. The book is aimed at medical/nursing students, and practising healthcare professionals, but would also be of interest to other allied disciplines.

In recent years, attention has been drawn to the fact that compassion towards the patient seems to have decreased, with events at certain healthcare settings showing alarming gaps in the humanity of the care offered, both in the UK and internationally. The focus on delivering good care and preventing factors that prevent it was propelled further by the recently appointed President of the UK Patients Association (www.patients-association.com), Robert Francis QC following his earlier inquiry and report on devastating events surrounding the care of patients at Mid-Staffordshire Hospital (Francis 2013). This report gained international attention by demonstrating that for many patients the most basic elements of care were neglected, including toileting, hygiene, nutrition, dignity, and lack of attention to pain. Furthermore, morale at the Trust was low, and while many staff did their best in difficult circumstances, others showed a disturbing lack of compassion towards their patients. This Francis Report coincided with the current compassion activities of the editors and contributors to this book, throwing work in this area into even more sharper focus.

In addition, a north-east London hospital was recently found to have a 'catalogue of failings' during unannounced inspections by the Care Quality Commission (CQC) (2013), whilst a report by Keogh (National Health Service 2013) has further drawn attention to the quality of care and treatment provided by 14 hospital trusts in England.

Evidence suggests that the component parts of compassion such as kindness, empathy, attention to basic needs, attention to dignity, are crucial in alleviating pain, prompting fast recovery from acute illness, assisting in the management of chronic illness, and relieving anxiety. Moreover, physiological benefits of compassion have also been reported in studies which show that kindness and touch alter the heart rhythm and brain function in both the person providing compassion and the person receiving it (Fogarty *et al.* 1999; Shaltout *et al.* 2012; *Science Daily* 2012).

A UK Department of Health Report (2009), states that in providing compassionate care:

> we respond with humanity and kindness to each person's pain, distress, anxiety or need. We search for the things we can do, however small, to give comfort and relieve suffering. We find time for those we serve and work alongside. We do not wait to be asked, because we care . . .
>
> Department of Health (2009)

Most people would agree that compassion and basic care delivery should form an important aspect of healthcare globally, and we have been hearing the word 'compassion' for some time now. But what is compassion, and what does it encompass and what does it actually mean? In order to understand compassion, what enhances it, and what prevents it from taking place, it is important to look at a whole range of concepts within the health care setting. For compassion to succeed is not just about the relationship between the health care professional (HCP) and patient, but extends to organizational, managerial and administrative staff. Team work, HCP self-care and understanding, and a compassionate approach between HCPs towards each other is also important. Everyone working in the health care setting (including administrators, porters, cleaners), ultimately has a responsibility towards the patient – the patient is the person who is most vulnerable at that moment in time. As Chris Manning (in general communication) points out 'a surgeon can wield cutlery brilliantly, as can a ward cleaner who gives someone hope'. In fact, quite often we witness acts of simple humanity and kindness from auxiliary staff, who have no training in such issues, but who naturally feel compassion towards the patient. We may also witness compassion and kindness given from one patient to another:

> A sociological observation by one of the editors, who was admitted to hospital via accident and emergency, was that fellow patients themselves, presumably because of a certain vulnerability, bonded together and offered each other help and support in lieu of any professional help that wasn't forthcoming. This one incident alone says an awful lot about how compassion can arise in far from obvious places and in places where people find themselves at their lowest ebb.
>
> Patient experience

Administrative errors in health care are quite frequently reported, and can have a knock on effect on all concerned in the health care setting:

> '. . . we drove 45 minutes to attend a pre-arranged hospital appointment. When we arrived we were told that the appointment had been cancelled – nobody had informed us. A different surgeon agreed to see me instead, but the knock on effect of this was that it made him late for his ward rounds where several patient and nursing staff were waiting or his instructions . . . a simple telephone call could have prevented this . . . '
>
> Patient experience

HCPs are often under strain themselves, from large amounts of paperwork, and other factors, and burn-out is a growing issue, with a recent GP study demonstrating a very high risk of burn-out in UK GPs (Pulse 2013). Thus if HCPs are not cared for or correctly supported themselves, it will naturally prove more difficult for them to show compassion towards their patients.

Health care is further affected by issues and policies outside the health care setting itself. In times of austerity, as many countries are currently experiencing, health care is deeply affected by cut-backs, and although compassion is even more required at such times, it can be difficult under such circumstances. As Stuckler and Basu (2013) remind us, recession can hurt but austerity kills. Thus in Chapter 12 of this book, attention is drawn to the health risks associated with austerity, in the hope that our readers will reflect on this and incorporate it into an overall view of how compassion can be sustained and how it can be introduced when it is most needed (for both the patient and the HCP).

This book aims to address the basic concepts surrounding the notion of compassion and we hope that it will contribute to broader discussions of such, within a wider setting whereby various socio-cultural contexts may have an impact on the definition and understanding of compassion. Within this book, we have attempted to draw together a number of pertinent issues related to compassionate health care, within four key sections: *introducing the concept of compassion; theoretical and therapeutic approaches to compassion; implementation and impact of compassion in health care; organizational issues,* plus a concluding section where 'teaching compassion' is discussed. Within the first section, we begin by discussing the historical origins and roots of compassion, to lead our readers in with a multidisciplinary approach to the concept. This is followed by a look at compassion in nursing history, and the importance of kindness. The second section then addresses neurological, psychological and experiential approaches, ending with current approaches to compassion and end-of-life care. In the third section, we introduce a focus on compassion in primary and secondary care, and with specific conditions such as dementia and diabetes. This section ends by looking at evidence during times of austerity which, as mentioned above, can affect health care systems, thus adding to pressure on HCPs, and ultimately affecting the care provided. The fourth section brings us into the field of organizational culture, whereby certain initiatives are presented, and the issue of burn-out and compassion fatigue is discussed.

A key question that is often asked is: can compassion be taught? Early work by Howard Becker suggested that values in healthcare may be taught out of medical students during their training (Becker *et al.* 1961). It is possible that the scientific nature of nurse/medical training may lead to a decrease in compassion. There is growing interest in including courses on compassion within the medical/nursing school curricula and some such courses are already in existence (Adamson *et al.* 2011; Lionis *et al.* 2011). Thus within the concluding section of this book, an example is presented on the benefits of teaching compassion.

All of our contributors have considerable expertise, covering compassion related issues such as historical backgrounds, nursing values, neurological perspectives, theories and therapies, caring for carers, compassion in primary and secondary care, organizational issues, and teaching compassion.

Thus we hope that our readers can gain much from this book either as a learning tool (for students), or as food for thought to incorporate in everyday practice (practitioners), as the concept of delivering compassionate health care is important in any situation, from treating a minor cold, to delivering palliative and end of life care.

In a changing world, we still have a long way to go in addressing the complex issue of compassion. But people are united in this quest, with Dr Robin Youngson (http://heartsinhealthcare.com) currently calling for a global movement within this field, and to whom we are grateful for providing the foreword to this book.

References

Adamson, E., Dewar, B. (2011). Compassion in the nursing curriculum: making it more explicit. *Journal of Holistic Healthcare* 8(3): 42–45.

Becker, H., Geer, B., Hughes, E.C., Strauss, A.L. (1961). *Boys in White: Student Culture in Medical School.* New Brunswick, NJ, and London: Transaction Publishers.

Department of Health UK. (2009). *The NHS constitution: The NHS belongs to us all.* (Online). Available at: hwww.dh.gov.uk/prod_consum_dh/groups/dh_digital-assets/documents/digitalasset/dh_093442.pdf (Accessed October 2013).

Fogarty, L.A., Curbow, B.A., Wingard, J.R., McDonnell, K., Somerfield, M.R. (1999). Can 40 seconds of compassion reduce patient anxiety? *Journal of Clinical Oncology* 17(1): 371.

Francis, R. QC. (2013). *Report of the Mid Staffordshire NHS Foundation Trust Public Inquiry.* House of Commons: Stationery Office (Vols 1–3).

Lionis, C., Shea, S., Markarki, A. (2011). Introducing and implementing a compassionate care elective for medical students in Crete. *Journal of Holistic Healthcare* 8(3): 38–41. (http://www.patients-association.com) (Accessed Novembver 2013).

National Health Service. (2013). *Review into the Quality of Care and Treatment Provided by 14 Hospital Trusts in England: Overview Report* (Professor Sir Bruce Keogh KBE, Chair) NHS, Leeds.

Pulse. (2013). www.pulsetoday.co.uk (Accessed September 2013).

Science Daily. www.sciencedaily.com/releases/2012/12/121203145952.htm (Accessed November 2013).

Shaltout, H.A., Tooze, J.A., Rosenberger, M.S., Kemper, K.J. (2012). Time, touch, and compassion: effects on autonomic nervouse system and well-being. *Explore* 8: 177–184.

Shea, S., Wynyard R., West, E., Lionis, C. (2011). Reaching a consensus in defining and moving forward with the science and art of compassion in healthcare. *Journal of Holistic Health Care* 8(3): 58–60.

Stuckler, D. and Basu, S. (2013) *The Body Economic: Why Austerity Kills.* London: Allen Lane.

Part I

Introducing the concept of compassion

This section discusses the concept of compassion, what we mean by the use of the word 'compassion' and how current definitions and usages of the term may have altered over time. Current attempts to define and conceptualize compassion will be briefly discussed. The two chapters included in this section attempt to lay the foundations on which the other sections of the book can be built. In its very nature health care does not follow a neat diachronically process in time, and compassion as a concept goes in and out of the thoughts of health care professionals depending on the social and cultural context existing at any one time. In this section, the historical origins of the concept of compassion are discussed, together with the implementation of compassion in nursing history.

1   Understanding compassion: the tangled roots of compassion: historical origins, modern day reflections and concerns: *Robin Wynyard*
2   Compassion in nursing history: attending to the patient's basic human needs with kindness: *Ann Bradshaw*

1 Understanding compassion: the tangled roots of compassion
Historical origins, modern day reflections and concerns

Robin Wynyard

Introduction

> I will use treatment to help the sick according to my ability and judgment, but I will never use it to injure or wrong them. I will never give poison to anyone though asked to do so, nor will I suggest such a plan.
> Hippocratic Oath – Hippocrates, 460–370 BC

As this leading quote shows, what might be deemed to be compassion has a long history. This chapter as an introduction to the book looks at the roots of compassion in history, philosophy and religion and how in the context of these the word compassion has somewhat tangled origins rather like the roots of an old huge, tangled tree.

Compati is a Latin word meaning to 'suffer with', and as a word it has been with us a long time. Having said that as a word it is not easy to conceptualize and to say whether it is always good, or whether it is sometimes bad. In exploring the tangled nature of the word compassion in this chapter, I am trying to unravel this tangled nature by looking at how history has used it as a word and concept, how philosophers have used it, how the modern social sciences have used it. Finally I want to show how the media as a very important player in bringing the nature of compassion to millions of people worldwide, has used the concept. This last point has become very important following the extensive media coverage following the revelations of Robert Francis QC (2013) leading to the publication of the Francis Report.

Looking at the history of compassion, it is something that held a fascination for both the ancient Greeks and the writers of the Bible. In both instances, it was not always seen as a force for good.

Before discussing this, I would like to mention a modern writer who spans both the medical and the sociological. Thomas Szasz in his book entitled *Cruel Compassion* (Szasz 1994). Has expressed some doubt on the way the concept of compassion has been used by the medical profession. Cruel compassion is a good example of oxymoron in which apparently contradictory terms appear in conjunction. Most of us assume that being compassionate is the exact opposite of cruelty. Szasz a psychiatrist shows how compassion has been misused by the psychiatric profession, where unintended consequences of its use have produced all sorts of effects to the detriment of the psychiatrist's patients. His argument is that compassion, which is often seen as a virtue, is no such thing at all: 'A little self-scrutiny would quickly show us that compassion is not always or necessarily a virtue' (p. 3). The major thrust in his argument is that far from restoring patients to a self-regarding equilibrium, it removes a person's free will thus placing the patient totally in the hands of the psychiatrist – 'guided by the light of the fake virtue of compassion, we have subverted the classical liberal conception of men as moral agent, endowed with free will' (p. 3). Through in-depth historical research he shows that there is a deep flaw in the way we view compassion precisely because history has always drawn a distinction between two groups of people who might be deemed worthy recipients (or not) of compassion. These are defined as the 'deserving' and the 'undeserving poor'. This fits with the history of British health care policy from the earliest to modern times, where distinctions have always been made as to who or who does not deserve compassion and thus help.

'Sturdy Beggars' was a term used throughout the Middle Ages describing those who were fit and able to work, but begged or wandered for a living instead. Such individuals were punished by being branded on the cheek and placed in the stocks for punishment. The Statute of Cambridge (1383) differentiated between sturdy beggars and the infirm i.e. those genuinely incapable of work and thus deemed worthy recipients of care from their local parish which provided a levy for such contingencies. Further Parliamentary Acts like the Vagabonds and Beggars Act (1495) sought to firm up this distinction. Historically where compassion is concerned morality always lurks in the background.

Compassion as a virtue considered by the ancient Greeks

Although not actually using the term 'compassion' the ancient Greeks were certainly interested in what we would deem to be component parts of compassion. In exploring the parameters of compassion they exposed much that was ambiguity, oxymoron and doubt surrounding its use. As Hannah Arendt said '... the ancients regarded the most compassionate person as no more entitled to be called the best than the most fearful. The Stoics saw compassion and envy in the same terms' (Arendt, quoted in Szasz p. 4). So according to the Stoics, compassion was not a virtue at all and might in fact do more harm than good.

There was a debate amongst the ancients, as there is today, as to whether virtues including compassion could be taught? Or did such virtues already exist inside us and simply need the right techniques to evoke them? Plato thought that virtues could not be taught and as far as compassion is concerned it is only known after an act has occurred whether compassion has taken place. Socrates in Plato's *Meno* in argument with the Sophist Protagoras illustrates that only by going through certain procedures of the act in particular circumstances, can we know if a particular act is good, virtuous or compassionate. Socrates demonstrates this via the slave boy, who is capable of answering a complex geometry problem because he already has the questions in his soul (Plato 2005: 118–120). As Socrates said: 'Well, all I can say is, I've often asked that question (can we be taught to be good?) . . . and for the life of me, I can't find the answer (p. 118).

So where Socrates appeared to argue that no one teaches virtues, Protagoras appeared to argue that everyone teaches them. In recent times Pence (1983) takes this argument further in saying that compassion can be taught in medical training. According to him 'whether compassion can be taught depends in part on what we take it to be'. It must not be confused with related but different moral qualities, for example, like pity. What needs to be instilled in medical training is we want doctors, nurses, HCPs etc. to be compassionate towards their patients where qualities such as imagination 'play a key role in compassion in achieving understanding of, and feeling for, suffering people'. Pence draws attention to the nature of 'Trust' as something else that is needed in the practitioner/patient relationship: 'honesty, and the time and willingness to listen'. Pence points out that although we can teach compassion in medical training, it isn't going to be easy! So unlike Protagoras the Greek who argued that everyone possesses it, the problem with compassion is that it has a structural dimension as well as a pedagogical one. This is something I mention later when I talk about compassion distance. Pence argues that we must change the medical system to incorporate teaching compassion. Existing compassion in students must not be undermined by their medical training and time must be made available during the training to allow students 'to pursue particular cases in which they are involved'. There must also be 'systematic acceptance by medical teachers that such activities and the moral qualities they develop are worth encouraging'. In teaching compassion, medical training must give importance to illustrations through films and literature, these are points strongly endorsed in this chapter and which will be returned to later.

Not all ancient Greeks would agree with Socrates about compassion not being taught, as many of them were astute in providing tools for interpreting compassion and unlocking the key to it within ourselves. In Greek plays by playwrights such as Sophocles the chorus interpreted the plot for the audience, more or less as a running commentary, informing the audience what should or should not happen and how outside influences affect the behaviour of the protagonists. Through technical devices like the role of the chorus the ancient Greeks cultivated inner values that made for a fuller humanity which presumably made for a more compassionate person.

In Greek literature, compassion is sometimes treated with in passing often bound up with religious ritual and spiritual and mental health care. Homer gives a good example of what passes for compassion in the Iliad. Basically the plot of Homer's *Iliad* is about mass slaughter and degradation of basic human values, but you can still find a moving example of compassion which seems so powerful as to subvert the nature of nastiness within the epic. King Priam of Troy's son Hector has been killed by the mighty Greek warrior Achilles. Achilles conducts a shameful and very non-compassionate act by tying Hector to his chariot and dragging his dead body around the walls of Troy in full view of Priam, Hector's father. Priam under the cover of darkness sneaks into Achilles tent to beg for the return of his son's body 'I put to my lips the hands of the man who killed my son . . . Those words stirred with Achilles a deep desire . . . To grieve for his own father ...' (Book 24 the *Iliad*). From this example we see the two-way nature of a compassionate act, what is instilled by the giver is returned in kind by the recipient. Hence we come back to the Latin definition of compassion cited earlier, by which we suffer together.

Compassion as dealt with in the Bible

Historically the Bible is a good source of quotes and treatment of compassion. It is interesting to compare the Old Testament with the New Testament. There is really very little that passes for compassion in the Old Testament and it is difficult to relate biblical quotes like the following with anything remotely related to a concept of compassion: 'Now go and smite Amalek, and utterly destroy all that they have and spare them not; but slay both men and women, infant and suckling, ox and sheep, camel and ass' (Samuel 15:3). In the New Testament on the other hand, the word compassion occurs on many occasions e.g. Mark 1:41; Luke 7:12; Luke 15:20 and in the quote that follows there is great feeling for spiritual leadership in compassion that can be provided by great religious leaders such as Jesus '... but when he saw the multitudes, he was moved with compassion on them, because they fainted and were scattered abroad as sheep having no shepherd' (Matthew 9:36). The imagery used here is of the compassionate person as a shepherd as an organizing force for the flock. In a religious context this had a very contemporary feel to it when the new Pope Francis spoke about certain skills that priests need, presumably inherent to the compassionate, where there is a need to 'smell the sheep in his flock ...' (BBC News 28 March 2013). Compassion is used by all 'people of the book' including Judaism, Christianity and Islam. The Koran acknowledges the role that the prophet Jesus plays in furthering compassion. Speaking of Jesus: 'we gave him the Gospel, and put compassion and mercy in the hearts of his followers' (Koran 17:27).

The difficulty of studying compassion is that the journey is full of twists and turns. We can see how the Old Testament which does not readily advocate 'turning the other cheek' differs in treatment to the New Testament which bursts full of the nature of compassion. But later on this is not necessarily seen as something to be praised. In the philosopher Nietzsche's critique of Christianity, he does not reject compassion (although it is difficult to find any support for it by him), but he does say that within a

Christian context, compassion is driven by feelings of hatred and resentment and applied in an unhealthy way. What he is saying is that compassion in Christianity (and Buddhism) is just as much about personal power and control as it is about selfless devotion to others:

> I regarded the inexorable progress of the morality of compassion, which afflicted even illness, as the most sinister symptom of the sinister development of our European culture.
>
> (Nietzsche 2008: 101)

Even more vitriolic: 'How many tons of sugary spirits of compassion . . . one would have to export from Europe today before the air began to smell pure once again' (p. 133).

As I have been arguing, historically the study of compassion is never straightforward and supporters and detractors of compassion are somewhat evenly balanced.

Perhaps a key point regarding compassion is that it does not exist as a free floating idea, but in fact it is closely related to societal variables connected with issues such as the state of the economy, and work availability. Lord Beveridge's Report of 1944, in laying the foundation for the British NHS, had in mind that the disastrous unemployment and the poverty engendered from it must never happen again. The Report contained the five 'giants': want, disease, ignorance, squalor and idleness. In Beveridge's time these five 'giants' needed a lot of compassion to overcome them. The Report was referring to the situation in the 1930s where Britain, with a much smaller population than now, saw 3 million unemployed and where soup kitchens were the norm to feed a starving population. Misery of one kind or another has always been with us and historically this has always existed side by side with compassion.

Thoughts from modern theorists on compassion

Modern day theorists in the social sciences, from fields such as social psychology, social anthropology and sociology of medicine have had an interest in stressing the importance of compassion in relation to health care. With developments in the social sciences the treatment of compassion has become more balanced with better observational techniques and the increasing ability to link the empirical with the theoretical. We can talk more now about a dynamics of compassion and what I would call compassion distance – i.e. structural barriers which prevent compassion taking place. Members of the medical profession, as this book aims to show, are now far more interested in the nature of compassion and how it may be imputed into their work with patients, and in this they are more readily prepared to draw on findings in the social sciences, the mass media and the arts.

There is also more of a tendency in modern day theory to more closely relate disciplines such as medicine and the social sciences and a good example of where such conjoint has taken place, lies in the work of Arthur Kleinman. Arthur Kleinman is Professor of Psychiatry at Harvard University where he is also Professor of Medical Anthropology in Social Medicine. In the light of problems that beset modern healthcare a fellow clinician has said of Kleinman's work that his world is one where he questions: 'how we can create forms of healthcare appropriate to resilient sustainable communities. This is a crucial set of issues given that Western biomedicine in its current form is not sustainable' (Dr David Peters personal correspondence 29 March 2012).

This non-sustainability has been highlighted recently by the 'lack of compassion' debate in healthcare. In terms of the nature of dynamics, for me, as well as for Kleinman the understanding of compassion lies in the nature of narrative construction. The key work of doctoring according to Kleinman lies in the interpretation of narratives of illness brought to him by the patient where illness narratives edify us about how life problems are created, controlled, made meaningful Kleinman (1988). For him, diagnosis is a thoroughly semiotic activity where words have meanings that stretch beyond their immediate objective reference. So showing, for example, compassion on the part of the practitioner lies in an understanding that illness has a meaning beyond its relationship to a particular part of the body and is bound up as a social construction and given a particular meaning in the patient's wider world. Healthcare decisions about a person involve a person attempting to change the behaviour of clinical outcomes of individuals or a group for the better. The argument is that this cannot be done without compassion on the part of the practitioner. Without knowledge of the patient's wider perspective how can you be seen to be treating the patient adequately as a person in his or her own right?

An example of this comes from Jonathon Miller, medical doctor turned opera director. He cites the example of when he was a young intern on a geriatric ward in a hospital. An elderly gentleman out of humanity and courtesy had got out of bed to show a female visitor the way out of the ward, totally forgetting that he had no pyjama bottoms on. Someone might use the word 'disgust' associated with this incident or just put it down to senility using such words to construct their social world of interpretation in which to situate this event. In Miller's approach 'compassion' can overcome disgust to bridge radically different worlds and radically different logics. And for the elderly gentleman on the ward it was part of his constant effort to show others and himself that he was no less human than they. This is precisely the compassionate world of thoughts and feelings in which Arthur Kleinman cites his approach and intervention to medicine and healing. Compassion is all part of a broader issue where Western style doctors often abdicate the healer's role when faced with problems that no longer respond to technologically based care.

As a sociologist I am convinced that understanding the root of compassion lies in understanding the dynamic nature of constructed narrative existing between caregiver and patient. And in what I call compassion
distance the structural barriers existing preventing satisfactory narrative
construction and hence compassion taking place. For Kleinman showing
compassion on the part of a practitioner lies in an understanding that illness has a meaning beyond its relationship to a particular part of the body
and is bound up as a social construction and given a particular meaning in
the patient's wider world.

Pre-dating the work of Kleinman, the sociologist Erving Goffman
(1922–1982) best exemplifies the later approach advocated by Kleinman.
Goffman's sociology like Kleinman's work aims to construct an explanatory
narrative of the behaviour of people in certain settings. For Goffman people
are engaged in an elaborate drama, in the study of which Goffman aims to
pinpoint the distinction between appearance and reality. In this Goffman
explores the parameters as to what constitutes the boundaries of compassion distance, that is, that compassion can only be given and received when
the correct and appropriate mores regarding it are seen to be in place. So
like actor's we play a role, which can and does involve different degrees of
sincerity, the nature of which may or may not be perceived by the recipients
of action:

> participants are required to be sensitive to the consequences of their
> conduct both for themselves and for others. Such sensitivity, argues
> Goffman, is difficult to maintain with exactitude . . . such competences
> rely on knowledge of the ritualized forms of interaction.
>
> (Drew and Wootton 1988: 68)

In a hospital setting, observation clearly shows that the proprietary ritual-
ized forms of interaction must be observed. Between staff and service users
between clinical staff and non-clinical staff, and between staff themselves.
Regarding the latter there is a clear distinction between surgeons who come
at the top of the bureaucratic tree down through non-surgical clinicians,
interns, nurses, health care assistants. At each level of the bureaucratic train
appropriate due deference has to be shown.

> The self . . . seen as something that resides in the arrangements pre-
> vailing in a social system for its members. The self . . . dwells . . . in the
> pattern of social control that is exerted in connection with the person
> by himself and those around him.
>
> (Goffman 1961: 154)

Regarding the giving of compassion, boundaries can be established, broken and reestablished again. As Goffman says: 'In every social establishment, there are official expectations as to what the participant owes the

establishment'. Goffman goes on to say: 'we find that participants decline in some way to accept the official view of what they should be putting into and getting out of the organization' (p.267).

A recent observed example of 'establishment of correct compassion distance', 'breakdown of compassion distance' and then 'reestablishment of compassion distance' is as follows:

> A patient with her husband is brought into a busy A & E screaming with pain. This lasts for some time. After a while a health care professional approaches the patient and says '*Can you stop screaming you are frightening the other patients*' to which the husband replies shouting '*Can't you see she is in pain and that's what people do when they are in pain*'. HCP: '*Don't you talk to me like that*'. Husband: '*I'm not talking to you like that; I'm simply stating a fact!*' At which point HCP calms down and correct distance is restored and she says '*I'll get some pain killers and help get her on to the bed in the cubicle*'.

I believe that compassion can be taught and in doing this the pioneering work of theorists like Goffman can be drawn on. In teaching compassion to HCPs I have made much use of Goffman's work (1961, 1963, 1974) and have constructed what Leget and Olthuis (2007) call a 'portfolio' which according to them is a collection of evidence culled from the mass media, literature, films and books, helping to illustrate insight and narrative for compassion as a basis for ethics in medical education. One of the components I use in the 'portfolio' are extracts from the film made in 1975 *One Flew over the Cuckoo's Nest*, starring Jack Nicholson and based on a book by Ken Kesey (first published 1962). The film acknowledges the work of Goffman whose fascination for total institutions took him to the National Institute of Mental Health in Bethesda Maryland where from 1954 to 1957 he conducted hospital field work.

In the film mentioned above, set in 1963, Randle Patrick 'Mac' McMurphy (Jack Nicholson) a criminal sentenced for statutory rape of a 15-year-old girl is transferred to a mental institution in Oregon for evaluation. Although he shows no signs of mental illness he hopes that a short stay here will be more conducive than serving out his time in a state prison. McMurphy's ward is run by Nurse Mildred Ratched who employs subtle humiliation, unpleasant medical treatments and an obsessive daily routine to suppress the patients. The fear the patients have for Nurse Ratched detracts from them being able to move easily into the 'outside world'. McMurphy quickly becomes the leader of his fellow patients, who include Billy Bibbit a shy, nervous and stuttering young man. And 'Chief' Bromden a silent American Indian believed to be deaf and mute. It is not long before a strong battle of wills develops between Nurse Ratched and McMurphy. Both from the start are portrayed as lacking compassion for any of Mac's fellow patients. Over the course of the film McMurphy's attitude to his fellow patients changes, particularly in regard to young Billy Bibbit towards whom he develops as a father figure.

Through his struggle with the Nurse, McMurphy learns that Ratched and the doctors have the power to keep him committed indefinitely. Planning to escape with the 'Chief', Mac returns to the ward in order to successfully help Billy. When Nurse Ratched finds out she humiliates Billy who in turn commits suicide. Attempting to kill Nurse Ratched, McMurphy is restrained and eventually lobotomized. His friend the 'Chief' cannot stand to see him in this state, and in an act of compassion he smothers him and then escapes the institution alone.

The film through a succession of five clips cleverly shows in the compulsory group therapy session how the main protagonist J.P. McMurphy (Nicholson) comes to realize, that the fellow participants in the group are not simply 'nuts' to be used for his own purposes but to be treated as individuals with a fair degree of understanding and compassion, but this eventually leads to his own downfall.

Constructing a teaching unit showing the dynamic involved in compassion distancing, using the film and Goffman's books, I have constructed a series of questions and answers. The task set from the unit is: 'imagine that you are a trained observer and you want to get to the core of the group dynamic which you suspect is compassion for your fellow patients'. The task is:

1   To identify the main characters and their relationships to each other.
2   After viewing the fifth and final sequence, attempt to stitch together the whole narrative, i.e. how has the group moved forward and what has changed regarding the nature of compassion?

Ethnography in sociological theory relates the part to the whole. It reveals the interpretation and negotiations needed to decontextualize observation situations and to reconstruct the 'others' point of view and therefore their culture.

This diagram shows participants in the compulsory therapy sessions in the film *One Flew over the Cuckoo's Nest*. Broken lines indicate non-verbal communication. Double arrowed unbroken lines indicate two-way verbal communication, single arrowed lines indicate one way communication from patient to Nurse Ratched. Over a period of time in the therapy sessions, McMurphy's (Nicholson)interpretation via interactions in the sessions with Nurse Ratched (Fletcher) leads him from viewing the other patients of the mental institution in Oregon as 'nuts' to a feeling of compassion towards them, particularly Billy Bibbit.

What this exercise hopefully illustrates to the students is how compassion gives rise to an active desire to alleviate another's suffering. But even this is not straightforward, as has been constantly argued throughout the chapter; compassion can go wrong, as in the case of McMurphy in the film. Although I would argue strongly that in any medical setting compassion benefits far

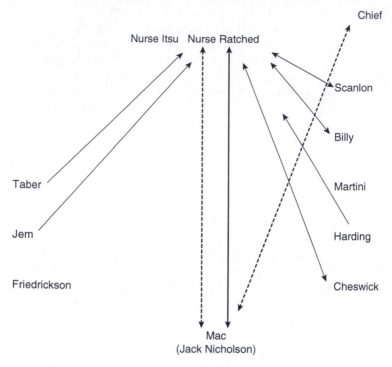

Figure 1.1 Diagram indicating communication between participants in the
    compulsory therapy sessions in the film *One Flew over the Cuckoo's Nest*

outweigh its negatives, the basis of compassion is unstable, because it is not
predictable.

   I use this film and the other examples of literature because I find them
particularly useful, of course, others attempting to teach compassion with
all its manifestations and twists and turns, can use examples pertinent too
them. Ideas for a portfolio often come quite casually. As an example of this,
I have often thought about using the hospital scenes in the TV drama *The
Singing Detective* (1986). This deals in a filmic way with serious subjects. It is
also enhanced by a clever use of music, like the song 'Dry Bones' which in
one scene all the nurses and doctors spontaneously burst into. The use of
music is one area that could be explored and its relationship to compassion,
something I haven't done!

Conclusion

The argument has been put forward in this chapter that compassion is an
essential component of any medical setting. But it is not always easy and
straightforward to give and receive because of the many variables needed

to identify it which I would see as its 'tangled roots'. Also teaching compassion directly is problematic as we the provider cannot always know that what we are giving is seen as compassion by others. In such a sense 'teaching' might be the wrong word and 'insights' and 'example giving' might be better words. Usually we know what we mean and as this book illustrates, the many definitions use always have considerable overlaps of key points.

I maintain that compassion' can, however, be talked about in a meaningful way providing we view it as more than a word, but return to it as a concept, where we examine the variables and events in which the concept of compassion is situated.

I believe that the social sciences and the various media can help the health care student or worker focus on understanding the concept of compassion in a medical setting, and understanding the nature of narrative construction and the barriers allowing compassion distance could be crucial for understanding compassion.

Care Experiences: a compassionate consultation

Craig (UK)

I have learnt that one of the most effective ways to help patients in general practice that have complex and seemingly intractable problems is to say nothing. They are given space to tell their story, and I listen in a non-judgemental attentive way. I keep my mind clear and free from wandering thoughts so that I am engaged and present for them. At the same time I am detached at an emotional level and do not get drawn into any of their negativity. As a healing practice I visualize myself as a conduit for a loving, kindly energy that source is like a huge ocean and passes through me and from my heart to the patient. At the end of the consultation patients often remark they feel better and thank me for my advice, although I have said nothing. This detached engagement is a subtle compassionate practice and it makes me feel good too.

References

Drew, P., Wootton, A. (1988) *Erving Goffman, Exploring the Interaction Order* Polity Press, Oxford.

Francis, R. QC (2013) *Report of the Mid Staffordshire NHS Foundation Trust Public Inquiry* House of Commons, Stationery Office (Vols 1–3).

Goffman, E. (1961) *Asylums* Penguin Books, London.

Goffman, E. (1963) *Stigma* Penguin Books, London and New York.

Goffman, E. (1974) *Frame Analysis* Penguin Books, Harmondsworth.

Homer (1990) *The Iliad* Viking Penguin, London.

Kesey, K. (2005) *One Flew over the Cuckoo's Nest* Penguin Modern Classics, London.

Kleinman, A. (1988) *The Illness Narratives* Basic Books, New York.

Leget, C., Olthuis, G. (2007) Compassion as a basis for ethics in medical education *Journal of Medical Ethics* 33(10), 617–20.

One Flew over the Cuckoo's Nest Dir. Milos Foreman. United Artists, 1975.

Nietzsche (2008) *On the Genealogy of Morals* Oxford University Press, Oxford.

Pence, G.E. (1983) Can Compassion be taught? *Journal of Medical Ethics* 9, 189–91.

Plato (2005) *Protagoras and Meno* Penguin Books, London.

The Singing Detective Television serial drama written by Dennis Potter in six instalments, starring Michael Gambon, 1986.

Szasz, T. (1994) *Cruel Compassion* John Wiley, New York.

2 Compassion in nursing history

Attending to the patient's basic human needs with kindness

Ann Bradshaw

Introduction

Although there may be other understandings of the term 'compassion', the Western shared understanding has considered it to be empathy for the suffering of others and help to overcome it. Care for the sick is where this understanding of compassion is most relevant, and since the nineteenth century, outside the family, the nursing profession has been the traditional province for such care – the nurse's care for the vulnerable stranger being one expression of this shared understanding.

Hence this chapter will focus on compassion related to nursing, and in particular the UK nursing profession, and consider what 'compassion' meant for the nursing profession historically, highlighting implications for modern UK nursing and for society more generally. Although the focus of this chapter is on UK nursing and health care, this has international relevance because of its worldwide historical influence and interest. Examples from North America and Greece will be used to underline this. However, before proceeding, it needs to be noted that the modern understanding of the term 'nurse' has in recent years become blurred in the UK as the nursing role is very often undertaken by the unqualified health and social care assistant.

In 2001 the late Lord Morris of Castle Morris wrote a Foreword to a book (Bradshaw 2001a) that charted the radical changes in UK nurse education from 1978 to 2000, which had remade British general nursing. He stated that 'Compassion is an inconvenient concept: it cannot be measured, rationed or costed. It cannot be planned or delivered, but it will not go away.' And he reprised the central message of the book that 'the contractual model has been unable to sustain the ethic of compassionate care' (Morris 2001).

Over ten years later the Mid Staffordshire NHS Foundation Trust Public Inquiry (the Francis Report 2013) found scandalous shortcomings in nursing care at a major UK hospital. The Francis Report posed two questions for UK nursing. The first is why too many nurses are not showing compassion to patients, and the second is why too many nurses are not attending to the fundamental needs of patients such as keeping their skin clean, preventing pressure ulcers developing, helping patients to eat and drink and use the toilet. These questions are not limited to the Mid Staffordshire Hospital Trust, but are widespread, according to the Care Quality Commission (2011), Parliamentary and Health Service Ombudsman (2011), the Patients Association (2012). Further worrying reports that followed the Francis Report, the Cavendish Review (2013), the Independent Review of the Liverpool Care Pathway (2013) and the NHS Review of 14 NHS Trusts conducted by Professor Sir Bruce Keogh (NHS 2013), reinforced these questions.

And it is arguable that these questions reflect a deep ethical tension about the nature of care for vulnerable human beings, and in particular the connection between compassion and praxis. This analysis will therefore seek to address this question by first, examining relevant findings in the Francis Report. Second, it will compare and contrast these findings with traditional teachings on compassion in the British nurse training system. Third, it will consider the effect of fundamental changes to these values. Fourth, it will connect traditional values to their roots and some conclusions drawn that will relate to the observations of Lord Morris (2001).

The Francis Report: implications for UK nursing

The Healthcare Commission was first alerted to high mortality rates at Stafford Hospital. An investigation followed, which led by a public inquiry chaired by Robert Francis QC. Although the report highlighted many findings, one of the most important was that a completely unacceptable standard of nursing care was prevalent at the Trust and that this 'caused serious suffering for patients and those close to them' (p. 1497). The report noted that nursing activity was often performed by staff, who were not registered nurses, and did not carry 'nurse' in their title. Nevertheless, a very significant proportion of complaints of poor care were due to poor nursing care. These were listed as inadequate staffing, poor leadership, poor recruitment, deficiencies in the nursing task and those who perform it and declining professionalism. The report concludes: 'It is clear that the nursing issues found in Stafford are not confined to that hospital but are found throughout the country' (p. 1499).

While the report did not want to deny that there was much high-quality, committed and compassionate nursing it also stated that:

> Until this scandalous decline in standards is reversed it is likely that unacceptable levels of care would persist, so this was an area requiring highest priority. There was no excuse because what was required were not additional financial resources, but 'changes in attitude, culture, values and behavior'.
>
> (p. 1499)

The report gives examples: nurses did not answer buzzers to help paralyzed or distressed patients. They did not take patients to the toilet. There was a lack of hydration and nutrition for patients, and a failure to help patients eat and drink. There was a negative attitude among some nurses, and relative who complained as being seen as difficult. A patient was left naked in bed, covered in faeces, 'her nails, her hands and all the cot side . . . and it was dried. It would have been there a long time. It wasn't new' (pp. 1499–1500).

The report considered that progress to degree level nursing had 'been at the expense of exposure to personal experience of the basic tasks that all nurses should be able and willing to do' (p. 1515). And the report considered that providing caring, compassionate, sensitive and thorough attention to the basic needs of patients is, and should remain, the highest priority of any nurse. It could not be taken for granted that all applicants to nursing were assessed for this, but now it was necessary to ensure that all those entering the profession were committed to providing basic care and were not 'too posh to wash' (p. 1516). Fundamental care, such as lifting or washing a patient, is not a 'simple' task but requires a high degree of attention, meticulous observation to help protect against pressure ulcers and detect early signs of deterioration in the patient's condition. And the report recommended a review of nurse training to ensure practical elements were incorporated, and a consistent, uniform standard, requiring national standards.

The Chief Nursing Office at the Department of Health, Dame Christine Beasley, admitted problems in standards of nursing in her evidence to the Inquiry. She attributed this to a lack of attention to 'values and behaviors' (pp. 1286–7). Beasley's successors at the Department of Health responded by publishing a vision statement for nurses. *Compassion in Practice* (DH 2012). These values were delineated as: care, compassion, competence, communication, courage and commitment.

This was taken up in the parliamentary Health Select Committee (2013a, 2013b) that followed publication of the Francis Report. Both the Director of Nursing at the Department of Health and the Chief Nursing Officer for the NHS Commissioning Board, were questioned (Health Select Committee 2013a). The MP Rosie Cooper expressed surprise:

> I really fear that a lot of what I have heard today is about what we 'should' do – 'we should be', 'the frontline should be' – and, if I were to leave you with a comment from me, it is not about what you should be doing but what you are actually doing, what you are doing day to day to make this change
>
> (Q97).

The Francis Report and the Department of Health both presume compassion and attention to patients' fundamental practical needs to be core requirements for nursing, enacted in practice, whoever actually did the hands-on nursing. For, as the Francis Report (2013) noted, much hands-on fundamental nursing care was now being given to patients not by qualified nurses, but by unqualified health and social care assistants. A follow-up report on health care assistants, chaired by Camilla Cavendish, confirmed the vital importance of particular values – 'value-based recruitment' – for all those working with patients, whether registered nurses or not (Cavendish 2013). What is clear is that all these reports and officials are assuming timeless core nursing values and acknowledging an absence. And it is an examination of the core values from history that will show the connection between compassion and practical action with regard to fundamental patient care.

Compassion and care: teaching in nursing 1860–1970

In the UK an entirely new nurse education system, Project 2000, was introduced in 1986. Until then nurse training was an apprenticeship, learned on the wards under supervision of the ward sister, with annual blocks of class-based teaching. The basic practicalities of care for patients, such as washing, feeding, toileting and pressure ulcer prevention, took primacy. Under this system textbooks were basic to nurse training. These were written by nursing tutors and matrons from the major UK hospitals, who were themselves still involved in the organization of clinical care of patients (Bradshaw 2001b).

These books, written from about 1860 to 1970, and published in updated editions, provide a rich source of data about how nurses were inducted into the profession. Examples of these are: Williams and Fisher (1877); Wood (1878); Voysey (1905); Ashdown (1917); Smith (1929); Fisher (1937); Pearce (1937); Houghton (1938); Gration (1944); Gration and Holland (1950); Darnell (1959); Houghton and Whittow (1965).

Each textbook has a similar format. The first chapter deals with the underlying values required of the nurse. Then follow chapters on fundamental care, for example, making a bed with a patient in it, washing and dressing, feeding and drinking, with subsequent chapters focusing on more clinical aspects, such as inserting a catheter, or performing a wound dressing. There was a presumption of practice, and the first chapter, which set a historical context for nursing, defined the purpose of the nurse, and delineated values she required. Compassion was considered to be the motivation to practical care. It was not a concept to be examined, a theory or an emotion, but a practical activity – a vocation to serve. And the term that is most often used by authors to describe the nurse's expected attitude to the patient is 'kind'.

The moral purpose of nursing was inseparable from its practical outworking; dealing with the intimate bodily needs of patients was a calling. Order, method and structure were vital to achieve good practical care. Tasks and procedures involved diligence and precision, the manner of performance was crucial. Nightingale (1882) described these tasks and procedures in minute detail. Seemingly unimportant and insignificant matters, such as how urinals should be washed out, how chamber utensils should always be kept covered when not in use and when carried, and that urinals should never be left under the bed but beside the patient and emptied immediately after use, were the vital details that differentiated good care from bad. Hygiene of the nurse's skin, including short nails, and careful washing and scrubbing of surgical instruments and dressing forceps were crucial to prevent infection.

In a letter to probationer nurses, Nightingale (1914: 11) drew on a biblical quotation to teach that a nurse should be intelligent in her service to the patient, giving it honestly from her heart with her strength and mind, and not pretending to care 'with deceitful evasion of service, or with careless eye service'. As she wrote in a medical textbook (Nightingale 1882: 1038–1049): 'The nurse must always be kind, but never emotional. The patient must find a real, not forced or "put on", centre of calmness in his nurse.'

The Lady Superintendent of the Hospital for Sick Children, Great Ormond Street, Catherine Wood, held a similar position (1878 p.v.). The duties of the nurse and the signs and symptoms of disease provided her focus for the textbook, but she stated her intention as primarily 'to place the standard of nursing on the very highest level, as being the Christian work of Christian women'. Like Nightingale, Wood (1878: 18) stressed that the nurse must think only of the patient's comfort, not of herself, and that she should be conscientious and diligent, unseen as well as seen. Painstaking attention to detail was for the sight of God, rather than for the praise and reward of doctors, and could not be feigned: 'Gentleness of the heart will teach gentleness to the hand and to the manners. I can give no better rule than to put yourself in your patient's place.'

Evelyn Pearce, a former Senior Nursing Tutor at the Middlesex Hospital and member of the General Nursing Council, wrote a standard nursing textbook from 1937 to 1971. In her introductory chapter she refers to the Nightingale nursing tradition, telling nurses to keep their vocation alive in order to serve: 'in the spirit which asks not what do you want? But what can I do for you? How can I help you?' (1949: 8–19). In a small supplementary book called *Nurse and Patient* she expands on the meaning of this, appealing to the inspiration of Christian values for the nurse to become compassionate and kind (1969: 73). She explained that a nurse is 'privileged to be an integral part of God's design'. For the patient this meant:

> The nearness of another human being helps tremendously. A nurse by kindly little attentions, such as gently adjusting the bedclothes and pillows, moving a shaded light, altering the patient's position in his bed or chair, provided that these attentions are performed with a genuine interest in him, will all help.
>
> (Pearce 1969: 39)

Cicely Saunders, the founder of St Christopher's Hospice (whose teaching methods are appealed to by the Francis Report) and the modern hospice movement, trained as a nurse at the Nightingale School in the 1940s. She commented in 1998 that her 'nurse training taught me attention to detail and courtesy to patients which has proved invaluable in my palliative care work' (Saunders 1998: 14). And she quotes verses from St Matthew's Gospel as the motivation for her work in founding St Christopher's Hospice: 'I was hungry and you gave me food, I was thirsty and you gave me drink, I was naked and you clothed me . . .' (Saunders 1986: 41).

No less significant were the opinions of nurses trained under the old system, at St Thomas's Hospital, interviewed by Wake (1998). Most were very proud of their training and were taught precision, discipline, attention to detail, authority, structure and hierarchy. A few felt this was painfully conformist but for most it was excellent. This approach to compassion as kind, careful, selfless, practical action is identified by a modern educationalist (Jarvis 1996: 193–197):

> The educator of nurses is more than just one who transmits nursing knowledge to new recruits; he/she is the guardian of a tradition about the meaning of nursing into which new nurses are inducted . . . 'Education worthy of the name is essentially education of character' and the character of the nurse is as important as the knowledge that she possesses.

A picture of this approach to compassion is painted by a physician at the Westminster Hospital and later the Hospital for Sick Children, Great Ormond Street, who observed what nursing work involved in 1880:

> the ingratitude of many patients, the actual violence of some . . . All this the hospital nurse endures week after week, with small money remuneration, limited prospect of promotion, scanty share in any credit which may accrue, and prompted only by a motive which, however it may find expression, is of the highest and noblest kind. The dignity of such service seems to me quite unequalled.
>
> (Sturges 1880: 1091)

'Is humanism enough'? Fundamental change to the ethic of care

Writing in 1967, Dame Muriel Powell, Matron of St George's Hospital and Chief Nursing Officer at Scottish Home and Health Department, was concerned that in an increasingly secular age, nurses should not forget those qualities of mind and spirit, compassion, integrity and tolerance, which had sustained British nursing. She wondered if these values remain without the ethical framework to sustain them?

In Britain the nursing profession has traditionally looked to the Christian religion for its concept of wholeness . . . If this framework is removed, will the rules still be relevant? It is commonly assumed that they will; but it is a question to which we have paid little attention; and it requires an answer. Is the humanity and the humanism of our age enough?

(Powell 1967: 581–584).

Powell was acknowledging that this approach to nursing, which continued from about the 1860s to the 1970s, was subjected to severe criticisms from the 1970s onwards, by theorists and UK nursing leaders, for failing to give the nursing profession standing (Bradshaw 2001a, 2001b). Values of altruism and vocation, and the focus on menial aspects of nursing, had hindered the development of the profession. It was repressive to nurses. These arguments persuaded UK politicians to overhaul the profession and have persuaded them to continue to move to a full graduate profession (Willis 2012). And it is a similar situation that existence 30 years ago in the United States (Newton 1999); which has surrendered the traditional role of the nurse for that of 'autonomous professional'.

Newton, in defending the traditional nurses, might cast some light on this. She originally wrote her article in the context of North American nursing in 1981. She suggests that the 'monolithic' consensus of the ideal of the 'autonomous professional' badly needed questioning. Her view that the traditional role of the nurse as 'skilled and gentle caregiver' may have had faults, but 'but we may perhaps also be able to see virtues that went unnoticed in the battle to displace it' (p. 562). Her arguments are pragmatic. She believes that the traditional nurse, under authority, is more suited to the hospital than the autonomous professional.

It is at least arguable that the traditional system of nursing has important lessons to teach the present, post-Francis. Indeed Newton argues that the traditional nursing role is crucial to humanise the hospital system, which 'will become a mechanical monster without her' (p. 569). Newton's analysis of North American nursing resonates with Francis's assertion that nurses should never be 'too posh to wash'. And in this context, it is ominous that, writing in 1981, she was puzzled by the then 'current crop of nursing graduates' who did not want a traditional nursing role (p. 568).

Lanara (1976), at the time Professor of Nursing at Athens University in Greece, makes similar criticisms of North American nursing to those of Newton. However, she differs from Newton in her rationale and in so doing resonates with Powell. She argues that the basis for the model of compassionate, practical care is rooted not in maternal instincts, as Newton thinks, but in the Christian ethic of care.

Both Newton's and Lanara's criticisms resonate not only with Francis, but also with the review of the Liverpool Care Pathway, which found the pathway dehumanised dying people by becoming a tick box technique:

Not surprisingly, this Review has uncovered issues strongly echoing those in the Mid Staffordshire Public Inquiry, notable among the many similar themes arising were a lack of openness and candour among clinical staff; a lack of compassion, a need for improved skills and competencies in caring for the dying, and a need to put the patient, their relatives and carers first, treating them with dignity and respect.

(Independent Review of the Liverpool Care Pathway 2013: 48)

It is arguable that these shortcomings are yet another example of failing to cultivate the roots of practical compassion which inspired Cicely Saunders to found the modern hospice movement and the speciality of palliative care.

Philosophical roots: compassion as a praxis

To gain an understanding of these roots, and their effects, it is helpful to turn to Martin Buber (1959); Emmanuel Levinas (1999) and Karl Barth (1960). Their understanding of the human being, and the nature of human life, is grounded in the same ethic that underpinned nurse training 1860–1970.

This concept of life as a gift is the starting point for Buber. It is the same starting point for Levinas, writing after experiencing the Holocaust. It is also the starting point for Barth, a near contemporary of both Buber and Levinas. And it is with this understanding of life as a gift that human beings have a responsibility towards each other. This responsibility involves a practical relationship. For Buber this is the I and Thou. For Levinas it is attentiveness to the other. For Barth, the basic form of human creation is relationality in which eye-to-eye contact and listening is the prelude to helping – that is – practical action.

Kitwood (1997), who has made famous a new approach to caring for the person with dementia, revolutionizing it, draws on Martin Buber to establish his position that people with dementia remain persons, and that personhood is the primary category of human life. This is not individual persons, but persons in relationship. This is the I and the Thou purpose of humanity. And he quotes Buber's main reference point, that this is a gift of 'grace' (1997: 11):

more than any of thee, the word that captures the essence of such meeting is grace. Grace implies something not sought or bought, not earned or deserved. It is simply that life has mysteriously revealed itself in the manner of a gift.

And this is the point: compassion is not separable from human ontology and a way of *being* in the world. It is about being the kind of person that *being* itself requires. Because human beings are autonomous this involves a free choice. People choose to become nurses, and in so doing make a free choice to become a certain person that *being* requires of them. According to Levinas, this is by attentiveness to the other person – in this case, the patient. But because this choice is free, some people, including some who choose to become nurses, choose not to become this certain kind of person. This gives rise to the problems that Francis has identified, and as his report states, such a person should not be recruited into nursing.

The sense of the nurse being a person of virtue, and hence living out a virtuous life, what Nightingale called 'a good woman', bears clear resemblances to MacIntyre's (1985) conception of virtue. This is being which results in doing rather than merely thinking. And it is not merely a cosmetic 'eye service', or 'put on' as Nightingale said. It is, as she said, real, not forced. It runs deeply and ontologically into the kind of person the nurse is and what she does, and the way she does it.

Hence, as Nightingale, Wood, Pearce and Saunders show, compassion is witnessed in attentiveness to the practical details of care, in which nothing is too much trouble, and nothing is too menial to do. It is about clearing away vomit, helping the person to the toilet, cleaning faeces off the skin, helping the person to feed and drink, and done willingly with kindness. It is a covenant vocation rather than a contractual duty. As Lord Morris recognized, it is not a quality that is quantifiable. It cannot be measured, rationed or costed. Neither can it be pretended. And as Sturges observed, it does involve a personal cost because it is motivated by a genuine self-giving response of one human being to another. It is at least arguable that it has provided the collective mind of nursing until about the 1970s. The Francis Report is assuming this when it calls for an urgent change in values, attitudes and behaviours to reverse this 'scandalous decline in standards'.

Conclusion

In 1967 the Matron of St George's Hospital surveyed the changing UK nursing profession and wondered whether secular values could support compassionate care. Nearly 50 years later, the Francis Report, as well as other reports, appears to answer her question. It may be that, as Powell acknowledged then, that it has become unacceptable to espouse traditional values, such as those held by Nightingale, Wood, Pearce, Lanara and Saunders, as a basis for compassionate care. Be that as it may, it seems unarguable that these beliefs and values once sustained nurses in their willingly given commitment to washing, toileting, cleansing and feeding patients, with kindness – often in the most difficult of circumstances. The loss of these values coincides with a loss of this service ethic and its practical outworking – and indeed the changed nature of the UK nursing profession which is delegating fundamental patient care to non-nurses. The past of nursing, and its moral basis, has much to teach the present nursing profession on compassionate care as the attitude of kindness. And modern society can also learn from this approach, and from writers as diverse as Levinas, MacIntyre, Barth and Buber: compassion is a gift of grace, a practical and freely given human response to the other person in need.

Care Experiences: hospital experiences

Linda (UK)

The paramedics were superb, but the hospital I was taken to had no emergency surgery facilities, thus a decision was made to transfer me. We waited 4 hours at hospital A, during which I was in considerable pain and initially had great trouble trying to obtain pain killers from the A & E staff. The staff at hospital A showed very little care or compassion, and very little interest in me or the other patients. I remember there was an old lady on a trolley who was calling out to me and John to help her but given my condition, there was nothing we could do. We felt so bad about this. Eventually the ambulance arrived to transfer me to hospital B, but it broke down on route and had to be replaced with another one. The A & E at hospital B was very busy and the staff were clearly over-worked, but I was seen and cared for quite quickly by a Portuguese male nurse who although very serious, was very very attentive and I felt very reassured by his presence. I was seen by two surgeons – both of whom were exceptionally kind to both myself and to my partner. Later on (still in A & E after a total of 17 hours), we realized that my partner, who has diabetes, had not taken his medication. He mentioned this fact to one of the surgeons, who explained that he also had diabetes, and he gently took my partners arm and led him away to find him some medication. Little things like this make such a big difference. Even the tea lady treated John with kindness, offering him a sandwich even though she was not supposed to do so.

Eventually I was transferred to a ward, where again the staff were very kind and attentive. When I was taken into surgery I begged the anaesthetist not to let me wake in pain (mainly because I did not want to disturb the other patients in the ward), and he totally reassured me.

I could not criticise the staff, they were doing their very best despite being bogged down with paperwork etc. I also noticed their extreme kindness to elderly people on the ward. I would also note the kindness of the people who delivered food to patients during meal-times.

One thing that also struck me was the compassion shown between patients themselves. When an elderly lady fell from her bed in the middle of the night, my instinct was to help her but I couldn't because I was wired up to an IV drip and oxygen, so I called 'help' which awoke another patient, who instantly went to fetch the nurses.

Hospitals are not good places to be in, obviously, constant sounds throughout the night (bleeps and alarms), patients in pain, etc. But basic kindness and compassion can make a very big difference to this experience.

References

Ashdown, A.M. (1917) *A Concise System of Nursing* London: Dent & Sons.

Barth, K. (1960) *Church Dogmatics* Edinburgh: T&T Clark.

Bradshaw, A. (2001a) *The Project 2000 Nurse* London: Whurr.

Bradshaw, A. (2001b) *The Nurse Apprentice* Aldershot: Ashgate.

Buber, M. (1959) *I and Thou* Edinburgh: T&T Clark.

Care Quality Commission (2011) *Dignity and Nutrition Inspection Programme* London: CQC.

Cavendish Review (2013) *An Independent Review into Healthcare Assistants and Support Workers in the NHS and Social Care Settings* (Camilla Cavendish, Chair) London: Crown Copyright.

Darnell, L.M. (1959) *Nursing* London: Robert Hale.

Department of Health (2012) *Compassion in Practice* London: Department of Health NHS Commissioning Board.

Fisher, E. (1937) *The Nurse's Textbook* London: Faber and Faber.

Gration, H.M. (1944) *The Practice of Nursing* London: Faber and Faber.

Gration, H.M., Holland, D.L. (1950) *The Practice of Nursing* London: Faber and Faber.

Health Select Committee (2013a) House of Commons Oral Evidence. Nursing. Uncorrected Transcript to be published as HC920 – i. January 22.

Health Select Committee (2013b) House of Commons Oral Evidence Report of the Mid Staffordshire NHS Foundation Trust Public Inquiry Uncorrected Transcript to be published as HC982 – i. February 12.

Houghton, M. (1938) *Aids to Practical Nursing* London: Baillière, Tindall & Cox.

Houghton, M., Whittow, M. (1965) *Aids to Practical Nursing* London: Baillière, Tindall & Cox.

Independent Review of the Liverpool Care Pathway (2013) *More Care, Less Pathway: A Review of the Liverpool Care Pathway* (Rabbi Baroness Julia Neuberger, Chair) London: Crown Copyright.

Jarvis, P. (1996) Commentary on a Case Study of a Patient-Centred Nurse In Fulford, K.W.M., Ersser, S., Hope, T. (eds) *Essential Practice in Patient-Centred Care* Oxford: Blackwell Science.

Kitwood, T. (1997) *Dementia Reconsidered: The Person Comes First* Milton Keynes: Open University Press.

Lanara, V. (1976) Philosophy of nursing and current nursing problems *International Nursing Review* 23(2), 48–54.

Levinas, E. (1999) *Totality and Infinity* Pittsburgh, PA: Duquesne University Press.

MacIntyre, A. (1985) *After Virtue* London: Duckworth.

Mid-Staffordshire NHS Foundation Trust Inquiry (2010) *Independent Inquiry into care provided by Mid Staffordshire NHS Foundation Trust January 2005 – March 2009* Volumes I and II (Robert Francis, Chair) London: Stationery Office.

Morris, B. (2001) Foreword *The Project 2000 Nurse* London: Whurr, pp. vii–x.

National Health Service (2013) *Review into the Quality of Care and Treatment Provided by 14 Hospital Trusts in England: Overview Report* (Professor Sir Bruce Keogh KBE, Chair) Leeds: NHS.

Newton, L.H. (1999) In Defense of the Traditional Nurse In Kuhse, H., Singer, P. (eds) *Bioethics* Oxford: Blackwell.

Nightingale, F. (1873–1897) Letters and addresses to the Probationer Nurses in the 'Nightingale Fund' School at St Thomas's Hospital and Nurses who were formerly trained there. Original Letters and Prints for Private Circulation London: University College library holdings.

Nightingale, F. (1882) Nurses, Training of; Nursing the Sick In Quain, R. (ed.) *A Dictionary of Medicine* 1st edn. London: Longmans, Green, and Co. pp. 1038–1049 (part II).

Nightingale, F. (1882) Nurses, Training of; Nursing the Sick In Quain R. (ed) *A Dictionary of Medicine* London: Longmans, Green and Co, pp. 1097–103.

Nightingale, F. (1914) *Florence Nightingale to Her Nurses* Nash, R. (ed.) London: Macmillan.

Parliamentary and Health Service Ombudsman (2011) *Care and Compassion?* London: The Stationery Office.

Patients Association (2012) *Listening to Patients Speaking up for Change* Harrow: Patients Association.

Pearce, E.C. (1937–1971) *A General Textbook of Nursing* London: Faber and Faber.

Pearce, E.C. (1969) *Nurse and Patient: Human Relations in Nursing* London: Faber and Faber.

Powell, M. (1967) The Challenge of Nursing Education *Nursing Mirror* March 17, pp. 551–554; March 24, pp. 581–584.

Royal College of Nursing (2012) *Report of the Willis Commission on Nursing. Quality with Compassion: The Future of Nursing Education* London: Royal College of Nursing.

Saunders, C. (1986) The Modern Hospice In Wald, S. (ed.) *In Quest of the Spiritual Component of Care for the Terminally Ill* New Haven, CT: Yale University Press, pp. 41–8.

Saunders, C. (1998) What Made the Nightingales so Special? *Nursing Times* 94(20), 14.

Smith, E.M. (1929) *Notes on Practical Nursing* London: Faber & Gwyer.

Sturges, O. (1880) Doctors and Nurses I *The Nineteenth Century* 7(40), 1091.

Voysey, M.H.A. (1905) *Nursing: Hints to Probationers on Practical Work* London: The Scientific Press.

Wake, R. (1998) *The Nightingale Training School 1860–1996* London: Haggerston Press.

Williams, R., Fisher, A. (1877) *Hints for Hospital Nurses.* London: Simpkin, Marshall and Co.

Wood, C.J. (1878) *A Handbook of Nursing for the Home and the Hospital* London: Cassell.

Part II

Theoretical and therapeutic approaches to compassion

Theoretical underpinning is often essential for the understanding of human behaviour. In this section, various theoretical approaches to explaining and understanding the receipt and provision of compassion are explored. In addition, therapeutic techniques that are currently in practice, demonstrate how theory can be applied. Here we deal theoretically with diverse subjects, all equally important in health care, such as neurological mechanisms, psychodynamics used in psychotherapy, and how connecting with spiritual approaches to values are related to compassion in health care.

3 Empathy, stress and compassion

Resonance between the caring and the cared[1]

George P. Chrousos

> He who has committed himself to the art of medicine must convert wisdom
> to medicine and medicine to wisdom.
>
> Hippocrates, 5th c BCE

Compassion, i.e. the ability of empathizing with other human beings – or
by extension with other living beings – and of expressing this empathy with
acts of mercy, is a virtue of the soul and one of its most exalted properties.
However, the feeling and expression of compassion can take a grave toll on
a person, when certain conditions are not met. Before going over these conditions, it would be of interest to define exactly what we mean by the term
compassion. The ability to empathize is a fundamental, deeply inherent and
necessary property of human beings. Missing the feeling of empathy is utterly
pathological for both the person that lacks it and for those around him or
her. Indeed, two human conditions, both individually and socially detrimental, that are characterized by deficient empathy, are autism and psychopathy.

Recently, the neurological substrate of inter-human communication and
attunement and, hence, socialization has started to be revealed. Special
neurons, the "spindle" or "von Ecomomo" neurons in the prefrontal, insu-
lar and anterior cingulate cortex subserve social interactions, while other
"mirror" neurons resonate between human beings in visual communication, a phenomenon which has been termed "resonance." I believe "consonance" would be a more accurate appellation.

"Em-pathy" is a Greek term meaning feeling inside another human being,
as opposed to "sym-pathy," feeling together or in parallel with another person, or "a-pathy," not feeling what somebody else feels at all. The Latin term
"com-passion" is a congener of "sympathy," however, over time it has come
to mean empathy combined with action based upon the feeling.

Expression of compassion means interaction between two emotionally
resonating stressed persons: the caring and the cared. The recipient of compassion is already the victim of some calamity, serious disease, trauma, loss,
etc., and, hence, by definition, in a state of distress. The caring compassionate human feels the victim's distress, vicariously, by empathizing, and is, thus,
also distressed. In both instances, distress is expected to take a toll. What can

be done to minimize the impact of distress in both the cared and the caring? The proper care of the victim is palliative and, hence, diminishing his or her distress. On the other hand, administration of care should not take a toll on the caregiver influencing his or her wellbeing and, naturally, because of this, potentially decreasing the quality of care provided. This is what we call "principled compassion." The caregiver empathizes with and achieves the best possible comfort for the cared without harming herself or himself in the process. Actually, and even better, the caring might transform the compassioned act into a positive experience arising from the feeling of altruism.

There have been many studies on caregivers, including relatives, or professionals, such as physicians, nurses and others involved in the care of the sick, all showing frequently the negative psychological and physical effects of chronic stress. These include increased psychiatric and cardiovascular morbidity and mortality and a curtailment of their life expectancy. Burnout, depression and post-traumatic stress disorder are common in caregivers and there is an increased risk of suicide. All of these are explained by the deleterious effects a chronically activated stress system and its mediators may have on the mind and body.

The genetically and constitutionally unsuitable and unprepared caregiver, who is distressed during the provision of care, usually provides suboptimal care to the already hurting subject. In that distressed person's behavior we can distinguish the three hardwired stress program options of a stressed subject: flight, fight or freeze. In his or her behavior we see the effects of an activated amygdala – fear and anger – and stress system-high levels of the stress hormones cortisol, adrenaline and noradrenaline – and a suppressed dopaminergic reward system, i.e. dysphoria or even anhedonia. Fear is expressed as avoidance or appearance of lack of caring, while anger may be associated with aggressive behavior toward the cared, her or his relatives, and/or the other caregivers, even against the self. Freeze or helplessness is expressed as emotional numbing. Lack of "reward" and, in fact, presence of actual "punishment," is expressed as anxiety, depressive feelings, anhedonia and guilt. Undesirable changes in appetite and sleep patterns appear, and the unwanted obesity, metabolic syndrome, and cardiovascular changes that accompany chronic stress gradually establish themselves. It is clear that people that have to provide optimal care to less fortunate human beings without suffering the consequences of their empathy must be prepared for this difficult task and this preparation comes down to "principled compassion," which is, in my opinion, proper stress management of the caregiver.

To decrease the effects of stress on our organism, we can take two not mutually exclusive actions: first, we can try to change the environment that causes the disturbance and, second, if this is not possible, to change our coping strategies towards the stressor. The former is frequently, but not always, unavoidable, while the latter is usually achievable. Empathy that damages the person that expresses it is an uncontrolled emotional response, activates the stress system, with all that this entails. The solution is empathy combined with emotional control and, hence, good stress coping or management, i.e. compassion. Such

principled compassion cannot only prevent the feelings and somatic consequences of distress, but can in fact provide the caregiver with the superior mental reward of service to others, altruism and other-centeredness.

While thinking on empathy and compassion and what they mean for the
caring and the cared, I realized that principled compassion can be natural
in a small proportion of fortunate humans that are this way because they
have the right combinations of genes and exposure to a propitious developmental environment. Unfortunately, the majority of human beings have to
struggle for long to achieve this equanimous state, which is a component of
or at least has many similarities with the exalted state of wisdom.

The qualities, which the Greek sages deemed present in every wise

person – pertaining respectively to the *logisticon, thymeticon, epithymeticon,
and dioraticon* – correspond in Latin to the four cardinal virtues of prudence,
fortitude, temperance, and justice. On the other hand, in his recent book
on wisdom, S. Hall (*Wisdom: From Philosophy to Neuroscience*, Vintage Books,
2011) summarized the ingredients of wisdom as follows: *fearless aggregation
of knowledge, emotional regulation, dealing with uncertainty, moral judgment, sense
of fairness,* and *other-centeredness,* including *principled compassion.*

After a long discussion with Joan Halifax, we re-classified these ingredients of wisdom into four categories: those pertaining to *eugnosia,* i.e. proper
attainment and use of knowledge; *euthymia,* i.e. proper emotional control;
eupraxia, i.e. proper behavior; and *eusomia,* i.e. good physical health. These
are summarized in Figure 3.1 and shown below:

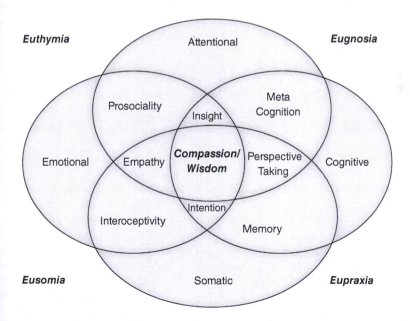

Figure 3.1 An integrated perspective of compassion/wisdom

Proper Emotional Regulation – Euthymia

Interoception

Dealing with Uncertainty

Patience – Delayed Gratification

Emotional Consonance – Empathy

Moral Reasoning

Good Somatic health – Eusomia

It is obvious that the attainment of wisdom requires time and effort. However, it is all worth it. Wisdom leads to feeling good and getting from life all life can give to a human being.

Let me close with the words of three wise men. Aristotle in his eulogy at his teacher's Plato funeral said of him:

> he showed with his deeds and the method of his logic that for somebody to be happy one has to be good.

On the other hand, John Mill gave a statement that summarizes the connection of *eupraxia* with happiness:

> Those only are happy, who have their minds fixed on some object other than their own happiness; on the happiness of others, on the improvement of mankind, even on some art or pursuit, followed not as a means, but as itself an ideal end. Aiming thus at something else, they find happiness by the way.

Finally, Epicurus, a totally misunderstood ancient philosopher, wrote a letter to his student Idomeneus on the last day of his life, showing that death is not necessarily stressful and that a wise person can temper his feelings and even be serene at those last moments of life:

> I have written this letter to you on a happy day to me, which is also the last day of my life. For I have been attacked by a painful inability to urinate, and also dysentery, so violent that nothing can be added to the violence of my sufferings. But the cheerfulness of my mind, which comes from the recollection of all my philosophical contemplation, counterbalances all these afflictions. And I beg you to take care of the children of Metrodorus, in a manner worthy of the devotion shown by the young man to me, and to philosophy.

I am convinced that the higher wisdom one attains in his or her life, the better it is for him, those around him and the society at large. Providing care to the severely ill is an act that can be associated with major distress that is expected to harm people who are not inherently "wired" or prepared mentally and emotionally to deal with it. Not all young physicians, nurses or patient relatives are born with the innate ability to control their emotions and provide care with principled compassion. All of us should be preparing for coping with stress and learn from others, and this is a life-long process. In the meantime, the general rules that help develop resilience to stressors should be followed: adequate sleep, proper diet, moderate bodily exercise, some form of brain exercise and being or doing good. Preparation for dealing with stress can convert even caring for a sick fellow human, a process which is usually associated with distress, into an ultimately positive experience, a process characterized by Hans Selye as eustress, i.e. stress with a good outcome.

Note

1 The edited summary of a lecture by Dr. Chrousos at the Library of Congress, Washington DC.

References

Chrousos, G.P. (2009) Stress and disorders of the stress system *Nature Reviews Endocrinology* 5(7), 374–381.

Hall, S. (2011) *Wisdom: From Philosophy to Neuroscience* New York: Vintage Books.

Halifax, J. (2012) A heuristic model of enactive compassion *Current Opinion and Supportive and Palliative Care* 6(2), 228–235.

4 Who cares for the carers? Keeping compassion alive in care systems, cultures and environments

A psychologically minded approach

Martin Seager

Introduction

It is an indisputable psychological law that care always involves a relationship and depends broadly upon an interaction (a × b) between:

a) care-giving qualities on the part of the care provider;
b) the receptivity and accessibility of the service user.

It is less recognised, however, that, whilst care relationships will always be unique interactions between individuals, they also depend upon:

c) environmental, cultural and systemic conditions that may support or undermine '(a)', '(b)' and the interaction (a × b) between them.

The idea that there is a '(c)' should be straightforward enough in 'common sense' terms. In this chapter I will focus on perhaps the most fundamental aspect of '(c)' which can be broadly defined as the *care and back-up that the care-giver receives.* I will also explore some of the science that explains why all carers regardless of their individual integrity, resilience and skill, need care and support to remain emotionally engaged, energised and receptive. In terms of the 'abc' model, described above, this means that '(a)' cannot be a fixed entity but also depends upon '(c)'. This also means that where '(c)' is ignored in designing care services, care providers will inevitably become stressed and burned-out, undermining the quality of care, increasing staff sickness and creating an unnecessary cost for our society in both human and financial terms.

If this '(a)' × '(c)' interaction makes *common* sense, then why is any recognition of this interaction so conspicuously absent in the design of care services in the UK and elsewhere? One explanation is that Western societies remain gripped by a materialistic model that reduces mind to brain and medicalises care relationships. This reductionist obsession with biological explanations for human experience has been termed 'neuro-mania' by Tallis (2011). Similarly, Seager (2006; 2013) has expanded Baron-Cohen's (1995) concept of 'mind-blindness' from its original specific application to autistic thinking to describe a wider lack of empathy and compassion that results from reductionist thinking across public policy in relation to care services. This thinking means that the inter-subjective, personalised and contextual nature of care-giving all too easily gets reduced to a set of objective 'skills', 'techniques' or 'competencies' that are seen as education-ally transferable, teachable, manualisable, packageable and reproducible. The 'heart and soul' of care-giving is therefore subtly disqualified and only seen at best as an unscientific and unquantifiable 'values base', the 'bath-water' rather than the 'baby' itself. I shall then conclude by showing how a more psychologically minded scientific approach such as the 'abc' model is needed to ensure that service systems, environments and cultures will keep compassion alive both in spirit and in practice.

Mind-blindness in traditional Western science

The capacity for compassion is one of the defining characteristics of our species and it constitutes the largest part of what we mean by 'care' in the first place. However, once compassion is looked at through the lens of tra-ditional Western science, it can only be seen as a 'soft' moral value or at the other extreme as a 'hard' skill or even as a biologically driven capac-ity resulting from brain development (measured, for example, in terms of 'mirror neurons')

Once compassion is looked at in these 'mind-blind' terms (i.e. we are lost. It becomes much harder for us as scientists of the human condition to see the dynamic, systemic and psychological processes that are obvious in our everyday lives and also to our artists, writers, film makers and spiritual thinkers. It becomes harder to see that compassion involves a *live meaning-ful identification or empathic connection with the suffering of another person* that can easily be registered subjectively 'in the moment' but cannot so easily be quantified by traditional scientific methods. Empathic connections can only be experienced subjectively by one mind connecting with another. Empathic connections and failures of empathy determine the outcome of all human interactions. This is not beyond the realm of science, but a sci-entific paradigm that tries to factor out subjectivity as a 'soft' subject for art alone is itself unhelpful and misguided. Indeed subjective observation is at the core of all science, even 'physical' science.

Within a materialistic scientific paradigm, however, only brain corre-lates of experience are legitimised and not lived experience itself. This also means that the universal concept of 'love' gets disqualified from science, being consigned to art and religion, even though the object of human psy-chological science is precisely our own personal and emotional life. The term 'compassion' is perhaps the nearest that a materialistic science will allow itself to get to the human spirit. However, by using such a mind-blind scientific model to study our own psychological nature, we are in dan-ger of being defeated from the outset by objectifying human beings and depersonalising phenomena which by their very nature are highly personal, spiritual and even sacred.

From a mind-blind towards a psychologically minded model of compassion

In a mind-blind society, therefore, the emphasis is placed almost exclusively on the pseudo-objective 'compassion quotient' of individual care-givers and on how to instil or teach it as a skill or competency. Professionals with duties of care to others are consequently also being blamed simplistically as individuals for failures of compassion when things go wrong in care organisations as if the maintenance of compassion was something that only required individual effort, competence and a 'moral muscle'. Conceptualising compassion in such an individualistic way is, however, more likely to kill it than create it. It also ignores the obvious truth that those who choose to undertake caring roles will by definition already be on average significantly more compassionate as individual personalities than those who do not. This is illustrated admirably by a poem called 'Nursing the Nation' delivered to the 2013 RCN Congress by a student nurse called Molly Case. The poem was her response to all the bad publicity that the nursing profession had been receiving and her attempt to voice the true vocational and compassionate mentality of the vast majority of nurses who each and every working day take on board the anguish, the suffering, the fears and the life and death struggles of strangers who are their fellow human beings. Here is an excerpt:

> One lady passing had no relatives to stay,
> We sang her to sleep, let angels carry her away.
> Were you there that day when we held her hand?
> Told her nothing would harm her, that there was a higher plan?
> Saw her face as she remembered a face she once held?
> Saw her breath in the room as she finally exhaled?

By reading this poem it is impossible for the empathic mind not to feel compassion for this lady in her last moments of life and appreciation for the value of nursing care at its best in honouring the sanctity of human life. This poem enables the reader or listener to *identify* with this situation in a way that would not be possible if the same situation was described in the language of traditional Western science which is deliberately *de*personalised. Poetry is therefore in many ways a better method for achieving a true description of human compassion than traditional Western science. Poetry and art generally invite us to *identify* with other human beings and the *meanings* of human situations. The meaning of a human situation can never be reduced to physics, biology, chemistry or mathematics.

There can therefore be no compassion without *personal identification*. How then does the capacity to identify with others develop in the human condition? The existing scientific evidence, most recently from the field of 'mentalization' (e.g. Fonagy *et al.* 2002), is already very clear that the empathic aspects of the human personality can only be nurtured in the context of human attachments and relationships. This means that an individual's compassion could never be either genetically predetermined or instilled through formal education. Our innate potential to identify with other human beings can only really be realised in one way – by the actual lived experience of being identified with by others. This usually happens during the developmental period of our species (childhood) from the first attachment onwards, when the individual personality is shaped. We reach adulthood having unconsciously internalised the cumulative impact of such successes, honourings, failures and violations of empathy over the course of personality development. Where first relationships fail and the child does not experience true identification, subsequent relationships (e.g. friendships, counselling, psychotherapy, fostering, mentoring and adoption) can potentially heal emotional damage and make up for the deficits in self-development.

Human beings can only therefore develop compassion as individuals to the extent that they themselves truly know what it is like to receive compassion. This is because compassion involves at its core an empathic identification with others and requires a sufficiently healthy personality that is self-aware and able to 'read the minds' and the communications of others accurately without major distortions. This vital importance of 'empathy, warmth and genuineness' was recognised long ago by humanistic psychologists such as Carl Rogers (1957) and before that by Sigmund Freud (1906) who said that 'psychoanalysis is in essence a cure through love'.

Recently (Seager 2010) I was asked by the national Samaritans to conduct a review of why talking helps (and fails to help) people. I looked at the psychotherapy literature, the arts, religion and also everyday life. The evidence emerged clearly and perhaps not surprisingly that accurate empathy and identification (in the context of a meaningful attachment) forms a major part of all successful psychotherapy regardless of its 'brand' or 'model' (see also Wampold 2001; Norcross 2002) and it also underpins the 'golden rule' of all world religions: 'treating others as we would wish them to treat us' (Seager *et al.* 2007). Similarly, in Harper Lee's 'To Kill a Mockingbird' (1960) Atticus Finch says:

> You never really understand a person until you consider things from his point of view – until you climb into his skin and walk around in it.

Designing care systems and cultures that nurture compassion rather than kill it

Accurate empathy based upon personal identification may be said to underpin all successful human relationships and endeavours. It is probably the most important element in civilisation itself. This means that above all else promoting and sustaining empathy and compassion should be the greatest priority of organisations whose core business is to provide care.

Organisations, however, are like families on a larger scale. They can be healthy or unhealthy. They will only promote empathy and compassion to the extent that those in authority transmit those human qualities themselves. From childhood onwards, we become and stay healthy only in response to the authentic enactment of empathy by those in authority over us, in other words the *congruity* and *authenticity* of their words and deeds rather than their words or slogans alone. This applies to any form of organised leadership. Mahatma Gandhi (1913) famously advised us all to:

Be the change that we wish to see in the world.

Even relatively healthy and empathic adult personalities, who have had a good emotional start in life, need to be sustained and nurtured by healthy relationships and healthy human environments. Let us take an obvious example. A loving mother who has no partner and gets no break from a demanding baby will quickly become tired, distractible, impatient and intolerant. That same mother, however, with the back-up of grandparents, an extended family and the support of a partner will be much more likely to sustain a high quality of attunement and care in relation to her baby. This is because the mother's own emotional needs are being met and her energies nurtured so that she can carry on caring. To sustain a caring role, carers also need ongoing care and support. In the well-known film *About a Boy* (2002) this was clearly demonstrated in the finishing sequence:

I don't think couples are the future; you need more than that – you need *back up*.

Within the psychoanalytic literature, this has sometimes been referred to as 'containing the container' (Bion 1959). More recently, taking these ideas even further, the need for professional teams, services and environments to be 'psychologically safe' (Seager 2006), 'psychologically informed' (Johnson and Haigh 2010; Seager 2011) and 'emotionally nourished' (Briggs 2012) has been outlined.

The obvious truth that a compassionate mind still needs to be sustained and nurtured in a compassionate culture has huge implications for how we should be designing care environments. The most important implication is that the quality of a care environment cannot properly be measured without considering the human attachments and relationships that it supports, not just between service user and provider but also within the 'professional family' (Seager 2006, 2008) of the care organisation. Without healthy attachments and supportive relationships, care-givers in any environment like single mothers will lose emotional energy, focus, attention and tolerance. Compassion cannot thrive in a psychological vacuum. When we add to this the fact that in mental health services at least, those being cared for have often already been neglected and abused as children and so will be even more complex and demanding, it becomes even more vital to optimise the supportive environment for the front-line professionals. We know, however, from numerous sources (including several public investigations, e.g. Francis 2013) that the culture of the NHS, for example, is still far from optimal in this respect and may be said in too many instances to be blind to such issues or even 'toxic'. Our most vulnerable citizens are therefore often presenting themselves to care-givers in our public services with a great potential for compassion but who are all too often drained, stressed, burdened, overworked, distracted, exposed, burned-out and lacking in support or nurturance. Instead of receiving the highest quality attention that they need, therefore, NHS patients and others in need of professional care may all too often find a care-giver who is not, to use Stephen Wright's (2011) terminology, 'clear-eyed' but 'glassy-eyed'. By this Wright means that those providing care can become emotionally detached and that those receiving care can sense this just from the glazed look in their eyes.

This has almost nothing to do with skill or moral goodness and almost everything to do with staff being emotionally supported to maintain a receptive state of mind.

In public care systems and environments, however, the emotional needs and energies of our professional 'single parents' with heavy caseloads can often be the last thing that gets thought about. All too often professional care-givers, so far from being supported, are undermined by impersonal performance targets, staffing shortages, bureaucracy and neglectful management cultures. Ironically, there is also a danger that compassion itself could become the latest focus for yet another set of unhelpful 'top down' performance targets.

There is already a wealth of literature, for example, on 'burn-out', 'vicarious trauma' and 'compassion fatigue' (e.g. Figley 1995; Wright 2010) but strangely almost no formal links have been made between this clear evidence and our policies and practices in relation to designing human care environments, system and cultures. This is essentially because the humanity of our care environments is still seen as an issue of moral values rather than one of practical science. However, there is nothing more practical in its implications than the obvious truth that a GP, however caring and skilled, who has already seen 20 people in one day without a break will be at risk of not really being able to listen properly to number 21. It should be obvious that there is a human limit to the sheer numbers of people that any one person can truly think about, care about, hold in mind and remember, especially when there is a time pressure and when the clients are complex, distressed and demanding. Regardless of their personality, training and experience, helpers need to remain in a *receptive* state of mind, if they are to attend to the complex needs of distressed people. Receptivity is affected by stress, tiredness, distractions and pre-occupations, motivational and support factors. Listening to distressed or traumatised people involves 'tuning in to' and identifying with painful feelings. This inevitably means getting a personal taste or 'dose' of the traumatic feeling. This 'vicarious traumatisation' is a normal part of care work (Figley 1995; Seager 2010) but if it is not *processed* (in regular supervision, managerial support, informal corridor conversations, debriefing, personal therapy, peer support and a supportive home life) it can become quite toxic, leading to 'burn-out' or emotional 'overwhelm'. Under such conditions, the helper will 'switch off' and cease to listen attentively to clients, partly out of an understandable need for self-preservation. This emotional 'burn-out' happens all the time, for example, amongst GPs in busy surgeries and nurses on frenetic psychiatric wards.

Reporting on measures of burn-out in GPs Dobbin (2013) states:

> The measure of burnout that impacted most on the patient satisfaction was depersonalisation, described as an 'unfeeling or impersonal response toward recipients of one's service, care, treatment, or instruction'. That is about as close a description of lack of compassion that I can think of. You cut yourself off from understanding your patient's viewpoint, from empathising with their position, seeing yourself in their position, mirroring their circumstances emotionally.

The work of Isabel Menzies-Lyth (e.g. 1960) also shows how nursing care systems in general hospitals can easily become defensive and depersonalised to avoid overwhelming anxiety and distress in the staff. Whenever this happens, however, clients may lose the empathy that they need from helpers and the helpers can only lose 'job satisfaction', morale, confidence and their own mental well-being. The ultimate result of such human processes can be staff sickness or absence and even at times suicide (see Daley 2013).

The helper's capacity to remain receptive to clients in an empathic way will therefore depend in a large part on the capacity of the helping organisation to provide an empathic or supportive culture, including in particular the right number of colleagues for the job, the opportunity to process toxic feelings (especially secondary or vicarious traumatisation), to 'sound off' to peers and colleagues, to debrief, to rest, to think, to be validated and to recuperate emotionally between periods of intense client contact. A patient or client's chances of getting an empathic experience depend therefore not just on the skills and empathic capacities of the helper, important though these are, but on the extent to which the organisational culture is empathic to the helper's own state of mind. Recently, the term 'psychological safety' (Seager 2006, 2008) was introduced to describe this concept of empathy within organisations and caring environments as systems or cultures.

From teaching compassion as a pseudo-skill towards creating the conditions that sustain it

There is therefore an urgent need for us as scientists of the human condition to investigate and articulate the universal psychological conditions that sustain the mental energies and capacities of human beings to maintain *empathic personal identifications* in care-giving relationships. In science the most important thing is not only getting answers but asking the right questions. Once psychologically minded questions are asked it does become possible to provide some preliminary answers from our existing human knowledge. Our knowledge base for compassion does not have to be drawn exclusively from 'empirical' studies. The world of art, film, literature, religion and everyday life provides a wealth of data in which some fairly obvious patterns can be observed. Science is simply the observation of patterns that unify and explain a range of individual observations. If our object of study is human compassion, then to ignore the vast wealth of observable data in the world of art, religion, human culture and history would be a true scientific failure.

I shall conclude therefore by setting out what I believe to be the most fundamental questions and psychological principles in relation to the maintenance of human compassion and to provide some preliminary answers where possible. These answers will also indicate some practical conclusions for the future design of our public care environments, systems and cultures. The questions fall into three broad areas.

Area (1): capacity factors

What are the limits of the capacity for compassion in the mind of a healthy human being?

This question is complex and must be considered along several dimensions.

Time dimension: the limits on time spent in continuous emotional attention and personal identification

How long can a healthy or resilient human being provide *continuous* emotional attention that involves identifying with another person in distress? There are certain clues. Psychotherapy arguably creates the most intense emotional connections between carers and clients and it can be observed that the 'therapy hour' has evolved as a universal pattern over different cultures and therapy models. It seems reasonable therefore to assume that a human being, even when highly trained, can probably only give active, intense, focused emotionally attuned attention to another human being in distress for about one hour continuously before needing a significant break to process the emotional impact and refresh the emotional energy-level. In a more passive role, for example watching an emotionally intense film or play and identifying with the suffering of characters, human beings can give attention on average for longer, perhaps 90–120 minutes. The capacity for such attention can be enhanced, however, by creating breaks and punctuations. In successful films, plays, stories and musical productions there are typically passages and moments of light relief or even intervals. In therapy sessions there too is a value in punctuation and taking breaks for reflection and emotional recovery as particularly pioneered within systemic family therapy approaches.

It also follows from this that even where care is being given in shorter bursts, for example in the working day of a general nurse or general practitioner, this will start to become a cumulative problem emotionally for every hour of caring work that is undertaken, if there has not been an opportunity to have a reasonable break to process the emotional impact and refresh the emotional energy-reserves before the next hour begins.

Number dimension: total limit on number of care-giving relationships that can be held in mind at any one time

The evidence from looking, for example, at patterns of caseloads (across different care professions) and classroom sizes across different settings and cultures would indicate that 20–30 is the 'magic' range for the number of relationships that a professional carer can take primary responsibility for. This seems to reflect how many people a professional carer can get to know in reasonable depth and hold in mind at any point in time. In primary care, where there is potential for a much wider range of relationships involving briefer contacts, the same figure of 20–30 can also be used as a guide for how many such contacts can be meaningfully sustained over any given working day before there is a total overload. The quality threshold for exceeding the proper number of care relationships can be simply measured psychologically: *that point is reached when the care-giver, during live encounters, is unable to hold in mind the basic story or identity of existing patients or clients.*

Energy dimension: care as a limited energy resource

Psychologically, it makes sense to assume that all human beings, however compassionate, resilient and skilled, have a finite emotional capacity (energy) to remain 'tuned in' to the distress of others. The more intense care-giving relationships are, the less of them can be sustained by any given care-giver over any given unit of time. This means that we can infer a *constant* (that can be called 'K') that is the product of multiplying these two factors (intensity × frequency) together and it follows from this that a care-giving system that regularly pushes individual carers beyond the threshold of 'K' will be ineffective and potentially damaging to all parties. Care systems that make no attempt to monitor the number and intensity of care-giving relationships therefore cannot be said to be 'psychologically safe'.

Area (2): burden factors

What are the core elements of emotional burden (aside from the cognitive and physical burden) that consume the available energy for compassion in carers? Clearly the following two elements must be included in any list.

Vicarious suffering through identification

'A problem shared is a problem halved.' If this proverb contains an emotional truth then care providers must at some level be 'taking on board' half of a problem that they didn't have before. Compassionate caring for other people involves empathy which in turn involves identification. Identification means using one's own life experience to imagine oneself in the place of another. When that other person is distressed, it follows that the carer who truly 'tunes in' must experience some level of vicarious distress (see Figley 1995; Seager 2010). It can be argued that without this resonance there can be no true emotional connection between human beings, so that caring has to have some emotional cost to be effective. Any care system therefore that does not make a clear and planned provision for compensating for this emotional cost is psychologically unsafe.

Burden of responsibility

Caring for others inevitably means feeling responsible for alleviating their distress. Regardless of the resilience of the carer, the burden of caring can become overwhelming under the following conditions:

- the greater the emotional attachment
- the greater the distress in the cared for persons
- the more irreversible the cause of the distress
- the greater the number of cared for persons
- the smaller the number of peers to share the burden of care with
- the less time that is available to process the emotional impact of caring
- the greater the 'top down' pressure on the carer to achieve imposed targets
- the less choice or freedom the carer has to escape from the care-giving role.

Area (3): support factors

What are the key factors that sustain (or in their absence deplete) the emotional energy required for compassion in carers?

Looking at the evidence from psychotherapy research, the arts, religion and everyday life, the universal primary five factors would appear to be:

1   Having *time* to *process* and reflect upon the emotional impact of one care-giving contact before moving on to the next (or at least 10 minutes processing time in every hour). This processing time does not always require the presence of another person. It can happen, for example, when a district nurse or social worker is driving between home visits.

2   Having a *secure attachment* to at least one trusted peer or colleague who can provide regular empathy and identification with the position of the carer. This can be part of supervision but equally could be much more informal.

3   Having regular *back-up* from and a sense of belonging to a healthy team or 'professional family'. The evidence relating to group therapy processes (e.g. Yalom 1995) indicates that where teams, or at least their meetings, get bigger than about 10 people, conversations become more impersonal and less empathic. The same principle also applies to the maximum size for a healthy human family.

4   Receiving regular *supervision (including peer)* that involves a secure attachment and values not just skill development but the need for emotional processing, empathy and identification.

5   Having the support of an *authentic management culture* that validates and honours the emotional burdens involved in care work and recognises the value of its professional expertise.

Conclusions and implications for future service design

I hope to have demonstrated beyond reasonable doubt that sustaining compassion goes well beyond the immediate qualities of individual care-givers, important though these obviously are. A psychologically minded approach to sustaining compassion involves looking at the wider system, context and culture of care-giving. I have proposed an 'a(b)c' interactive model where I hope to have shown that '(a)' which refers to the quality and receptivity of care provided by an individual care-giver is also dependent upon and dynamically related to '(c)' which refers to the quality of the support and back-up that the carer is receiving. Whilst it would not be valid or psychologically minded to impose rigid guidelines based on this model, it can still be used in highly practical and creative ways to define general quality standards that can help reduce the human and financial cost of care by optimising:

a)   caseload sizes and staff-patient ratios
b)   the design and working practices of care teams
c)   psychological safety in care environments
d)   the outcomes of care interventions
e)   staff and service user satisfaction, morale and well-being
f)   working patterns for people with caring roles
g)   supervision and management practices in support of professional care providers.

Only by applying psychologically minded principles (based upon empathy and identification) to carers themselves can compassion be optimised in any care environment for any given level of human resource. We have to care for our carers too if we want our service users to get the best care.

Care Experiences: the importance of little acts of kindness when dealing with a depressive condition

Derek (UK)

In the text that follows, Derek recalls the background to a depressive illness which has been with him from childhood to adult life. Derek shared with the editors correspondence from the children's hospital that initially treated him in the 1950s. His stories drew attention to lack of attachment to his parents who were very busy in their respective occupations at that time. One letter in particular, from the children's hospital refers to 'inadequate housing, poor schooling, and an unsatisfactory relationship between the boy and his parents'. The letters portrayed his thoughts with regards to the then military service whereby Derek had stated that he 'did not like killing though he was quite willing to do his military service'. The key point in the story that follows, is how little acts of kindness, can make a world of difference to somebody who has a history of depression from childhood to adulthood.

In personal correspondence, Derek shared the following story with the editors:

> *Here is an outline of my mental health problems from an early age to the present time – my memories of moments which I feel are milestones through life, and as I reflect on them, many of my actions I recall with shame and regret. However, the clock cannot be turned back.*

At the age of about seven years old and running around with the other children at school during playtime I fell over and hit my head on the playground tarmac. Our GP suggested I'd suffered mild concussion which led to nightmares I suffered during the few years following the fall and led to him referring me to a specialist children's hospital.

The nightmares followed the same pattern every night. Sounds became louder and louder, in particular the tick of the clock and my parents' voices also, until unbearable as the sounds got louder so all objects appeared to get closer and closer and by then I was screaming in fear. At its crescendo so the sounds decreased and objects appeared to move farther away until I could barely hear the sounds or see the objects which led to further fear and anxiety, this situation would continue from start to finish over and over again each and every night. Since those days I've never been able to sleep without a light on, or background noise, such as a radio.

(continued)

(continued)

We moved back to Dartford in 1952 and the nightmares ceased and I was discharged from the hospital. Following this I developed a violent temper which would flair up for no apparent reason and I would break and destroy my most prized possessions, yet, not offering aggression or violence to people, only to my own special objects. I'm ashamed to say this trait stayed with me until about 2005.

Since my formative years I've been dogged by anxiety states and my medical records will bear this out. However, in my mid thirties I suffered my first full bout of depression and I was off work for over four months, at this time our GP told my wife I was not to be left alone as he felt I was suicidal. I will add I have never had a desire to take my own life however low my state of despair has been. Over the next twenty years I had treatment for depression on many occasions, you name the anti-depressant – I've taken it!

In my mid fifties it came to me that medication only helped get you through the stage until you could cope with life again. I realised there was always a catalyst which turned me around and it was at this point that I ceased to visit the doctor and take anti-depressants. I still get depressed and weighed down with despair and these bouts will last from three days up to three months or more, but, always something will happen to give me a kick start back to reality.

I'm offering this as an example: when depression sets in I'm consumed with a feeling of utter despair and want to be in company yet wish to create a barrier, so I see people, but, I do not wish to converse with them. In this mood it creates difficulties for me in my local pub, as my friends must feel I'm snubbing them yet it's not the case, I need them there for the support I gain from their presence. Today I'm just over two weeks out of an eight week depressed state. The catalyst on this occasion was young Alice who serves behind the bar – (her dad also suffers with depression) when she approached me and she just put her arm around me gave me a peck on the cheek and said 'cheer up'.

Derek (UK)

References

Baron-Cohen, S. (1995) *Mindblindness: An Essay on Autism and Theory of Mind* Boston, MA: MIT Press.

Bion, W. (1959) Attacks on linking *International Journal of Psychoanalysis* 30, 308–315.

Briggs, A. (2012) Under-nourishment and clinical risk: Two concerns of CAMHS clinicians *Journal of Social Work Practice: Psychotherapeutic Approaches in Health, Welfare and the Community* 26(4), 427–441.

Daley, M. (2013) Social worker killed herself after restructure caused workload to increase, *Community Care*. Available at: www.communitycare.co.uk/articles/12/

02/2013/118909/social-worker-killed-herself-after-restructure-caused-workload-to-increase.htm?cmpid=NLC%7CSCSC%7CSCDDB-20130213-GLOB%7Cnews (accessed 6 February 2013).

Dobbin, A. (2013) We have to be compassionate – to ourselves *Scottish Review* (21 May).

Figley, C.R. (Ed.) (1995) *Compassion Fatigue: Coping with Secondary Traumatic Stress Disorder in Those who Treat the Traumatised* New York: Brunner/Mazel.

Fonagy, P., Gergely, G., Jurist, E.L., Target, M. (2002) *Affect Regulation, Mentalization and the Development of the Self* New York: Other Press.

Francis R. (2013) Report of the Mid Staffordshire NHS Foundation Trust Public Inquiry. Available at: www.midstaffspublicinquiry.com/sites/default/files/report/Executive%20summary.pdf (accessed 6 February 2013).

Freud, S. (1906) Letter to Jung as quoted in Bettelheim, B. (ed.) *Freud and Man's Soul* New York: Knopf, 1983.

Gandhi, M.K (1913) *Collected Works*, Volume 13, chapter 153, p. 241.

Johnson, R., Haigh, R. (2010) Social psychiatry and social policy for the 21st century: New concepts for new needs – the 'psychologically-informed environment *Mental Health and Social Inclusion* 14(4), 30–35.

Lee, H. (1960) *To Kill a Mockingbird.* Philadelphia, PA: J.B Lippincott & Co, Chapter 3, p.30.

Menzies-Lyth, I. (1960) Social systems as a defence against anxiety *Human Relations* 13, 95–121.

Norcross, J.C. (ed.) (2002) *Psychotherapy Relationships that Work* New York: Oxford University Press.

Rogers, C. (1957) The necessary and sufficient conditions of therapeutic personality change *Journal of Counselling Psychology* 21, 95–103.

Seager, M. (2006) The concept of 'psychological safety' – A psychoanalytically-informed contribution towards safe, sound & supportive mental health services *Psychoanalytic Psychotherapy* 20(4), 266–280.

Seager, M., Orbach, S., Samuels, A., Sinason, V., Johnstone, L., Fredman, G., Hughes, R., Antrican, J., Wilkinson, M., Kinderman, P. (2007) National advisory group on mental health, safety & well-being: Towards proactive policy: five universal psychological principles [unpublished paper available on request from the author].

Seager, M. (2008) Psychological safety: A missing concept in suicide risk prevention, chapter 17 in *Relating to Self-Harm and Suicide* London: Routledge, pp. 210–223.

Seager, M. (2010) How can talking help people feel better? A review of the psychological evidence for the National Samaritans [unpublished paper available on request from the author].

Seager, M. (2011) Homelessness is more than houselessness: A psychologically-minded approach to inclusion and rough sleeping *Mental Health and Social Inclusion* 15(4), 183–189.

Seager, M. (2013) Attachment theory as a basis for informing service systems, cultures and environments, chapter in *Attachment Theory in Adult Mental Health* London: Routledge, in press.

Tallis, R. (2011) *Aping Mankind: Neuromania, Darwinitis and the Misrepresentation of Humanity* Durham: Acumen Publishing.

Wampold, B.E. (2001) *The Great Psychotherapy Debate: Models, Methods and Findings*, Mahwah, NJ: Lawrence Erlbaum Associates.

Wright, S.G. (2010) *Burnout: A Spiritual Crisis on the Way Home* Redmire, Cumbria: Sacred Space Publications.

Wright, S.G. (2011) The heart and soul of nursing *The Nursing Standard* 25(30).

Yalom (1995) *The Theory and Practice of Group Psychotherapy* Scrantan, PA: Basic Books.

5 Experiential learning and compassionate care

Encouraging changes in values, beliefs and behaviour

Craig Brown

Summary

This chapter outlines a training programme in compassionate care for healthcare workers. It is based on the 'Values in healthcare – a spiritual approach' (vihasa) training programme that was designed specifically for healthcare professionals. Experiential learning in small groups is suggested as the main educational approach to bring about a change in values, beliefs and behaviour necessary to make compassionate care central in all healthcare practice.

Introduction

> Be the change you wish to see in the world.
>
> Attributed to Gandhi

It is obvious to those working in the healthcare sector that for years there has been a lowering of morale and increase in stress levels in staff which is detrimental to patient care.

Dealing with others suffering can be draining on healthcare workers and it is not uncommon for them to find it difficult to maintain their ideal of being compassionate. They can suffer from exhaustion, depression and low self-esteem (Maslach and Schaufeli 1993) with the result patients receive poor care. The causes are multiple and complex and include a heavy workload, poor support and rapid organisational changes. Excuses such as being too busy, having more important things to do, completing forms are often cited as reasons that compassionate care cannot be delivered.

It often takes a crisis to draw our attention to the situation and for the public and media to demand something is done. As a result there may be a flurry of enquires and recommendations by various bodies. However the change required will only happen when individuals are motivated to change at a personal level first.

Despite being clearly stated in many medical and nursing codes of practice, values and in particular compassion are not adequately covered, if at all, in many of the professional educational programs. If values' training is included in a teaching programme it is usually as part of a series of lectures on ethics, or as a separate session for students with a special interest. To bring about the attitudinal and behavioural changes needed to improve compassionate care it is the author's opinion that the most effective training is facilitated experiential learning in groups.

Experiential learning

> I hear and I forget. I see and I remember. I do and I understand.
>
> Confucius, Chinese philosopher and reformer (551–479 BC)

Two and half thousand years on it still holds true that the best way to learn is through 'doing'. Lectures, presentations and seminars are useful for learning information or new skills, but having the experience makes it stick so that we remember and understand what is being taught.

In the past learning from experience has meant learning on the job and in the case of professional values it has been by observing the behaviour of teachers and senior colleagues. Unfortunately they do not consistently set a good example and are rarely explicit about how their actions are values based enabling students to learn from them.

Experiential learning can be thought of as consisting of two elements. One is learning by reflecting from one owns experience of life and work, relationships, etc. The other element is having an awareness of one's own thoughts and feelings. It gives the individual the time to integrate the new learning to suit his or her own personality and circumstances.

Groups

Training in groups empowers individuals while also encouraging a team approach, which is more open and inclusive. Although larger groups can be managed when learning about values, a small group of 8–12 students is the optimum learning environment for a group session.

'Values in healthcare, a spiritual approach', is a training programme designed for health professionals as a holistic approach with the emphasis on promoting the self-care of the practitioner as the way to improve patient care (Figley 1995; Janki Foundation for Global Health Care 2004). It has been used successfully in other professional groups and mixed groups of staff from all levels (Brown 2003). The training pack has been translated into nine languages and used in over 30 countries. There are seven modules, peace, positively, values, cooperation, compassion, self-care and spiritual care. Each module is designed for a days training, but is flexible enough to run as a shorter session.

The group needs to be a safe, respectful and a confidential space for students to be able to share their experiences and insights freely. Ensuring adequate introductions of each participant, encouraging the group to create their own ground rules and setting their objectives contributes to a successful session.

The activities in the group are designed to encourage students to be curious and consider the many aspects of delivering compassion care. Students are invited to reflect on their own experience and share their story with others in the group. Initially sharing with one or two people allows for more intimate exchanges, before the essence of their sharing can be fed back to the whole group to broaden their experience and build knowledge of the subject. As a final activity in the session they are invited to consider how they can apply what they have learnt in practical ways in their work.

Consideration should be given to the environment for the training such as noise, lighting, heating and the general comfort including the seating. The learning in a small group is enhanced is by having quiet time for reflection, playful and creative activities and stretch breaks. Most importantly the success of any group will be dependent on the facilitator's skills.

Facilitation and feedback

A facilitator's role in a session is to guide the group of individuals to discover and learn about themselves and not to impart knowledge or teach anything (Eagger *et al.* 2005). The facilitator needs to be non-judgemental and encouraging and know not to play the expert. They should try to be flexible and creative and be sensitive to the group dynamics and energy. The emphasis is that the learning is through participation. It is acknowledged that there is no perfect facilitator and that each facilitator has their own style and will bring their own experience and stories to the group. Finally the facilitator should model compassion in the sessions and in their work, as this is a powerful way for students to learn.

It is useful for the facilitator to be familiar with the appreciative Inquiry approach (Cooperrider *et al.* 2000; Cooperrider *et al.* 2003). It is used in organisations to focus on what works well rather than correcting what does not work. Facilitators can use this appreciative approach by making positive observations that highlight what students have done well in the group and emphasise their individual qualities. This acts as a model of how they can use this kind of appreciative feedback in practice. Besides giving positive feedback to students the feedback should focus on what and how they are learning. Observation rather than judgement is the approach taken. Examples of questions are, 'What have you learnt?' and 'How would you do things differently?' This encourages self-awareness, and curiosity about their core values and develops good communication skills with colleagues and patients.

There are specific three day trainings run by the Janki Foundation charity in the vihasa style of facilitation with ongoing support for the facilitators through a website (Janki Foundation 2013). The participants are usually people who have had experience of training and wish to introduce the training into their own healthcare setting.

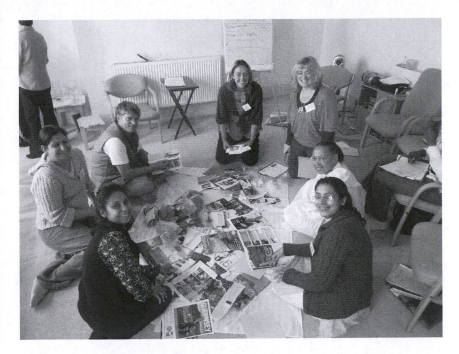

Figure 5.1 A creative group exercise: making a poster of 'values at work' from cut outs from magazines

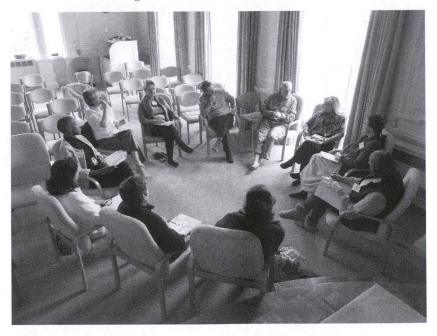

Figure 5.2 Sharing stories in a group. Notice the attentive listening of some of the participants

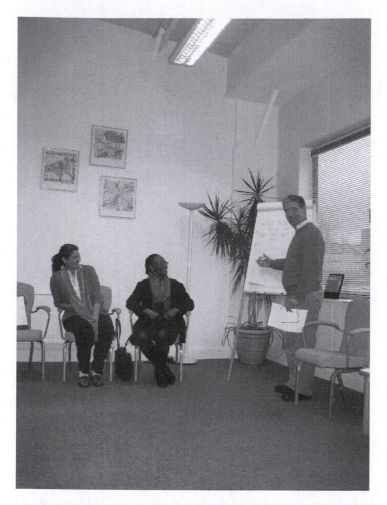

Figure 5.3 The facilitator collecting feedback on a flipchart from participants to share with the whole group

The process of the sessions

It is helpful to have a structure to each training session that includes: introductions, the exercises, action planning and breaks. However each session should be flexible enough to suit the group. Compassion is essentially a spiritual quality and although much can be learnt at a cogitative level with information and discussion one needs also to include an inner experience. This is described as 'a spiritual approach' where time is made for silence and reflection. Spirituality can be described as that awareness of our inner being and reaching out to connect to others and the environment and possibly some greater consciousness. Developing an inner stillness is helped with visualisation and meditation exercises that are included in every training session. Being creative and playful is also a means of participants exploring their own spirituality as can poetry, stories and artwork that relates to compassion. Creative writing is another way of helping students explore compassion in depth (Holder 2010).

The word compassion

Compassion is a soft, gentle word that has a deep strength and richness. It is kindness in action. Compassion is a feeling that rises up in response to another's difficulty and urges one to act to alleviate their discomfort. Compassion is the most humane of qualities.

Words such as 'sympathy' and 'empathy used in the caring context do not reach that full emotional soul felt response of compassion. 'Sympathy' is when we acknowledge another's suffering and 'empathy' is an understanding of the patient's situation, perspective and feelings. There has been some useful reported work using these words in healthcare. Morse *et al.* in a literature review describes four components of empathy; emotive, cognitive, behavioural and moral (Morse *et al.* 1992). Mercer *et al.* suggest that empathy in a clinical setting involves an ability to understand and check its accuracy, and to act on that understanding with the patient in a helpful (therapeutic) way (Mercer *et al.* 2002). However, tying words down to a working definition can be limiting as we all use words in different ways to describe how we feel and what we mean, and the meaning can vary in different settings.

The content of the sessions

Compassion the word

As an exercise students can be asked to reflect on the word 'compassion' and ask what they consider it means. This is not done as a test of whether they can construct a definition but more a way of reflecting and exploring it for themselves. One method is to write the word compassion on a blank page then write as many words as they can that are associated with it. They can do this by working on their own or in pairs, then sharing their ideas with the group with the purpose of developing a discussion and a language around compassion.

Imagine being in a care home

Students are invited to use their imagination by visualising themselves as an elderly person in a care home. Invite the students to sit comfortably and relax and to close their eyes if they wish. Read the following slowly to them:

'Imagine you are in a care home. You are sitting in a large sitting room with many other elderly people and you are not entirely sure where you are. You are a bit frail and your hearing is not very good and your memory is not clear. You are not sure why you are here. You notice a person in a white coat approach you to come and talk to you. How would you like them to behave towards you?'

Invite the students to open their eyes and write for several minutes about the sort of person they would like to care for them. What do they say? What to they do? What are they like? They can share what they have written with a partner, and then the essence of their story with the whole group. This will give the students a personal experience of what sort of care they would like for themselves and what makes good compassionate care for their patients.

Box 1   An example of imaginative writing

I am in sitting in this place and am a bit wary and anxious as she approaches. She draws up a chair and sits next to me. 'Hello', she says 'I am Alice your occupational therapist and I am here to help you if I can. She smiles easily and pauses waiting for a response. I shift in my seat uneasily. 'Can you hear me ok?' and I respond with a raspy, 'Yes I am not deaf.'

'Would you like some water?' and reaches over for the water jug and starts to pour me a glass and guides it to my lips. I take a refreshing gulp and thank her. She smiles again and takes the glass holding my hand for a few seconds.

She asks where I come from, what was my job and about my family. I notice she listens easily without interrupting and is genuinely interested. We share a few stories and I find for the first time in ages I begin to tell her my worries: how I cannot remember things so well, how the corridors in this place are confusing and how embarrassed I am that I dribble when I eat.

Compassion to ourselves

The stress of the job and risks of burnout and compassion fatigue needs to be acknowledged by the facilitator in a brief discussion with the group before considering self-compassion.

However, the emphasis of this exercise is to take a constructive approach by enquiring what the students already do as individuals to care for themselves. The benefit of this exercise is that it focuses on the students' needs and supports the principle that healthy workers produce good care. This can be done with the students as a reflection on sheets of paper headed 'All the things I do to look after myself', with the sub-headings: physical, mental, emotional, spiritual and social, and for them to make a list. The findings are shared as feedback with the group so there is learning about various strategies that they can be used to be more compassionate to themselves.

Compassionate listening

Most students will have had communication skills training and others may have learnt and practised specific counselling methods. Non-judgemental attentive listening is the key skill to be compassionate, and it is worth practising. Ask them to 'set aside' their previous training and experience, and instead focus on the following when in the 'listener' role:

- Maintain an inner stillness and a sense of peacefulness.
- Be fully present for the speaker with no interruptions, including making encouraging noises, facial expressions, etc.
- Listen from the heart and be non-judgemental.

Invite the students to choose a partner and remind them that everything said to them in this session is held in confidence. For 10 minutes each person has the chance to talk about a current issue such as a professional problem, a relationship problem, or conflicts between the job and home life. The listening person should not comment, interrupt or prompt even when a silence occurs. When the time is complete they can change over from being the talker or listener. In the group they can share the process of how it felt to talk and to listen in this way. The facilitator can then draw on the groups experience to share the learning.

Visualisation: a compassionate work place

The facilitator explains the process and reads the script slowly with gaps between the phrases.

> 'Sit comfortably on a chair so that your body can relax . . . Place your feet on the floor and rest your hands on your lap. Feel the tension release from your muscles and your breathing become even and regular . . . Allow your thoughts to slow down and become calm.
>
> 'You are going to think about work and create a picture in your mind . . . Think of your workplace and how you would like it to be truly compassionate. How would it be if everyone were working well together . . . ? That patients were treated with kindness and the staff were caring and supportive to each other. What comes up in your ideal workplace . . . ? What is it like . . . ? What is the atmosphere . . . ? How are people behaving . . . ? What are they saying . . . ? What feelings are they sharing in their interactions . . . ? What qualities are they showing . . . ?

'You may get pictures, feelings or words coming to you . . . colours, sounds, a texture . . . let your mind wander freely . . . is there a symbol or particular image . . . ?

'What would it be like at your workplace if everyone is acting with compassion? Observe what emerges for you.

'When you are ready, become aware of your body sitting on the chair. Feel your feet on the ground . . . begin to deepen your breathing . . . and in your own time, open your eyes.'

Students can share their thoughts or just sit silently for a few minutes. Sometimes it can be useful to draw the images or write down thoughts or words.

Meditation experiencing compassion

First, invite students to sit upright, with hands held loosely in their laps, and feet on the floor. Speak in a soft, calm voice, pausing at ellipses (. . .) to allow participants to follow you in a relaxed state.

'Sit comfortably and relax. Become aware of your feet on the ground. Feel the connection to the earth. Allow the muscles of your shoulders and neck to relax . . . Allow the tension to dissolve and move down into the ground.

'Let the muscles of your arms feel calm and relaxed . . . next your legs . . . now your face . . .

'Now focus your attention on your breathing . . . let it find its own calm rhythm . . . breathe in peace and breathe out any negative feelings . . . gently breathe in peacefulness and calm.

'Allow your mind to slow down . . . try to watch your thoughts . . . do not judge them as good or bad . . . they are just thoughts . . . acknowledge them and let them go . . . they are like clouds in the sky that you can watch drifting past. Beyond the clouds is the deep blueness of the sky . . . feel that deep calm of the blue sky.

'Now focus on your own inner calm . . . that place that is deep within yourself . . . that is peaceful . . . where your inner compassion lies . . . here you are patient . . . tolerant . . . generous . . . understanding . . . all these qualities are here which make up your own inner compassion. Experience the feeling of compassion . . . feel it within you . . . and see it focused as a point . . . a point of light . . . (long pause).

'Now raise your awareness beyond yourself . . . to a place of infinite peace . . . see it first as a small point of light. As you move towards it, it becomes brighter . . . it is like an ocean of peace . . . a space of calm, of love, of compassion . . . you feel connected . . . part of that ocean of deep peace and love . . . it surrounds you like a cloak, it fills you up, absorbing every part of you with a comfortable warmth.

'Rest in that feeling of being loved . . . it is like energy . . . a vibration . . . a light filling you . . . until you overflow . . . (pause for 8 seconds).

'Now, slowly you move away from the ocean – as a point of light. You still have that memory of being loved . . . and can reconnect at any time you wish . . .

'Gradually become aware of your body. Feel your feet on the ground . . . begin to deepen your breathing . . . and in your own time, open your eyes. When you feel ready, stand up and have a stretch.'

Introducing training sessions to organisations

It will require a change in attitudes at all levels in organisations to introduce compassionate training to healthcare professionals and staff. Following the Francis enquiry (there has been much discussion as to how best to bring about change (Francis 2010; 2013; Davies and Mannion 2013)). Before introducing a training programme on compassionate care into any organisation it is important to have discussions with people at all levels of the organisation; the executive board, the management team who will be commissioning the training, the professional bodies, the training team and facilitators, the ward or community teams and as many of the staff representatives as possible. There are some simple questions that need to be explored. See Box 2.

Box 2   Questions when introducing compassion training

Why do you want/need compassionate training?

What are your expectations?

On completion of the training how do you think participants will be doing things differently?

How is the training going to be evaluated?

How will those that have had the training be supported?

What provisions are made for ongoing learning?

Are there teams that could be models of good compassionate care?

The training needs to be planned either within professional training, part of mandatory training for all staff or as part of an induction programme for staff. Organisational infrastructure must be in place that includes the learning space and training of facilitators, with specific times set aside that ensures proper cover for the trainees if the training is done in work time.

Leaders that are enthusiastic determined and committed need to be identified to drive and ensure the programme is introduced and changes are imbedded in practice. This is no easy task but a vital one to improve health care and very worthwhile for patients and practitioners.

Evaluation

At a personal level we know when we have provided compassionate care; the patient is content, the relatives are appreciative and we feel satisfied that what we are doing is worthwhile. We are aware that the team works well, there is cohesiveness in the organisation and there is an atmosphere of purpose and caring. It is a challenge to capture such changes on questionnaires and although evaluation can be challenging it is preferable to have a broad range of assessment of the possible consequences of the compassionate training. See Box 3.

With the vihasa training itself we make time for completion of evaluation forms from the participants at the end of each session and do the same in the sessions for training the facilitators. The evaluation is quite detailed and something that is constantly developing using rating scales and open questions. The last four training sessions for facilitators 48 people were trained and on a rating scale of 1–6, 14 scored 5 (very good), and 29 scored 6 (excellent), with 3 non-completers. Some of their comments are in Box 4 and Box 5.

The facilitators are encouraged to reflect on what went well in their sessions and anything they would do differently in the future and share their comments with an online vihasa learning community of facilitators.

Box 3   Evaluation assessment

A vision statement on values developed by all staff

Strategy for embedding the vision statement in all levels of practice.

- Professional codes of practice: known and adhered to.
- Staff well-being assessment: sickness rate, recruitment, retention, staff questionnaires, staff rotas, staff facilities, staff support, staff concerns.
- Environment: eating and rest facilities, cleanliness, friendliness.
- Patient satisfaction: questionnaires and complaints procedures.
- Visibility of board and senior staff: openness, accountability.
- Performance date allows the inclusion of compassionate care.

Box 4   Comments from participants of vihasa training

'It was an opportunity to share ideas in a supportive environment.'

'Help me realise that I have a lot of inner qualities that I can draw on.'

'The periods of silence are something I will do more of.'

'It helped me look at my life–work balance.'

'It was the first time in my training that I felt I seemed important.'

Box 5   Comments from facilitators training

'An inspiring and supportive training.'

'I found it to be a balanced and a practical approach.'

'It was informative and fun.'

'It helped build my self-confidence.'

'I appreciated the non-judgemental and positive approach.'

Conclusion

It is acknowledged that in organisations there needs to be a clear intention, leadership and determination for compassionate care to become central in all healthcare practice. Patients are becoming more assertive in their demand to be treated with kindness and good care and it cannot be left to governments to be prescriptive in bringing about change. Healthcare workers need to reflect on how they can be more compassionate and small group experiential learning is considered by the author to be the most effective educational method to consolidate core values as part of health care practice and bring about better healthcare. It needs people passionate about providing such care, have the self-awareness that they need to change, and to be models of compassionate care, that can bring about the necessary changes at a local level with simple and creative initiatives.

Compassion

Craig (UK)

Now your grief is an aching, empty chasm.

The commotion surrounding the resuscitation is over

And your husband's corpse lies on the pontoon.

(continued)

(continued)

The smell of rosemary and pine drift down the hillside,

The moon light dances on the water

And the cool south wind offers some relief.

Death visits on any occasion

Starting the long sorrow.

Waves gently lap against the side of the boat.

I am the moon, the fragrances and the wind.

My compassion reaches out to the stranger.

(Tying up at a small harbour in Croatia next to a boat we notice the family is anxious as someone is ill. The paramedics arrive and as he is taken off the boat he collapses. Many people help and cardiac massage is carried out for 30 minutes before his body is left on the pontoon for the coroner to arrive. I walk past his wife sitting alone on a bench).

References

Brown, C.K. (2003) Low morale and burnout: Is the solution to teach a value based approach? *Complementary Therapies in Nursing and Midwifery* 9(2), 57–61.

Cooperrider, D., Sorensen, J.P., Whitney, D., Yaeger, T. (2000) *Appreciative Inquiry: Rethinking Human Organization toward a Positive Theory of Change* Champaign, IL: Stipes Publishing.

Cooperrider, D., Whitney, D., Stavros, J. (2003) *Appreciative Inquiry (AI) Handbook* Bedford Heights, OH: Lakeshore Communications Inc.

Davies, H.T., Mannion, R. (2013) Will prescriptions for cultural change improve the NHS? *BMJ* 346, f1305.

Eagger, S., Desser, A., Brown, C. (2005) Learning values in healthcare? *Journal of Holistic Healthcare* 3, 25–30.

Figley, C.R. (1995) *Compassion Fatigue: Coping with Secondary Traumatic Stress Disorder in Those who Treat the Traumatized* New York: Brunner/Mazel.

Francis, R. (2010) *Robert Francis Inquiry Report into Mid-Staffordshire NHS Foundation Trust*. London: Stationery Office.

Francis, R. (2013) *Report of the Mid Staffordshire NHS Foundation Trust Public Inquiry: Final Report* London: Stationery Office.

Holder, J. (2013) *49 Ways to Write Yourself Well*. Hove: Step Beach Press.

Janki, D. (2013) Values in healthcare: A spiritual approach. Available at: www.janki-foundation.org/values_in_healthcare/index.jsp (accessed 6 June 2013).

Janki Foundation for Global Health Care (2004) *Values in Healthcare: A Spiritual Approach*. 449/451 High Road, London NW10 2JJ.

Maslach, C., Schaufeli, W.B. (1993) Historical and conceptual development of burn-out. In: W.B. Schaufeli, C. Maslach and T. Marek (eds) *Professional Burnout: recent Developments in Theory and Research* New York: Taylor & Francis, 1–16.

Mercer, S.W., Reilly, D., Watt, G.C.M. (2002) The importance of empathy in the enablement of patients attending the Glasgow Homoeopathic Hospital *Journal of the Royal College of General Practitioners* 52, 901–5.

Morse, J., Anderson, G., Bottorff, J., Yonge, O., O'Brien, B., Solberg, S.M., McIlveen, K.H. (1992) Exploring empathy: A conceptual fit for a nursing practice? *Journal of Nursing Scholarship* 24, 273–80.

6 Compassionate care
The theory and the reality

Alys Cole-King and Paul Gilbert

Summary

This chapter outlines the development of an emerging new approach to compassion based on aspects of human evolution and neuroscience and a review of some of the evidence for the compassionate approach. The authors also acknowledge some of the current barriers to delivering compassionate care and highlight the importance of identifying and minimising such barriers in order to enhance patient outcomes and promote clinicians as facilitators of healing.

Introduction

The NHS Ombudsman's report *Care and Compassion* which gives an account of ten investigations into NHS care of older people makes difficult reading. For example 'Hospital staff at Ealing Hospital NHS Trust left Mr J forgotten in a waiting room, denying him the chance to be with his wife as she died.' We suggest that improving clinical governance will not improve patient care unless systemic and widespread changes enable compassionate care to be delivered. The recent Care Quality Commission Report *Dignity and Nutrition* reviewing care in some of the hospitals identified in *Care and Compassion* found that some of the problems still remained.

The *Point of Care* document published in 2009 by the Kings Fund suggests actions that could promote compassionate care in acute medical settings. We suggest that they are also relevant in primary care. *Nothing personal: Disturbing Undercurrents in Cancer Care* by Mitzi Blennerhassett (2008) outlines her cancer treatment and her experience, at times, of a lack of compassion. Compassionate care can enhance staff efficiency, help elicit better patient information, and so inform treatment plans which lead to better recovery and increased satisfaction (Matthews *et al.* 2006; Halpern 2001; Sanghavi 2006).

A science of compassion?

Compassion is commonly misunderstood as being only about traits such as warmth, kindness and gentleness. These are important of course, but compassion is much more than that. Paul Gilbert's 'compassionate mind' approach integrates the scientific study of compassion and affiliative behaviour with the use of compassion in health and mental health fields (Gilbert 2009). This approach suggests that compassion is an aspect of the same abilities that primates evolved for parenting and for developing the affliliative and cooperative relationships that enable group survival. These abilities are evident in many species: all mammalian mothers are sensitive to distress in their infant and will try to reduce that distress. Bowlby's model of attachment developed out of his animal studies and infant observations, and led to important insights into how we form (and break) affiliative relationships. More recently, the neurobiological substrates of affiliative relating and empathy have been revealed (Porges 2011; Baron-Cohen 2011).

Today we might define compassion as 'a sensitivity to the distress of self and others with a commitment to try to do something about it and prevent it'. This sensitivity implies that awareness, attention and motivation are all involved. 'Doing something about it' would require commitment, courage and wisdom; indeed it is difficult to think of compassion without these qualities. Compassion is not synonymous with pity: it does not depict one person as being weak, inferior or lesser in comparison with another. Compassion is an important aspect of the Institute of Medicine's definition of patient-centred care (Committee on Quality of Health Care in America 2001).

There is now a large and growing literature on the psychology and neurophysiology of affiliative relating (Depue and Morrone-Strupinsky 2005). For example oxytocin and opiates are known to be biological mediators of care affiliation, with oxytocin linked particularly with feelings of affiliation, trust, soothing and calmness (Gilbert 2009; Carter 1998). Oxytocin receptors in the amygdala influence threat-processing and important modifications of sympathetic and parasympathetic activity which have enabled mammals to engage in close personal relationships and soothe each other (Porges 2007). Therefore it would be a serious misunderstanding of science to dismiss compassion as too 'woolly' a concept for serious study or application.

Of course there is more to compassion than hormones and mammalian affiliation. Humans are unique to the extent that our compassion depends on a number of other abilities such as empathy and the ability to stand back, think and reflect. Compassion is more than just caring: we can care for the family car or a beautiful painting but we can't have compassion for inanimate objects: the only object of compassion is another sentient being. In fact it seems the skilful use of compassion fundamentally depends on humans having evolved to interact and understand the minds of others.

Paul Gilbert's 'compassionate mind' approach builds on this basic idea, namely that specific abilities and skills go into developing compassion; that it is not something as simple as an emotion or motivation, but rather a

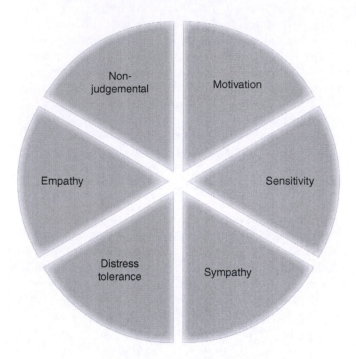

Figure 6.1 Adapted from P. Gilbert (2009) *The Compassionate Mind*, with kind permission Constable Robinson

complex combination of attributes and qualities. Gilbert suggests that in the light of current research, the human capacity for compassion appears to involve two 'different' psychologies: on the one hand for awareness and engagement, on the other for skilled intervention in action. Hence the inner ring of *attributes* in the Figure 6.2 below are the core attributes necessary for the sensitivity to engage with, and understand suffering. The outer ring relates to the skills required to (skilfully) do something about that suffering.

We can look at the key attributes in more detail.

Motivation. The initial stage requires the *motivation* to be caring, supportive and helpful to others. This is the 'commitment to try to do something about it' aspect of compassion which can operate at particular points of time, but also represent a set of values which define how we would like to be in our roles and also as human beings. Motivation is the fundamental component that shapes compassion's other attributes. For example, empathy without motivation to help could be exploitative – the advertising industry uses a certain kind of empathic insight to manipulate our desires. The motivational system is what provides the focus, the purpose and point of all the other abilities. (Motivation is referred to as 'care for well-being' in Figure 6.2). Individuals who are motivated to help others rather than

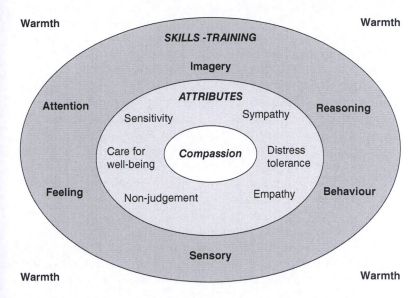

Figure 6.2 The compassion circle: Key attributes of compassion (inner ring) and the skills needed to develop them (outer ring)

From P. Gilbert (2009) *The Compassionate Mind.* With kind permission Constable Robinson

having ego-focused goals have better social relationships, less conflict and greater well-being.

Sensitivity is the capacity to be sensitive and to maintain open attention – it enables us to notice when others need help. It is the opposite of 'turning a blind eye'. All being too preoccupied to be able to notice – or to aware that one 'doesn't have time to notice' and so gradually one doesn't measures.

Sympathy is our emotional response to distress. Compassion requires an ability to be moved emotionally by another's distress. Sympathy is the sort of 'emotional connectedness' that happens when we see a child who is playing happily falling over and hurting themselves. The spontaneous feeling of being moved to help would be familiar to most of us. So sympathy is linked to sensitivity plus an urge to relieve suffering.

Distress tolerance is our ability to bear difficult emotions both within ourselves and in others. People who feel overwhelmed by another's distress may feel psychologically unable to face it and so have to turn away. Alternatively because the suffering feels too distressing, they have to act as rescuers under compulsion to turn off the other's distress as fast as possible. Being able to bear distress and cope with it allows us to *be with* distress: actively remaining present to listen and feel able to work out with the other person what might be helpful for them.

Empathy has both emotional (affective) and cognitive (thinking) aspects. It requires not simply an ability to recognise another human being's feelings, motivations and intentions, but also to make sense of their feelings and our own emotional responses. For example when we see somebody who looks tearful we register this at an emotional level, and we also try and understand that they may have experienced some kind of loss. The process is less automatic than sympathy, and requires the effort and time to imagine what it might be like to be that person in their predicament: 'to be in their shoes'. Empathy also enables us to predict the effects of our actions on others. For example an empathic nurse sees that a patient needs their water to be moved within reach, or that one patient needs a lot of information while another may not want it. Empathy can allow us to understand another's needs even when they may be unaware of them or in denial: the shy or proud person who doesn't want to ask for help may be left alone because they never 'cause a fuss', although they have important needs they feel unwilling to express. Empathy allows us to understand and respect the importance of a patient's dignity and, even though their body is decaying, deformed, disfigured or malodorous, to honour it.

The nature of empathy and its importance in social relationships now has a substantial grounding in neurobiological research which has shown that it depends on distinct pathways in and between certain distinct areas of the brain. It has become clear too that when these areas are damaged the capacity for empathy may be greatly reduced and certain states of mind can block or disrupt empathic processing. Some neuroscientists are beginning to suspect that a lack of empathy may underpin poor caring or even cruelty (Baron-Cohen 2011; Liotti and Gilbert 2011).

Non-judgement means not judging a person's pain or distress, but simply accepting and validating their experience. Compassion also involves being non-judgemental in the sense of not condemning. Some clinical encounters may make us feel frustration (or anger, fear, disgust, sadness and so on), but if we don't find ways to work these feelings out and deal with them, they will hinder empathy. Feeling angry about a situation we cannot influence or control undermines compassion, lowers morale and makes us more vulnerable to burnout.

The compassionate skills shown in the outer circle in Figure 6.2 are the ways in which we go about helping. For example *sensitivity* in the inner circle is to do with openness to suffering, whereas *attention* in the outer circle means paying attention to what can be helpful. Using compassionate imagery and sensory focusing can be especially valuable when we stop and just imagine what a person is going through, or what might be genuinely helpful to them emotionally and physically. Or we might try imagining the relief somebody could experience if we were able to help them. Hence the feelings of the outer circle tend to be more positive – taking pleasure in our ability to be helpful and share a moment with our patient.

These interconnected elements enhance one another, and all are infused with an underlying warmth towards others, rather than detachment. For example, think what might happen to your compassion if any one of these inner ring attributes were missing: you might be motivated but lack empathy; you might want to help but find it difficult to understand other people well enough; or you might work on (say) a children's cancer ward but get so upset that you lose sleep and become depressed; such compassion fatigue is well-recognised.

Becoming compassionate

The evolution of attachment and affiliative behaviour helps explain how it is possible to be emotionally invested in others, motivated to care for them and moved by their distress, yet be able to maintain empathy and make sense of it (Seager 2006). Based on this understanding, we propose that there may be ways to maximise health professionals' ability to access and operate from a compassionate mind position whatever their personal situation.

Seager suggests that having secure attachments and relationships is one of the most important contributors to empathy, but that some people (or that people in certain situations) will have a greater capacity for empathy. A personal quality that influences this capacity is *self-compassion*, a concept which Kristin Neff – using a Buddhist model of self-compassion – has been at the forefront of developing (www.self-compassion.org) (Neff 2011). Her model focuses on three major dimensions:

- *kindness* – understanding one's difficulties and being kind and warm in the face of failure or setbacks rather than harshly judgemental and self-critical;
- *common humanity* – seeing one's experiences as part of the human condition rather than as personal, isolating and shaming;
- *mindful acceptance* – awareness and acceptance of painful thoughts and feelings rather than over-identifying with them.

Buddhist approaches and Gilbert's compassionate mind training can provide techniques for developing self-compassion and for working through various forms of personal resistance to it.

The inescapable facts of life are that we are born, flourish for a while and must then decline, decay and die. Medicine and nursing are confronted by the darkness of the human condition, but the reality that life entails suffering and limitation is not an easy one to embrace. So although these professions will always be intimately linked with compassion, it is understandable that many of those who work on medicine's front line find it easier to focus on the objective mechanics of healthcare, than to engage with the anguish that will sometimes surround them.

It seems that the capacity for compassion is associated with certain psychological and social factors. Hope and especially feeling cared for and cared about are among the more prominent. For instance in one study of an emergency room compassion-intervention, 133 consecutive homeless individuals received a hot drink and a caring conversation. Perhaps surprisingly, this significantly *reduced* the likelihood of their repeatedly returning (Rendemeier *et al.* 1995). Men have a death rate 40 per cent higher than normal in the year after they have been widowed (Parkes *et al.* 1969). Self-compassion can be effective in protecting against and relieving concomitant depression, as one RCT of an online intervention supporting optimism and self-compassion exercises has shown (Shapira *et al.* 2010). And, because patients are more likely to disclose concerns, symptoms and health behaviours to compassionate healthcare professionals, empathic staff could ultimately be more effective at delivering care (Larson and Yao 2005)

There is growing evidence that compassionate clinical relationships have significant physiological effects, including prevention of health problems and faster recovery from various conditions (Hamilton 2010). Cortisol and oxytocin for instance, which have far-reaching impacts on the immune system, are among the many hormonal determinants of resilience and recovery, that stress and attachment profoundly affect (Lutz *et al.* 2008). Furthermore compassionate care also plays an important part in creating satisfying physician-caregiver relationships and better patient-and doctor-experiences (Darren *et al.* 2003). Patients appreciate consistently compassionate physicians and rarely forget their 'spontaneous acts of kindness and generosity' (Graber and Johnson 2001). A scientific understanding of such relationships and their profound physiological (or conversely, patho-physiological) effects ought to make compassionate care a more central concern in medical training and practice.

There is a relatively small subset of medical practices and procedures where 'fixing' is the most appropriate approach to take. For example, we can fix broken bones or remove cataracts and replace joints; immunisation and anaesthetics are undeniably great gifts to humankind. Moynihan, however, suggests that we have 'over-medicalised' patients, and that doctors who focus only on treating and 'fixing' are in fact scientifically and clinically limited (Moynihan 2002). People with chronic long-term disease, or relapsing illnesses, or 'medically unexplained symptoms', or whose lives are ending, are all definitively 'unfixable' if approached only from a mechanical point of view rather than an emotional and personal perspective. In our fascination and deserved admiration with medical 'magic' it is all too easy to lose sight of the Hippocratic tradition that we should attend not just to the disease, but also to the person who has it. If medical science is to be wisely employed we must use it in context. Therefore, since the context is the whole person, our ever-present question should be 'how do we create the conditions for healing to happen?'

What gets in the way?

Organisations shape the way health services are delivered, in as much as they either support or militate against certain styles of working. Many kinds of constraint on compassionate care have been cited: reward systems, time demands, bureaucratic (often defensive) paperwork and various aspects of organisational culture are among them (Darren *et al.* 2003). Others have blamed 'shackles of routines and ritual', which hinder flexible, individual-ised and creative delivery of patient-centred care (Kelly 2007). More specific barriers such as autonomy clashes and end-of-life values and preferences have also been implicated (Cornelison 2001).

It is widely believed that nurses who are empathic and caring are more prone to absorb the traumatic stress of those they help (Joinson 2010). Eventually this 'compassion fatigue' is said to impair such nurses' performance and make them prone to burnout. On the other hand Graber noted, after interviewing highly praised compassionate physicians, that their compassion or empathy appeared to sustain and support, rather than tire or weaken them (Graber *et al.* 2001). In our model empathy is one of the attributes of compassion. But without the motivation to be helpful and the skills to do it, empathy can become far less benign: an empathic torturer is worse than a non-empathic one; the ultimately cold and calculating psycopath may in fact score extremely high for empathy; and empathy is very important in marketing for working out how to attract or manipulate people and 'push their buttons'. So what may be sustaining these individuals is the effective combination of empathy plus their commitment (motivation) and their skills for helping. Whether their compassion ultimately helps or harms the carer may also depend on whether the organisation they work in encourages compassionate action or stifles it. Burnout is more likely when people feel constrained from acting compassionately, because of work–culture constraints. An exploratory study of emergency care physicians and nurses found three barriers to quality improvement and compassionate care: the patient being looked at as an object; physicians and nurses belonging to dif-ferent organisational cultures; and hospital internal organisation, if it hinders optimal working with patients and improvements in quality (Lown et al. 2010).

Moving forward

Several professional bodies which have recognised how organisations can inhibit compassion are now actively working to promote more patient-centred care. They include the RCGP RCPsych Primary Care Mental Health Forum, and the College of Medicine. The college describes itself as a new force bringing together patients, scientists and all healthcare professionals to redefine what good medicine means by promoting 'the traditional val-ues of service, commitment and compassion.' In fact, in many parts of the world our colleagues are exploring ways of developing a compassionate ori-entation towards oneself and others. (See for example Paul Gilbert's www.compassionmind.co.uk; the Center for Compassion and Altruism Research and Education http://ccare.stanford.edu; Hearts in Healthcare www.hearts inhealthcare.com.)

Wales Mental Health in Primary Care (www.wamhipc.org.uk), an action group of the RCGP Wales, has developed three 'gold standard' hallmarks – excellent communication, trust and person centeredness – to enable excellent patient care. Managerial approaches to healthcare reform are very valuable, provided they are informed by a deeper understanding of what influences individual motivation towards compassionate practice, and what facilitates compassionate behaviour. The Schwartz rounds are one such initiative. During an inpatient stay on a palliative care ward in the United States, Kenneth Schwartz observed that staff were experiencing emotional difficulties of their own – perhaps with attachment issues, grief or pain – and that this would sometime interfere with their providing compassionate care. For example a professional looking after a terminally ill man who reminded them of their father might find it reawakening feelings of loss and grief. In the light of his insights Schwartz established the Schwartz Rounds Centre in 1995, his assumption being that compassionate care required a compassionate setting and therefore that staff needed to attend to their own emotional health and the well-being of their team. Here once again we see self-compassion in action (Lown *et al.* 2010).

The Schwartz rounds are a way of encouraging multidisciplinary teams to acknowledge and share the emotional impact of working with very distressed patients, and manage their team dynamics. They are in effect a form of psychological supervision that would be familiar to GPs who have benefited from membership of Balint groups. The rounds aim to improve relationships between members of the many disciplines involved in high-pressure multidisciplinary palliative care teams. But are they effective? Recent research into Schwartz rounds in acute hospital care suggests that by setting aside time to come together and talk through their feelings about patients, clinical teams can improve morale and provide better patient care (www.theschwartzcenter. org). But how rarely do most clinical teams meet in this way to think about the compassionate care they deliver? A recent evaluation by The King's Fund regarding the impact of team supervision on patient outcomes is awaited. Meanwhile some clinical teams in Betsi Cadwaladr University Health Board in Wales who have been engaging in Schwartz rounds for several years report very positive feedback from the staff involved.

Dr Rita Charon, director and founder of the Program in Narrative Medicine at Columbia's College of Physicians and Surgeons has another approach. She has found that encouraging medical staff to write about their patients' and their own experiences in a 'parallel–chart' enhances staff levels of compassion. In a recent study, 82 per cent of the participating students rated this 'parallel-chart' method as beneficial, both as a therapeutic outlet for the emotional trials of residency and as a more effective way of preparing for conversations with patients and their families (www.colum bia.edu/cu/alumni/Magazine/Fall2003/artofhealing.html).

Toxic organisations

We know the nature of compassionate actions and feelings, and we know how we can train staff to develop these capacities within themselves. But the systems and structures in which health professional have to operate may prove more problematic. Though it would be a great relief to think that the poor care identified in the NHS Ombudsman report *Care and Compassion* applied only to isolated incidents perpetrated by flawed individuals, many of us suspect this is not the case. But if – despite the NHS brimming over with examples of excellent care – there is also widespread failure of care and even outright abuse and bullying, why should this be? Psychological and organisational research tells us that very often it is the organisations themselves and their structures that are the problem, because people who work in negative work cultures will tend in time to adapt to them. Just as individual practitioners can create the conditions for healing, so organisations can create conditions that facilitate compassion, or its opposite.

If cost-efficiency and 'numbers seen and processed' are the main criteria for quality assessments, it is not difficult for managers to convince themselves that they are creating highly efficient organisations. But these environments can be extremely unpleasant and draining to be in, both for patients and staff. Bowed down and wound up by work pressure and target chasing, we are more likely to experience our more complicated or complaining patients as a source of irritation; pushed for time, it gets easier to overlook the needs of patients who are quiet and uncomplaining, but all the more difficult to behave compassionately towards them. These are not criticisms, simply well-recognised observations of time-pressured working and the complexities of non-compassion-facilitating environments. If we are honest, we may to some extent have already lost control of our workplaces, and allowed target-driven bureaucracy and cost-limitation to take precedence. In a world were healthcare trusts must now become competitive businesses, efficiencies and targets are all too likely to be over-emphasised. Furthermore, in our efforts to squeeze ever greater efficiencies in, and bad practice out, our healthcare systems may be spreading fear and shaming as motivating mechanism for change. Yet though it might be tempting to believe that the more frightened people get the more they will conform, we are playing with fire by catalysing such anxieties, and risk creating cynical, defensive, burned out staff who long only for retirement.

The individual skills that enable compassion are increasingly well known. It is also very clear that social groups and cultures greatly influence practice and values. Therefore in order to grow compassionate patient-centred healthcare we will also have to look beyond the individual. In his forthcoming book *Caregiver stress and staff support in illness, dying and bereavement* (Youngson 2010) Robin Youngson describes his cultural and socially focused model for enabling compassionate care. It integrates three elements: inner resources (for compassionate caring); a sense of togetherness; and a sense of place. He also shines a light on the powerful forces that are already disintegrating humane and compassionate caring in our modern health services:

- The disease focus, reductionism and super-specialisation can overshadow our humanity and hinder the development of our inner resources for compassion, leaving us feeling powerless and overwhelmed.
- The traumatisation of young professionals in their training and early practice, the widespread bullying in healthcare, and our unresolved emotional responses to human suffering and loss all lead to distancing and isolation rather than to trusting relationships with our patients and colleagues.
- When we create a humane and supportive work environment we can develop the inner resources for compassionate caring (Kearney *et al.* 2009). When we make mistakes we need to have the courage to acknowledge them, apologise, be honest and make amends.

Studies of what facilitatoes pro-social behaviour in children have shown they need *role models* to guide them, to be *shown skills* that can be practised and developed, *offered rewards* for pro-social behaviour, in the context of *relationships that support* pro-social values. It seems that in developing pathways towards compassionate care in the NHS, these qualities will also prove to be central (Eisenberg 2002).

Compassion for the patient can be thought of as operating through another series of circles.

In the outer ring are the qualities, values and demands of institutional settings which may facilitate or inhibit compassionate support systems. In the middle ring are health providers who may or may not succeed in achieving genuinely compassionate mindsets, depending on whether their training and work environments support them. And at the centre is the patient who receives the compassionate care.

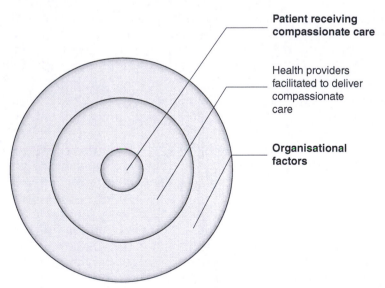

Figure 6.3 Compassion for the patient operating through a further series of circles

Conclusions

Clinicians who aspire to the highest medical standards and knowledge must understand that the therapeutic interpersonal relationship has very important effects on physiological regulation. At one level this is straightforward because in the absence of compassionate care people are frightened, upset, stressed, confused and even depressed. In the healthcare setting, all the technical, mechanical tools may be well enacted, yet delivered in such a rush of impersonal interventions, barren of time for kindness, and sensitivity to the fears of disease, injury pain and at times death, that in the outcome is a type of medicine none of us would wish for ourselves, our loved ones or anyone under our care. Yet how often do we find ourselves caught up in exactly such a rush. Consequently, for compassionate clinicians to become facilitators of healing processes rather than simple body mechanics, certain facts need integrating into our science of care: that our brains and bodies evolved to function optimally under conditions of safeness, affiliation and care; that therefore compassion has very powerful neurophysiological effects; that compassion makes our interventions more clinically effective, and therefore competent care must also be compassionate care. But if suffering is our concern. then surely all aspects of the person's (and family's) suffering need to be addressed – emotional as well as physical – for clearly these interact. And so we, and the organisations we work in, must aim to provide more than mere 'tick box' technically competent care at an ever faster rate.

There is science enough to prove that compassion is not some woolly add-on we can afford to dispense with in our frenetic resource limited times: it is the creator and hallmark of quality care. It helps heal us, both in body and mind, and to come to terms with disability and impairment, or die in peace. By developing health care systems that facilitate compassionate care, our patients' experiences and clinical outcomes will be better, our own risks of burnout or litigation will be less, and our job satisfaction will be considerably greater. Above all, the presence of compassion and its primacy as an organisational value would give us confidence that when we or our loved ones fall sick or are dying, we and they will be well cared for physically and emotionally.

Three perspectives from the real world

'*The very nature of being a doctor attracts students for many reasons; some because of the academic challenges, others through a family tradition or the promise of status and control, some because of experiences of suffering they feel they must relieve. Whatever draws people into medical career, it is to be hoped that some of their motivation grows out of a genuine desire to be a healer.*' Paul Gilbert (personal communication)

(continued)

(continued)

The following perspectives are from three different viewpoints but with the common thread of the authors having been Cardiff University 5th year medical students undertaking their Senior Clinical Project in Compassionate Care under the supervision of Alys Cole-King and the Senior Lecturer, Dr Philip Banfield, North Wales Clinical School. They are very grateful to the support and assistance they received from the North Wales Clinical School and staff in the Betsi Cadwaladr University Health Board who assisted them, particularly, Jill Newman and the Modernisation Team, Professor Matt Makin, Jilly Wilcox-Jones and colleagues, Sister Jenny Jones and colleagues in the Emergency Department and the Audit Department. Their reflections clearly demonstrate a desire to deliver compassionate care but also some of the 'real word' challenges of doing so.

Mo Hu MBBCh, BSc (hons) Doctor, Royal Gwent Hospital, Newport

I am a foundation year doctor working in Paediatrics, with a special interest in Cognitive Neuroscience. I have studied the importance of compassion in determining healthcare outcomes, and its practical delivery in NHS settings. The interplay between mind and body has always interested me, and I firmly believe that providing holistic healthcare is an integral part of the healing process. Although there are barriers to providing compassionate care, I have been struck by some of the negative attitudes of healthcare professionals to such a vital component of care.

A Paediatric Foundation Year 1 perspective

Compassion is a vital component of responsible medical practice. It can be pivotal in determining patient outcome and can shape patient experience. Working as a junior doctor I feel that the medical model often sidesteps compassionate care. On reflection, I have been struck by the lack of awareness amongst my peers regarding the benefits of providing compassionate care. Our reward systems are too heavily focused on quantifiable academic achievements rather than the qualitative aspects of treating patients holistically. Without support, I have found it difficult to strike a balance in providing the appropriate level of compassionate care that is consistent with my developing professional identity and individual values. I believe that more teaching and peer reflection on the quantifiable benefits of compassionate care, as well as staff reward systems, may increase the effortful practice of compassionate care. While I am finding it difficult to temper a professional relationship with a compassionate one, I believe that with experience and reflection I will become a better clinician. It would be foolish not to recognise that long hours, pressure and challenging patients can impact whether compassionate care is provided. I think it may be time for clinicians and managers to actively question their priorities.

Alexandra Lloyd, 5th year medical student at Cardiff University

I decided to contribute to this article due to personal experiences throughout my life where I have witnessed and received both good and bad care, in many situations. One particular moment was in Malawi, where out of hundreds of people, a Malawian woman who spoke no English was the one who reached out to me in a time of distress; showing me that you can do so much for people with small gestures, and that being a doctor extends far beyond the medical knowledge we have. Having seen people in both medical and non-medical situations gaining huge benefit from just one person reaching out and going that one step further, I strive to be compassionate and caring from every angle in my personal life, and throughout my medical career.

A medical student perspective

As medical students we are trained from very early on how to be compassionate with our patients, we are taught communication skills, go through role plays, analysing everything from the words we use, to our body language, and the importance of giving patients time to talk, no matter what their ailment is. The General Medical Council provides medical students with the guide *Tomorrow's Doctors* which has a section devoted solely to communication with patients, stating we should be able to:

'*Communicate clearly, sensitively and effectively with individuals and groups regardless of their age, social, cultural or ethnic backgrounds or their disabilities, including when English is not the patient's first language.*' *Tomorrow's Doctors*, GMC, p. 12.

I wanted to be a doctor for many reasons, but one key element was wanting: to be able to care for others with new skills and competencies, along with providing these people with someone to turn to, talk

(continued)

(continued)

to and trust, and to care for them in a holistic manner, providing each and every one of them with a high level of compassion. To me compassion means treating patients with respect, hearing and understanding situations from their perspective, and acting appropriately, and never making anybody feel they are wasting my time, no matter how busy I am. This, combined with medical schools teaching on compassionate care throughout the course, means it is difficult for me and others as fifth year medical students to be able to see how these seemingly basic qualities can fall below par, and in particular become a huge issue within the media. The reality of being a doctor will soon become real for me and whilst I can see how endless patient lists, shortages of staff and a feeling of being overwhelmed with the new responsibility, I hope to never lose my caring attitude and desire to give patients the empathetic care they deserve.

Yvonne Honstvet

I became interested in compassionate care as 4th year Cardiff Undergraduate Medical Student following attending both the Connecting with People 'Compassionate Care' and 'Suicide Awareness' training modules as part of my undergraduate psychiatry placement at the North Wales Clinical School. I work as a junior Foundation Year 1 doctor in a London teaching hospital and now have 'hands on' experience of the day to day challenges and rewards of delivering compassionate care.

A compassionate reality in a teaching hospital?
A Foundation Year 1 perspective

The wisdom goes that the longer time spent in service, the less compassionate doctors become. As a medical student I empathised closely with patients. I felt like a bridge between lay person and doctor; not yet confident enough in my medical knowledge, I found that providing an encouraging nod, listening ear, or a hand to squeeze came naturally. I admired compassion when demonstrated by my seniors, I silently promised myself to do better when I encountered less than compassionate care. I am now one of the newest members of the profession – an FY1 doctor on a busy firm, having undergone transition from idealistic student to the reality of 90-hour weeks. I endeavour to be compassionate, but am very aware of the obstacles faced in everyday practice: time pressure, an incessant bleep, forty patients to investigate, cannulate and prescribe for daily, with no time to eat or drink on duty. However, I remain optimistic that compassionate care is achievable. I have tried to build compassion into my style of work; that way it becomes the norm. As juniors we see our patients every day, and we have the benefit of building a rapport with them. I recently stayed back from a morning round to question why a patient did not seem his usual self. He announced he was contemplating suicide. I was able to get him the help he needed. This emphasised to me the importance of a compassionate interaction, no matter how brief. I cannot categorically state that every single one of my encounters with a patient or relative has been empathic. Yet neither can I recall one that I look back on and regret showing a lack of compassion. I hope that day does not come. My attitude has changed from my medical school days but for the better: I can now practice with compassion in my own right.

Acknowledgements

We would like to thank the following for their helpful comments regarding the drafting of this chapter: Robin Youngson (founder of Hearts in Healthcare), Mitzi Blennerhassett, Chris Manning and Martin Seager (members of the RCGP RCPsych Primary Care Mental Health Forum and the *College of Medicine) and Jocelyn Cornwell, Director, Point of Care project, The King's Fund*. Thanks also to Yvonne Honstvet, Mo Hu and Alexandra Lloyd, Cardiff University undergraduate medical students who contributed to part of the literature review.

References

Baron-Cohen, S. (2011) *Zero Degrees of Empathy: A New Theory of Cruelty* London: Allen Books 2.

Blennerhassett, M. (2008) *Nothing Personal: Disturbing Undercurrents in Cancer Care*. Abingdon: Radcliffe Publishing.

Carter, C.S. (1998) Neuroendocrine perspectives on social attachment and love *Psychoneuroendocrinology* 23, 779–818.

Committee on Quality of Health Care in America (2001) *Crossing the Quality Chasm: A New Health System for the 21st Century* Washington, DC: National Academy Press.

Cornelison, A.H. (2001) Cultural barriers to compassionate care – patients' and health care professionals' perspectives *Bioethics Forum* 17, 7–14.

Darren-Thompson, D., Paul, S., Ciechanowski, P.S. (2003) Attaching a new understanding to the patient-physician relationship in family practice *Journal of the American Board of Family Medicine* 16(3), 219–26.

Depue, R.A., Morrone-Strupinsky, J.V. (2005) A neurobehavioral model of affiliative bonding *The Behavioral and Brain Sciences* 28, 313–95.

Eisenberg, N. (2002) Empathy-related emotional responses, altruism, and their socialization In: Davidson, R., Harrington, A. (eds) *Visions of Compassion: Western Scientists and Tibetan Buddhists Examine Human Nature* New York: Oxford University Press.

Gilbert, P. (2009) *The Compassionate Mind: A New Approach to the Challenge of Life* London: Constable & Robinson.

Graber, D.R., Johnson, J.A. (2001) Spirituality and healthcare organisations *Journal of Healthcare Management* 46, 39–52.

Halpern, J. (2001) *From Detached Concern to Empathy: Humanizing Medical Practice* New York: Oxford University Press.

Hamilton, D.R. (2010) *Why Kindness Is Good for You* London: Hay House.

Joinson, C. (1992) Coping with compassion fatigue *Nursing* 22(4), 116–22.

Kearney, M., Weininger, R., Vachon, M., et al. (2009) Self-care of physicians at the end of life: Being connected. A key to my survival *JAMA* 301(11), 1155–64.

Kelly, J. (2007) Barriers to achieving patient-centred care in Ireland *Dimensions of Critical Care Nursing* 26, 29–34.

Larson, E.B., Yao, Y. (2005) Clinical empathy as emotional labour in the patient-physician relationship *JAMA* 293, 1100–6.

Liotti, G., Gilbert, P. (2011) Mentalizing, motivation, and social mentalities: Theoretical considerations and implications for psychotherapy *Psychology and Psychotherapy: Theory, Research and Practice* 84, 9–25.

Lown, B.A., Manning, C.F. (2010) The Schwartz Center rounds: Evaluation of an interdiscipilinary approach to enhancing patient-centered communication, teamwork and provider support *Academic Medicine* 85, 1073–81.

Lutz, A., Brefczynski-Lewis, J., Johnstone, T. et al. (2008) Regulation of the neural circuitry of emotion by compassion meditation: Effects of the meditative expertise *PLoS ONE* 3, 1–5.

Matthews, D.A., Suchman, A.L., Branch, W.T. (1993) Making 'connexions': Enhancing the therapeutic potential of patient-patient-clinician relationships *Annals of Internal Medicine* 118, 973–7.

Moynihan, R. (2002) Too much medicine? Almost certainly *BMJ* 324, 859–60.

Muntlin, A., Carlsson, M., Gunningberg, L. (2010) Barriers to change hindering quality improvement: The reality of emergency care *Journal of Emergency Nursing* 36(4), 317–23.

Neff, K. (2011) *Self-Compassion* New York: William Morrow.

Parkes, C., Benjamin, B., Fitzgerald, R. (1969) Broken heart: A statistical survey of increased mortality amongst widowers *BMJ* 1, 740–3.

Porges, S.W. (2007) The polyvagal perspective *Biological Psychology* 74, 116–43.

Porges, S.W. (2011) *The Polyvagal Theory: Neurophysiological Foundations of Emotions, Attachment, Communication, and Self Regulation* New York: Norton.

Rendemeier, D.A., Molin, J.P., Tibshirani, R.J. (1995) A randomised control trial of compassionate care for the homeless in an emergency department *The Lancet* 345, 1131–4.

Sanghavi, D. (2006) Beyond the white coat and the johnny: What makes for a compassionate patient-caregiver relationship? Findings from a national conversation sponsored by the Kenneth B. Schwartz Center *Joint Commision Journal on Quality and Patient Safety* 32(5), 283–92.

Seager, M. (2006) The concept of 'psychological safety' – A psychoanalytically-informed contribution towards safe, sound & supportive mental health services *Psychoanalytic Psychotherapy* 20(4), 266–80.

Shapira L.B. and Mongrain, M. (2010) The benefits of self-compassion and optimism exercises for individuals vulnerable to depression. *The journal of Positive Psychiatry* 5(5), 377–89.

Youngson, R. (2010) Taking off the armor. *Illn Crises Loss* 18(1), 79–82.

7 Compassionate journeys and end-of-life care

Sue Shea

Introduction

In a beautiful little book entitled *Leaves Falling Gently*, Susan Bauer-Wu (2011) reminds us that:

> No matter how old you are or how hardened your heart has become, you can always revive the lovely flower within you. And in doing so, you open the door to healing within and you create warmth and spaciousness that unites you with others.
>
> (Bauer-Wu 2011: 75)

The human life cycle has a beginning, a middle and an end, the final stage of the life cycle being end-of-life. End-of-life care refers to care of those with a terminal condition which is incurable and advanced, and the care of frail elderly patients and those in the final days or hours of life. Palliative care represents an important aspect of end-of-life care, assisting in relieving symptoms, and providing psychological, social and spiritual support to patients and their families/carers.

All patients deserve the right to be treated with compassion and humanity, whatever their age or circumstances and we are aware that such care can relieve symptoms and anxiety, promote faster recovery, and assist in the management of long-term illness. But how can we fully understand the needs and thoughts of patients reaching the end of the human life cycle? If we have a long-term disorder, we may gain support from others in the same situation, and if we are recovering from acute illness we might discuss this with other people who have experienced the same or similar illness. However, end-of-life is something very personal and individual, particularly at the final stages, and although it is the one thing in life that all of us can be certain of, how do we understand it if we have never experienced it? Thus, compassion towards the dying patient is essential to relieve suffering and to try to make their exit from this world as pain-free and comfortable as possible. This chapter aims to provide an introduction to approaches in end-of-life care and to summarize certain initiatives and practices.

Addressing the subject of 'end-of-life'

End-of-life is a topic that many of us have trouble discussing or coming to terms with, and most of us would find it problematic discussing our own end-of-life care, or the care of family and friends, either amongst each other or with health care professionals. As Ngo-Metzger *et al.* (2008) suggest, although physicians are in an appropriate place to assist and discuss patients' diagnosis or terminal illness, they may not feel equipped to discuss end-of-life care, possibly due to lack of training and discomfort when communicating bad news.

A survey conducted by the Kings Fund (2009), revealed that GPs themselves find it difficult to discuss preferences for their own end-of-life care with their doctor, family or friends. Sixty-three per cent of the GPs taking part in the survey believed that 'their personal attitudes towards death will inevitably affect the advice they give patients about end-of-life treatment'. The study by the Kings Fund demonstrates that health care professionals need to feel confident when talking to patients regarding preferences for end-of-life care, and that this is of importance to ensure high-quality care.

Davison (2010) in a study of preferences for end-of-life care amongst 584 chronic kidney disease patients found that patient needs such as pain management, psychosocial and spiritual support, were not currently systematically integrated into their care. Whilst Sampson *et al.* (2011) report on the problems associated with addressing the needs of people with dementia, stating that as people with severe dementia lack the capacity to make decisions about their care, this can have a profound impact on providing the vital components required for good end-of-life and person-centred care. Sampson *et al.* conclude that models to improve end-of-life care need to take into account the large range of settings as well as cultural and staff factors, taking into consideration what works best for whom and in what circumstances. Of course when discussing the subject of end-of-life care, we are not only referring to patients with terminal conditions, but also those who are naturally approaching the end of the life cycle such as frail or elderly individuals. Müller-Mundt *et al.* (2013) remind us that frail elderly people represent a major patient group, although little may be known about their needs. Thus in a proposed study, these researchers aim to address the needs of this patient group, and to explore their service utilization and experiences, integrating perspectives of patients, care-givers, family physicians and other health professionals.

End-of-life care is a sensitive and personal issue, requiring a multidisciplinary approach, wherein patient preferences represent an important aspect. Hannon *et al.* (2012) conducted a study to obtain the views of general practice staff regarding whether a single incentivized indicator to record the preferred place to receive end-of-life care could improve quality, but concluded that the appropriate time to ask a patient about end-of-life care is subjective and patient specific, and therefore does not lend itself to an inflexible single indicator. In 2011 Forbes *et al.* conducted a study aimed at exploring healthcare professionals' views on factors which influence good quality end-of-life care within acute settings. Through the use of a specifically developed end-of-life tool, a number of themes were identified, including difficulties in diagnosing dying, role of the doctor, changing role of nursing staff, hospital culture and environment. These authors conclude that the factors identified should be taken into account when trying to improve care for dying patients and in facilitating the use of end-of-life care pathways.

An earlier qualitative study by Singer *et al.* (1999) which aimed at obtaining perceptions of patients regarding end-of-life care, identified five domains of quality end-of-life care: receiving adequate pain and symptom management, avoiding inappropriate prolongation of dying, achieving a sense of control, relieving burden and strengthening relationships with loved ones. Taylor and McLaughlin (2011) emphasize the importance of a safe place for patients facing death, to explore their anxieties and relationships thus at a time of great uncertainty, creating positions of 'safe' uncertainty. Additionally, clinicians who care for the dying are thought to be at risk of both burnout and compassion fatigue, thus clinician self-care is important and may enhance the well-being of both the clinician and the dying patient (Kearney *et al.* 2010).

As Elliot (2011) reminds us, death is an inevitable part of living and how do we come to terms with it? Although death is often considered a 'taboo' subject, quality end-of-life care is essential for both the patient and their loved ones and carers. Thus models or therapies that can enhance such care, taking into account the sensitivity of the subject and the importance of compassion are therefore important to consider.

Huffman and Stern (2003) draw on real-life examples and clinical experience of the difficulties faced by clinicians in terms of the amount of information to give to a terminally ill patient, and in addressing the issue of evaluating depression. They state that a majority of patients appear to want to know the full truth about their condition, and that those who are told their diagnosis in a clear manner have better emotional adjustment. Clarifying to the patient that everything possible will be done to assist them can reduce patient anxiety and elicit trust. Huffman and Stern also draw attention to the fact that grief and depression share a number of features – both being associated with sadness, withdrawal and loss of energy – however, grief is characterized by waves of sadness which can be balanced by the patient's ability to experience pleasure. In looking at how clinicians can help patients who are terminally ill, Huffman and Stern suggest four approaches: aiding the psychological and spiritual coping process, assessing and treating psychiatric illness, maximizing treatment and treating the carers and family members.

In the guidelines suggested by Ngo-Metzger *et al.* (2008), a focus on patient-centred approaches is presented. These authors emphasize that 'when delivering bad news, it is important to prioritize the key points that the patient should retain', and that 'physicians should assess the patient's emotional state, readiness to engage in the discussion, and level of understanding about the condition'. They also stress the importance of sensitivity to the patient's cultural and individual preferences and that all involved in the patients care need to coordinate key prognosis points to avoid giving mixed messages and confusing the patient. Listening to patients' beliefs and values can help prevent misunderstanding and promote trust.

The above suggestions relate strongly to the development of the palliative care approach within healthcare where the following interventions are identified as core:

- offering a support system to help patients live as actively as possible until death;
- offering a support system to help the family cope during the patients illness and in their own bereavement;
- using a team approach to address the needs of patients and their families, including bereavement counselling, if indicated.

(WHO accessed at: www.who.int/cancer/
palliative/definition/en/)

The nature of suffering

Chochinov (2007) describes compassion as 'a deep awareness of the suffering of another, coupled with the wish to relieve it'. The term 'suffering' is frequently utilized when we speak of compassionate care, and is particularly important to consider when addressing end-of-life care. Cassell (2004) says that attendance to the suffering person should be a primary goal of medicine, and defines suffering 'as the state of severe distress associated with events that threaten the intactness of the person', stating that 'the obligation of physicians to relieve human suffering stretches back to antiquity. Despite this fact, little attention is explicitly given to the problem of suffering in medical education, research or practice'. Schulz *et al.* (2007) have looked into the fact that despite the evidence of how illness of a close relative causes distress in family members and increased vulnerability, little research has been conducted which has focused on 'patient suffering' as an independent contributor to care-giver outcomes. They propose that focusing on the concepts of suffering and compassion can enrich researchers' views of caregiving. Their primary interest has been on how the manifestation of suffering in others impacts on the perceiver, i.e. family/carer. In discussing available literature, Schulz *et al.* conclude that suffering can be seen as having three components: physical, emotional and existential, but there are individual differences in the way in which people suffer because of individual tolerance and perceptions of disease. Schulz *et al.* suggest that it should be possible to assess the effects of perceived patient suffering on involved family members and that if data is collected from both patient and care-giver it should be possible to identify which elements of suffering are most strongly related to care-giver outcomes. To this end, Schulz *et al.* have developed a conceptual framework linking patient suffering to care-giver compassion to serve as a basis for further discussion, and to promote empirical research on this topic. However, empirical research may not always be possible, and as Hunter (2010) asks 'What happens if we turn toward the very elements of death and loss that seem to frighten us most and ask their permission for us to look them in the eye, with a humble, gentle attention, supported by the right balance of compassion and courage?' 'In personal communication, Hunter suggests the following:

> maintaining a self-compassionate perspective allows us to set aside time-tables and agendas; we engage the pain of our grief in the spirit of 'just this much', thawing the numbness of grief, feeling and releasing the pain that is held there, only to the extent that we feel safe and able at any given time and place. We do not have to get through the rest of our life; we only have to live this very moment, as attentive and caring as we can be. A self-compassionate stance allows us to honour the natural wisdom of even our shock, numbness and hesitancy.
>
> (Brad Hunter, personal communication, 2013)

As Halifax (2011) suggests, we could perhaps utilize the term 'total care' to refer to compassionate care which exemplifies care that addresses ' . . . physical, spiritual, psychological, and social pain and suffering of dying people and caregivers . . . '. She suggests the use of spiritual and contemplative perspectives that might foster greater resilience in those who care for the dying. Such approaches may assist us in having the 'strength and perspective to acknowledge the pain and suffering in others and ourselves and develop an appropriate and transformative relationship to suffering through insight and the regulation of our emotions'.

Bauer-Wu (2011) also emphasizes a mindful approach, drawing our attention to the fact that even with a life-limiting illness, living more fully and openly than before is possible through living in the present moment, being reflective, and deepening connections with friends and family.

Such approaches may increase well-being and quality of life thus relieving suffering for both patients and loved ones.

Ferrell and Coyle (2008) have also looked into the nature of suffering, within the context of the goals of nursing in cancer care. The authors discuss issues in relation to the onset of acute illness of diagnosis of cancer, and how individuals seek reassurance and understanding from nurses, as a human connection in the 'overwhelming reality of health care'. Nurses witnessing the suffering of others, provide an important testimony for the experiences of people in their most vulnerable and broken states. Utilizing descriptions of suffering identified from the literature, and narrative data from interviews with care-givers and nurses, Ferrell and Coyle suggest a step towards supporting nurses who care constantly for those who suffer, focusing on the unique relationship between nurse and patient. They conclude that nurses recognize that witnessing suffering is a part of their daily work, yet they seek to understand each person who is suffering as a unique individual.

Dignity and care

A word that we often hear in association with compassion and care for those nearing end-of-life is that of 'dignity', but what do we mean when we use this word, and can we understand and enhance its purpose? The Royal College of Nursing (http://www.rcn.org.uk/__data/assets/pdf_file/0003/191730/003298.pdf) describe dignity as being 'concerned with how people feel, think and behave in relation to the worth or value of themselves and others' and that 'to treat someone with dignity is to treat them as being of worth, in a way that is respectful of them as valued individuals'. In 2004, Jacelon *et al.* (2004) conducted a concept analysis to develop a definition of dignity in older adults, reporting that dignity is an inherent characteristic of being human, it can be subjectively felt as an attribute of the self, and is made manifest through behaviour that demonstrates respect for self and others. Dignity must be learned, and an individual's dignity is affected by the treatment received from others. Dwyer *et al.* (2009) report that although dignity is a concept often used in end-of-life care, its meaning is rarely clarified. In a study to explore nursing home staff experience of what dignity means to patients and themselves, Dwyer *et al.* found that nursing home staff members deal with a moral conflict between the care that they would like to deliver, and the care that they are able to provide, concluding that to promote older people's dignity, there is a need to take account of staff members' work situation. Antiel (2012), conducted a study to describe beliefs regarding the concept of dignity, and to describe clinical scenarios in which the concept is believed to be relevant; 1,032 physicians from different specialties participated in the study, with 90 per cent reporting that dignity was relevant to their practice. The authors concluded that US physicians view the concept of dignity as useful, and that their views are associated with their judgements about common end-of-life scenarios in which dignity concepts may be relevant.

Over several years of study, Harvey Chochinov and his team at Manitoba (http://dignityincare.ca/en/research-team.html), in collaboration with researchers from Australia, the UK and US, have looked into the importance of dignity in care. Their findings show that:

- People working in health care can have a huge influence on the dignity of those who use health care services, which in turn can improve the patient experience and increase satisfaction with health care.

In 2002 Chochinov reported on a new model of palliative care, known as Dignity-Conserving Care. He states that:

> The term 'dignity' provides an overarching framework that may guide the physician, patient, and family in defining the objectives and therapeutic considerations fundamental to end-of-life care.
>
> Chochinov (2002)

And that:

> Dignity-conserving care offers an approach that clinicians can use to explicitly target the maintenance of dignity as a therapeutic objective and as a principle of bedside care for patients nearing death.
>
> Chochinov (2002)

Chochinov (2007) considers that the more that healthcare providers are able to affirm the patients' value – seeing them as the person they are or were, rather than just the illness, the more likely it is that the patients' sense of dignity will be upheld. In his work, Chochinov refers to a simple memorable framework underpinning the fundamentals of critical care. This he refers to as the 'A, B, C and D of Dignity Conserving Care' which is applicable to all types of health problem and all kinds of patient. The A, B, C and D included in this model refer to the following:

Attitude – the need for healthcare providers to look into their own attitudes and assumptions towards patients and to be aware of these, as these will shape their interaction with the patient who may look towards the health care provider as a mirror seeking a positive image of themselves, and their sense of worth.

Behaviour – small acts of kindness, noticing the needs of patients, and encouraging them to disclose personal information.

Compassion – defined by Chochinov as 'a deep awareness of the suffering of another, coupled with the wish to relieve it' that can be conveyed by any form of communication (spoken or unspoken) that shows some recognition of the human stories that accompany illness.

Dialogue – considered as a critical element of dignity-conserving care. 'At its most basic, such dialogue must acknowledge personhood beyond the illness itself and recognise the emotional impact that accompanies illness.'

Chochinov concludes that:

> this model may be readily applied to teaching, clinical practice, and standards at undergraduate and postgraduate levels and across all medical subspecialties, multidisciplinary teams, and allied health professions. For anyone privileged to look after patients, at whatever stage of the human life cycle, the duty to uphold, protect, and restore the dignity of those who seek our care embraces the very essence of medicine.
>
> Chochinov (2007)

With the importance of dignity in mind, the Dignity in Care Research team at Manitoba Palliative Care Research Unit conducts research on psychosocial, existential and spiritual dimensions of palliative end-of-life care with the primary goal of improving quality of life and easing the suffering of dying people and their families through research (http://dignityincare.ca/en/Cat-1/dignity-explained.html).

Dignity Therapy

Various work and research has been conducted with regard to 'life stories' in health and social care (McKeown *et al.* 2006). An important aspect of this includes Dignity Therapy which is a psychotherapeutic intervention for those near to end-of-life (Chochinov 2005). The content is informed by the dignity model of palliative care, which provides a framework for the intervention which is aimed at decreasing suffering, enhancing quality of life, and providing a sense of meaning, purpose and dignity. Underpinned by Dignity Conserving Care, Dignity Therapy invites patients to discuss issues that matter most to them, and what they would most like to be remembered. It involves sessions in which patients are invited to talk about their lives and to tell their own life story recording meaningful aspects of life that can be recorded in a document and passed onto family and friends as a valuable souvenir and memory of the patient's life.

The therapy is intended to reduce psychosocial and existential distress. It has been shown to be feasible for use in a number of settings including care homes (Hall *et al.* 2009), and across different cultures (Houmann 2010; Akechi 2012), and is found to be effective in addressing existential distress, enhancing quality of life and providing a sense of meaning.

Chochinov (2005), in a study to examine the feasibility of Dignity Therapy, and its impact on measures of psychosocial and existential distress among terminally ill patients in Canada and Australia identified significant improvements in patients following Dignity Therapy. These included reduced depressive symptoms, a lessened sense of suffering and an increased will to live; 81 per cent of patients also reported that the therapy had or would be of help to their families. In a qualitative study by Hack *et al.* (2010), using Dignity Therapy transcripts, it was revealed that the most common values expressed by patients included 'family', 'pleasure', 'caring', 'a sense of accomplishment', 'true friendship' and 'rich experience', illustrating the defining role of values in our lives. Perceptions of advanced cancer patients and their families regarding the benefits of Dignity Therapy revealed that the therapy helped them in many ways, although patients in the control group sometimes perceived similar benefits from taking part in the study, highlighting elements of Dignity Therapy that are common to dignity-conserving care (Hall *et al.* 2013). In addition, McClement *et al.* (2007) report that the therapy moderates bereavement experiences in patient family members.

The role of primary care practitioners and nurses in end-of-life care

In Chapter 8 of this book, the role of primary care and general practice in the provision of compassionate care is discussed and the core features of general practice are highlighted. Continuity of care has been recognized as a fundamental characteristic of effective primary care and the role of GPs as providers of continuity of care has been discussed in a qualitative study conducted by Michiels *et al.* (2007). This study outlines perceptions of terminally ill patients that may guide both undergraduate medical education and vocational training in the current world. There is a current debate about the lack of information and skills in both communication and management of dying people and there is an agreement that primary care personnel require more training in terms of end-of-life issues. The RCGP has also recognized the importance of end-of-life care and in a statement in 2009 it was defined as a key priority. Recently, the RCGP (2013) issued the Commissioning Guidance in end-of-life care in order to:

> be used to help GPs in their practices consider how they can influence the system around them to provide quality care for people nearing the end of life, along with other imperatives such as care for those with multiple long-term conditions, frailty and dementia, and reducing avoidable hospitalization.
>
> RCGP (2013)

The primary care physician is often seen as the key person involved in delivering bad news and making arrangements for end-of-life care. However, as Hebert *et al.* (2011) state, 'end-of-life nursing encompasses many aspects of care: pain and symptom management, culturally sensitive practices, assisting patients and their families through the death and dying process, and ethical decision making'. These authors refer to the concept of 'advocacy' in nursing in that although physicians remain the gatekeepers of information and are usually the ones to break bad news to patients, such as the diagnosis of a terminal condition, they may be hurried and not always sensitive to the needs of patients and their families. If the physician has not engaged with the patient, the relationship is technical rather than personal. Alternatively, nurses as advocates take on the role of communicator.

End-of-life as part of the medical/nursing teaching agenda

Although there are favourable changes taking place in the UK and elsewhere, the subject of end-of-life care is not so visible in academic departments and clinical practice where either teaching skills to take care for those nearing their end-of-life or providing palliative care maybe considered as a second priority. Providing compassionate care in the nursing/medical teaching curricula may enhance end-of-life care which may currently be receiving a low priority. As Hebert *et al.* (2011) tell us:

> challenges exist, such as limitations in nursing school curricula on the death and dying process, particularly in multicultural settings; differing policies and practices in healthcare systems; and various interpretations of end-of-life legal language . . .
>
> Hebert *et al.* (2011)

Thus, further attention to training in end-of-life care and compassion could prove beneficial to patients and their families/carers and could assist in reducing the discomfort experienced by health care professionals when delivering bad news.

Concluding remarks

Hebert *et al.* (2011) remind us that the need for better understanding of end-of-life care has never been greater than in today's healthcare climate, and that compassionate end-of-life care which is appropriate and in accordance with the patient's wishes is essential.

Whilst it is not within the scope of this current chapter to cover this important subject in any depth, I have attempted to introduce the topic and look at various approaches and current thoughts in this field. End-of-life is something very personal and individual, requiring greater understanding, but often viewed as difficult to approach and perhaps seen as a taboo subject. Providing quality patient-centred care, taking into account patient and family preferences, and individual values and beliefs is essential in order to assist in relieving suffering and providing dignified care. Certain models and therapies are in existence, such as Chochinov's Dignity Therapy which can be of great help to patients and relatives. It is also important to consider the role of the GP and nurse as primary sources of care for people with long-term and terminal conditions. Thus, greater focus on compassion and end-of-life care within the teaching curricula may assist health care professionals in obtaining greater confidence and overcoming the discomfort which may be experienced in addressing end-of-life care. This may in turn enhance the patient and carer experience.

In conclusion, dying is a part of life, and perhaps we should remember the 'flower' within us as noted in the opening quote of this chapter. Remembering the nature of the flower which starts as a bud, and then opens up into a beautiful flower giving hope and joy, then eventually withering and dying, but leaving us with the wonderful remembrance of its presence.

Care Experiences: hearing and touch – the last senses that leave us . . .

Kathi (Greece)

Jean was a 87-year-old widow, living alone but assisted by a house help, who came twice a week and her son's family. Jean took care of her small house, watched TV from dawn to night 'it just keeps me company, I don't watch it!', she used to say . . .

After her three grand-children had grown up, visits to her son's family became scarcer. Jean was taking good care of herself, but she was starting to forget and her frequent falls at home greatly worried her family. She suffered some uneventful falls before the critical one: hip fracture.

The operation was successful and although the recovery period took many months, she recovered. She recovered well from the operation but she was no longer exactly the same person. Suddenly, her family realized that she had 'changed', she looked now very much her age, she was often absent-minded, she would not engage in a conversation.

Her son attributed the change to the shock of the fall, the operation, the post-operative adjustment period. Until one day, getting out of bed, she fell and was not able to get up, she had difficulty speaking and communicating. At the emergency where she was taken, she was diagnosed with an internal brain bleed and at her age and general condition, it was not advisable to operate. The physicians suggested a wait and see approach hoping that the hematoma might shrink and not press the brain.

During the first days, Jean had some lucid moments, when she could connect with nurses, doctors, while even lethargic, she could feel her son coming and suddenly awake. One would say that she was living only for those times when her son visited her. Slowly, day after day, her brain withdrew, and she never came back.

(continued)

(continued)

Jean lay for days, eyes shut, without any sign of communication with her environment, not reacting to her family members talking to her, taking care of her, except for the moment her son arrived.

Jean was treated in the pathology clinic of an old public hospital in the same room with six other elderly patients. The medical staff limited and available only till 2p.m., after which the interns took over. The nurses were scarce, with only two nurses at night for 35–40 patients, many of them in critical condition such as Jean. In such circumstances, in the public hospitals, if a patient does not have relatives or friends to take care of him/her, he/she will bitterly experience the results . . .

Jean was lucky to have at all times someone at her bedside to wash, change, rub, talk to her. Her family took shifts at her bedside day and night. They had noted that the nurses, be it overwork or indifference, would hardly responded to calls to change bedsheets, check on an IV or for other assistance. What the daughter-in-law had noted was that the nurses never addressed the patient or looked at him/her . . . When she would ask one to come to Jean's bedside to help turn her on the other side or check some abnormal symptoms, they would always answer 'I come in a minute, I have to dispense medicines' the 'minute' usually lasted from half an hour to more than one hour and more visits to the nursing station.

The only island of caring 'care', besides that of her relatives, was offered to Jean at night, by the private nurse from Bulgaria, whom the exhausted family had hired to get relief at night. Sofia, the Bulgarian private nurse, not only knew exactly how to take care of critically ill patients but most importantly she performed her services, not only skilfully, but with real 'care', respect and without noise. Her professional attire, the expertise that her delicate but decisive movements in handling the patient, the soft tone of her voice talking to Jean and explaining to her what she was doing, eased the anxiety of the family, who felt relieved to go home to rest.

Sofia would arrive punctually five minutes before her shift, would put on her white robe and would come to the bedside to greet Jean, while holding her hand. 'She can't hear you', a family member remarked. 'Yes, she can perfectly hear and feel us, but she can't answer. Jean needs to hear us and feel our touch. These are her safety lines . . . ' Sofia would proceed gracefully to the night routine for the patient: bed bath, massage, change of gown, all the while speaking softly to Jean explaining what she was doing.

Jean continued to lay comatose for more than five weeks, the doctors in their morning and afternoon rounds passed by their bed, looked at her chart, and they would go to the next patient.

Despite the efforts of her relatives, who took shifts at the patient's side, to speak to her, to tell her stories in an effort to keep her 'alive', to touch her to make her feel they were at her side, expecting some sign of communication, Jean was drifting further away every day.

What was amazing though is that whenever her son came, he would tell her 'Mom, it's Marc, I am here, how are you today? If you hear me, press my hand' . . . and miracle, Jean who lay unconscious would imperceptibly press her hand against that of her son . . . It was heart breaking to watch and more than once, it brought tears to the eyes of the other patients and family . . .

It happened that Jean passed away a night when Sofia had arrived for her shift. The intern who came hastily wanted to apply CPR, one relative dared to say that it was not necessary given her condition, but the other members of the family urged the intern to proceed . . .

Sofia stood by the bedside and offered to assist the doctor, while she hushed the family gently to the corridor. It's not known what happened behind the closed door, but after a few minutes the door opened and the doctor announced the death of Jean.

Sofia came to the corridor to comfort and hug the family and asked their permission to take the last care of Jean and prepare her for her long trip. The family felt they should offer the last care to Jean as per their religious ritual, but Sofia assured them that as a member of the same faith, she would deliver the proper care and do everything that is customary; besides she had foreseen the event and had with her all necessary supplies for such a circumstance. With a motherly tone, she asked the family to trust her and go home to rest and that she would keep Jean company that night . . .

Even though I do not give a detailed account of all the nursing care details that Sofia was dispensing to Jean, Sofia for me is a living example of what compassionate, professional, respectful care is . . .

What I should mention is that Sofia had no interest whatsoever in being a good nurse, she was not an employee at that hospital, she could not expect a salary raise or promotion for excellent services. She was an independent nurse, called in whenever a patient would need extra nursing care paid privately. She did not expect a word of mouth reference, since patients come and go . . . She was just doing her job as best as she could, she told once . . . but was it only well performed nursing care? Of course not, it was compassionate nursing care delivered very professionally . . .

Care Experiences: personal note from ER doctor written after woman's death goes viral

By Eric Pfeiffer | Yahoo! News

An emergency room doctor at New York Presbyterian Hospital has touched the hearts of millions after a personal letter he wrote about the death of a patient went viral on the Internet. The letter was first published on Reddit by the son of the deceased woman, who reportedly died of breast cancer in December 2012. In the letter, the doctor explains that this is the first such note he has written in 20 years of ER work.

The letter has already been viewed by more than 2 million users on Reddit, with thousands leaving comments. The doctor's letter:

Dear Mr (removed),

I am the Emergency Medicine physician who treated your wife Mrs (removed) last Sunday in the Emergency Department at (hospital). I learned only yesterday about her passing away and wanted to write to you to express my sadness. In my twenty years as a doctor in the Emergency Room, I have never written to a patient or a family member, as our encounters are typically hurried and do not always allow for more personal interaction.

However, in your case, I felt a special connection to your wife (removed), who was so engaging and cheerful in spite of her illness and trouble breathing. I was also touched by the fact that you seemed to be a very loving couple. You were highly supportive of her, asking the right questions with calm, care and concern. From my experience as a physician, I find that the love and support of a spouse or a family member is the most soothing gift, bringing peace and serenity to those critically ill.

I am sorry for your loss and I hope you can find comfort in the memory of your wife's great spirit and of your loving bond. My heartfelt condolences go out to you and your family.

The 24-year-old man who posted the letter said in an email interview with the Huffington Post that the outpouring of support from Reddit users has helped him cope with the passing of his mother.

'If my mother were alive to see this, she would want readers to reflect on the power of showing compassion toward a total stranger,' he said in the interview. 'The support I got from Reddit was amazing – doctors, nurses and other Redditors who have lost their mothers to cancer were all shocked and amazed that the doctor took the time to write such a heartfelt, meaningful letter.'

http://news.yahoo.com/personal-note-from-er-doctor-written-after-woman's-death-goes-viral-000236336.html?cac

References

Antiel, R. M., Curlin, F. A., James, K. M., Sulmasy, D. P., Tilburt, J. C. (2012). Dignity in end-of-life care: Results of a national survey of U.S. physicians, *Journal of Pain and Symptom Management* 44 (3): 331–339.

Akechi, T. (2012). Dignity therapy: Preliminary cross-cultural findings regarding implementation among Japanese advanced cancer patients, *Palliative Medicine* 26 (5): 768–769.

Bauer-Wu, S. (2011) *Leaves Falling Gently.* Oakland, CA: New Harbinger Publications.

Cassell, E. J. (2004). *The Nature of Suffering and the Goals of Medicine.* Oxford: Oxford University Press.

Chochinov, H. M. (2002). Dignity-conserving care: A new model for palliative care helping the patient feel valued, *JAMA* 287 (17): 2253–2260.

Chochinov, H. M., Hack, T., Hassard, T., Kristjanson, L. J., McClement, S., Harlos, M. (2005). Dignity Therapy: A novel psychotherapeutic intervention for patients near the end of life, *JCO* 23 (24): 5520–5525.

Chochinov, H. M. (2007). Dignity and the essence of medicine: The A, B, C, and D of dignity conserving care, *BMJ* 335: 184.

Davison, S. N. (2010). End-of-life care preferences and needs: Perceptions of patients with chronic kidney disease, *Clin J Am Soc Nephrol* 5(2): 195–204.

Dwyer, L. L., Andershed, L. L. B., Nordenfelt, L., Ternested, T. B. M. (2009). Dignity as experienced by nursing home staff, *International Journal of Older People Nursing* 4: 185–193 http://dignityincare.ca/en/research-team.html (accessed 30 August 2013).

Elliot, H. (2011). Lets talk about it, *Journal of Holistic Healthcare* 8 (1): 4–7. http://www.kingsfund.org.uk/blog/2009/11/who-wants-talk-about-it-future-delivery-end-life-care (Accessed July 2013).

Ferrell, B. R., Coyle, N. (2008). The nature of suffering and goals of nursing, *Oncology Nursing Forum* 35 (2): 241–247.

Forbes, K., Gibbin, J., Burcombe, M. E., Bloor, S. J., Reid, C. M., McCoubrie, R. C. (2011). Healthcare professionals' views on factors influencing end-of-life care in hospitals, *BMJ Support Palliative Care,* 1: A19. doi:10.1136/bmjspcare-2011-000020.55.

Hack, T., McClement, S. E., Chochinov, H. M., Cann, B. J., Hassard, T. H., Kristjanson, L. J. (2010). Learning from dying patients during their final days: Life reflections gleaned from dignity therapy, *J Palliat Med* 24 (7): 715–723.

Halifax, J. (2011). The precious necessity of compassion, *Journal of Pain and Symptom Management* 41 (1): 146.

Hall, S., Goddard, C., Speck, P. W., Martin, P., Higginson, I. J. (2013). "It makes you feel that somebody is out there caring": A qualitative study of intervention and control participants' perceptions of the benefits of taking part in an evaluation of Dignity Therapy for people with advanced cancer, *Journal of Pain and Symptom Management* 45 (4): 712–725.

Hannon, K. L., Lester, H. E., Campbell, S. M. (2012). Recording patient preferences for end-of-life care as an incentivized quality indicator: What do general practice staff think? *Palliative Medicine,* 26 (4): 336–41.

Hebert, K., Moore, H., Rooney, J. (2011). The nurse advocate in end-of-life care, *The Ochsner Journal* 11: 325–329.

Houmann, L. J., Rydahl-Hansen, S., Chochinov, H. M., Kristjanson, L. J., Groenvold, M. (2010). Testing the feasibility of the Dignity Therapy interview: Adaptation for the Danish culture, *BMC Palliative Care* 9: 21.

Huffman, J. C., Stern T. A. (2003). Compassionate care of the terminally ill, *Primary Care Compassion J Clinical Psychiatry* 5 (3): 131–136.

Hunter, B. (2010) Relinquishment of Certainty: A Step beyond Terror Management, in Harris, D. L. (ed.), *Counting Our Losses*. London: Routledge, pp. 127–13.

Jacelon, C. S., Connelly, T. W., Brown, R., Proulx, K., Vo, T. (2004) A concept analysis of dignity for older adults, *Journal of Advanced Nursing* 48 (1): 76–83.

Kearney, M. K., Weininger, R. B., Vachon, M. L. S., Harrison, R. L., Mount, B. M. (2010). Care of Physicians Caring for Patients at the End of Life "Being Connected . . . A Key to My Survival", in McPhee S. J., Winker, M.A., Rabow, M.W., Pantilat, Z (eds), *Care at the Close of Life*. New York: McGraw-Hill Medical, pp. 551–563.

McClement, S., Chochinov, H. M., Hack, T., Hassard, T., Kristjanson, L. J., Harlos, M. (2007). Dignity Therapy: Family member perspectives, *J Palliat Med.* 10 (5): 1076–82.

McKeown, J., Clarke, A., Repper, J. (2006). Life story work in health and social care: Systematic literature review, Article first published in *Journal of Advanced Nursing online*, DOI: 10.1111/j.1365–2648.2006.03897.x.

Michiels, E. (2007). The role of general practitioners in continuity of care at the end of life: A qualitative study of terminally ill patients and their next of kin, *J Palliat Med.* 21 (5): 409–415.

Müller-Mundt, G., Bleidorn, J., Geiger, K., Klindworth, K., Pleschberger, S., Hummers-Pradier, E., Schneider, N. (2013). End of life care for frail older patients in family practice (ELFOP): Protocol of a longitudinal qualitative study on needs, appropriateness and utilisation of services, *BMC Family Practice* 14: 52.

Ngo-Metzger, Q., August, K. J., Srinivasan, M., Liao, S., Meyskens, F. L. (2008) End-of-life: Guidelines for patient-centered communication *Am Fam Physicians* 77(2), 167–74. www.rcgp.org.uk; www.rcn.org.uk/dat/assets/pdf file/003/191730/003298.pdf.

Sampson, E. L., Burn, A., Richard, M. (2011). Improving end-of-life care for people with dementia, *The British Journal of Psychiatry* 199: 357–359.

Schulz, R., Hebert, R. S., Dew, M. A., Brown, S. L., Scheier, M. F., Beach, S. R., Czaja, S. J., Martire, L. M., Coon, D., Langa, K. M., Gitlin, L. N., Stevens, A. B., Nichols, L. (2007). Patient suffering and caregiver compassion: New opportunities for research, practice, and policy, *The Gerontologist* 47 (1): 4–13.

Singer, P. A., Martin, D. K., Kelner, M. (1999) Quality end-of-life care: patients' perspectives, *JAMA* 281 (2): 163–168.

Taylor, R., McLaughlin, K. (2011) Terror and intimacy unlocking secrets at the end of life. *Journal of Holistic Healthcare* 8 (1): 12–17. (WHO http://www.who.int/cancer/palliative/definition/en/ (Accessed September 2013).

Part III

The implementation and impact of compassion in healthcare

Within this section, the practical implementation of compassionate care within various healthcare settings is discussed. Experiences and research efforts are reviewed, including the importance of considering how compassion can be delivered to people with chronic conditions. Experiences and research efforts are explored, including compassionate approaches to vulnerable groups such as people with dementia and mental health problems.

8 Encouraging a focus on compassionate care within general practice/family medicine

Christos Lionis and Sue Shea

The good physician knows his patient through and through, and his knowledge is bought dearly. Time, sympathy, and understanding must be lavishly dispensed, but the reward is to be found in that personal bond which forms the greatest satisfaction of the practice of medicine. One of the essential qualities of the clinician is his interest in humanity, for the secret of the care of the patient is in caring for the patient.

Francis Peabody (1927)

Introduction

When we speak about compassion, or lack of compassion, there is a tendency to refer to bad reports and publicity regarding hospital/secondary care settings. However, compassionate care is equally important in general practice (GP)/Family Medicine (FM), where the physician is responsible for a range of conditions, including management of chronic conditions, assistance with mental health issues and health promotion. In many countries, the GP often acts as a 'gate-keeper' to specialist care. The GP is often the first point of contact, dealing with a wide range of consultations and offering a broad spectrum of care (Allen *et al.* 2002). GP/FM services are essential – they can help to prevent unnecessary hospital admissions, and can assist in the prevention of long hospital stays by treating the patient in his/her own environment following discharge from hospitalization. 'Traditionally' FM was intended to encompass the treatment of a patient based on personal knowledge of the person, and taking into consideration the patient's biological/psychological needs, within the context of knowledge of his/her family/community. As such GPs are trained to treat patients of any age and sex to levels of complexity that are defined by each country (Allen *et al.* 2011). The concept of 'compassion' can be viewed as a crucial aspect of this process, and as Barry and Edgman-Levitan (2012) state 'Caring and compassion were once often the only "treatment" available to clinicians'. We are reminded that over time, advances in medical science have provided new options and although these can often improve outcomes, they may also inadvertently distance physicians from their patients. Thus, we might be working with a health care environment in which patients and their families are often excluded from important discussions and are left confused and unsure with regard to how their problems are being managed and how to understand the overwhelming array of diagnostic and treatment options available to them. Taylor (1997) argues the importance of compassion as a necessary value for GPs, calling for the resuscitation of 'The Personal Doctor', to whom 'general practice without compassion was as therapeutic as air without oxygen'. In a study by Tarrant *et al.* (2003), designed to examine patients perceptions of the future of personal care in general practice, and how far these are shared by healthcare providers, it was revealed that patients, GPs, primary care nurses and administrative staff hold similar views on the meaning of personal care. In addition, care providers felt that compassion was important from the stage of entering the reception, stating that this is the first stage towards the doctor and if this experience is off-putting, patients may adopt a defensive attitude when they see the doctor. Mercer (2012) refers to the key role that empathy (a component of compassion) may play in primary care settings, and in a recent systematic review by Derksen *et al.* (2013), it was concluded that the general outcome seemed to be that empathy in the patient–physician communication in general practice is of unquestionable importance. In an American study reported in *Science Daily* (2012), the conclusion was drawn that the doctor–patient relationship does not only develop greater trust and empathy, putting patients at ease, but it also changes the brain's response to stress and increases pain tolerance. Whilst Stevenson (2012) argues that patient-centred care exerts a positive influence on health outcomes and is especially applicable in general practice, providing an efficacious and compassionate response to suffering.

In 1952, the Royal College of General Practitioners (RCGP) (http:// www.rcgp.org.uk/) was developed in the UK to address the fact that general practice is a specialism in its own right and thus requires its own professional body. RCGP has a global outlook, relying on experiences from the UK and other parts of the world. Its purpose is to deliver education, training and development to GPs and primary care professionals, and to encourage research in the field of family medicine. In 1965, RCGP introduced the MRCGP Exam, which is designed to test clinical knowledge, and consultation and caring skills. During this process, candidates are examined by GPs who are at the forefront of knowledge, regarding the sorts of clinical and social issues experienced by patients.

With a growing interest in the concept of compassion, RCGP recently organized a one-day conference to address this issue, and to discuss and debate the challenges faced in providing compassionate primary healthcare. The conference looked at a number of issues including practitioner altruism, patient engagement and empowerment, and patient safety and health outcomes. The conference also addressed the issue of GP burn-out which has been recognized as a growing issue in the UK, as evidenced by a survey conducted among 2,000 GPs by the College of Medicine, Pulse, and RCGP (Pulse 2013). One participating GP reported that '... the stress would pile up and by 10am you've already reached rock bottom. I was very sad I couldn't express my care for patients how I used to ... '. Thus, compassion towards GPs themselves, and across the primary care team involved in family medicine is also an important issue if compassion towards the patient is going to be sustainable.

Additionally, the subject of compassionate care within primary care and general practice has recently received prompt attention by the UK National Health Service (NHS). The Care Quality Commission (CQC) has announced that general practitioners (GPs) will be rated for their compassion and values, and CQC inspectors will interview GPs and their patients to measure how caring and compassionate individual practices are (www. telegraph.co.uk/health/healthnews/10118620/GPs-will-be-rated-for-their-compassion.html and www.pulsetoday.co.uk/your-practice-topics/regulation/gps-to-be-interviewed-to-measure-their-compassion-says-cqc-lead/).

Is compassion and compassionate care lacking from the definition of GP/FM originated from Europe?

In 1972, the World Organization of Family Doctors (WONCA) was established, with the aim to maintain and improve the quality of life of the peoples of the world through defining and promoting its values, and by fostering and maintaining high standards of care in general practice/family medicine by promoting personal, comprehensive and continuing care for the individual in the context of the family and the community, encouraging and supporting the development of academic organizations of general practitioners/family physicians, providing a forum for exchange of knowledge and information between member organizations of general practitioners/family physicians, and representing the educational, research and service provision activities of general practitioners/family physicians before other world organizations and forums concerned with health and medical care (http://www.globalfamilydoctor.com).

WONCA comprises seven active regions. However, in focusing on the WONCA Europe region, we identified that the concept of compassion was not discussed extensively within the European Society of General Practice/Family Medicine (WONCA Europe) when the WONCA Europe region was working on a definition of general practice/family medicine (GP/FM) to serve the development of a strategic thinking cap in the European setting (Allen *et al.* 2002; Lionis *et al.* 2008).

The emergence of a new definition of GP in Europe has been considered as a high priority for the agenda of WONCA Europe since 2000 and the new definition was approved in 2002 (Allen *et al.* 2002; Richards 2003). The definition highlights 12 characteristics of the discipline of GP/FM, clustered into six independent categories of core competence: primary care management, person-centred care, specific problem-solving skills, comprehensive, community orientation and holistic approach (Allen *et al.* 2011) (See The WONCA Tree, Figure 8.1). The characteristic 'patient empowerment' has been added to the new version (Gay 2013). Up until now, certain translations in different languages have been reported (http://www.woncaeurope.org), while this definition has affected the educational policy of many colleges and associations (Lionis *et al.* 2008) and currently guides the research and educational agenda of WONCA Europe (Hummers-Pradier *et al.* 2009).

Core competencies such as patient-centredness and comprehensive care and the newly added characteristic patient-empowerment may be associated with the concept of compassion; however, there seem to be certain gaps remaining.

This raises the question as to how patient-centredness and comprehensive care can be achieved without humanity and compassion. As stated by Robert Rakel (2000), 'compassion is an essential component of high-quality medical care in today's technological world of medicine'. However, the concept of empathy has been largely utilized in the literature and

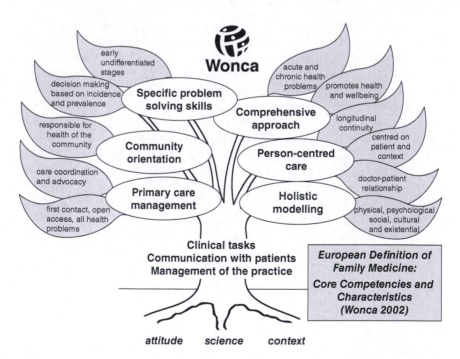

Figure 8.1 European definitions of family medicine: core competencies and characteristics

Source: Ueli Grueninger, MD Executive Director, Swiss College of Primary Care Medicine and WONCA Europe (permission obtained).

its clinical dimension has been denoted as a crucial component of the physician–patient therapeutic relationship (Jani *et al.* 2012; Larorain *et al.* 2013). As mentioned previously, it is also noted in the systematic literature review published by Derksen *et al.* (2013) that patients' perceptions of the doctors' empathy seem to be of key importance in patient enablement in general practice consultations. Likewise, a Scottish cross-sectional study conducted in high and low deprivation areas (Mercer *et al.* 2012) revealed similar findings in terms of the importance of empathy in general practice.

We can assume that compassion may incorporate other concepts frequently utilized in GP/FM including patient centredness and empathy. However, there is still much room for GP to place more emphasis on non-pharmacological treatment and to emphasize a crossroad of medicine with other disciplines, particularly the psychological and social sciences. This could open new therapeutical opportunities to this clinical and academic discipline where initiatives such as compassion-focused therapy (Gilbert 2010) could be in introduced, building on a range of cognitive-behavioural therapies and other therapies and interventions.

A focus on the importance of compassionate health care has caught the attention of both the public and health policy makers internationally, following the final report of the independent inquiry into care provided by Mid Staffordshire NHS Foundation Trust in the UK (2013). In this report Robert Francis QC gathered evidence from over 900 patients and families who provided information for the report.

A further report chaired by Professor Sir Bruce Keogh published a short time after the Francis report focused on the quality of care and treatment provided by 14 hospital trusts in England: overview report (NHS 2013). The key themes that were considered in the design of the review as core foundations of high-quality care for patients were patient experience, safety, workforce, clinical and operational effectiveness, and governance and leadership. Professor Sir Bruce Koegh in a recent interview said:

> People still need to be in hospital but I'm not sure we always have people in the right hospital with the right expertise,' he says. 'In many of our hospitals, if we had better community care and social services, we could get 25 per cent of patients out. It's that order of magnitude.
>
> (*The Independent*, Saturday, 10 August 2013.
> www.independent.co.uk/news/people/profiles/
> sir-bruce-keogh-raising-quality-reducingcosts-
> why-running-the-nhs-is-like-selling-pcs-8735619.html).

Professor Sir Bruce Keogh's words send a key message to GPs that in a period where there is a budget crisis affecting the public health care sector in many countries, emphasis should be placed on improving the quality and safety of primary care services, in order to prevent unnecessary hospital admissions that might add to the pressure of accident and emergency services. To what extent is this feasible? Is it possible to encourage GPs to be more compassion driven and mobilized by a patient-centred approach? What is the role of WONCA in assisting in the formulation of a strategy which is more focused on compassion? In this chapter, we attempt to elucidate some of the essentials of this effort.

Compassionate care in the undergraduate medical education

The above section draws attention to the potential lack of clarity regarding focus on compassion in the definition of general practice. Indirectly, this may be reflected in the residency programmes that the definition needs to guide. However, it can be explained mainly by the lack of focus on constructs related to compassion within GP/FM undergraduate medical education as reported by Soler *et al.* (2007). These authors recommend the teaching of communication skills within primary care doctor–patient encounters and exploration of new ways of teaching and enhancing the doctor–patient relationship.

Up until recently, the subject of compassionate care has rarely been discussed with regard to undergraduate medical education, although some academic settings have successfully introduced courses on this topic, for example, University of Crete (Lionis *et al.* 2011). Certain medical schools do teach courses on doctor–patient relationship where clinical empathy covers an important part. However, earlier work by Mercer and Reynolds (2002) reported that clinical empathy cannot be understood without a behavioural action component. Teaching doctor–patient communication and clinical empathy may be a good 'passage' for introducing the subject of compassionate care in undergraduate medical education. This could be particularly relevant in times of austerity where many people exist in isolation usually without continuity of care and access to a personal physician, and where there is an increased risk of depression and co-morbidity.

Compassionate care and family practice research

In addition to GPs, other health care professionals, for example nurses, often form part of the primary health care setting, playing a key role in disease management and other aspects of primary care. However, a narrative search in PubMed has revealed only a few publications with the MeSH (Medical Subject Headings) term 'compassion' with a link to primary care or general practice. It is not certain whether this result is due to negligence on the subject by GP, the lack of appropriate training either in the undergraduate or vocational training or the lack of strong evidence that compassionate care has an effect on physicians, health care professionals or patients. The lack of training modules on compassionate care within European universities may have an impact on the minimal academic and clinical research within this field. However, the effects of the current financial crisis on health care in many countries offer a suitable frame within which research on compassionate care could be further developed, particularly as at such times humanity, compassion and attention to basic needs may be even more crucial, and may assist in the prevention of and attention to various mental health issues. Certain factors such as the currently available methodological tools to measure compassion and the evidence of the biological effect of compassionate care should be elucidated as a result of this focus of research within GP/FM. The utilization of European funds is a good opportunity to start researching this issue, alongside other funding opportunities that could be explored. The role of WONCA is crucial towards this effort and previous positive experiences where global organizations have had strong involvement in such efforts, could be appropriately utilized.

Compassionate care and quality of care and patient safety in GP/FM

Quality of care and patient safety are two interrelated disciplines that have received prompt attention by GP/FM Europe and a core network, the European Rural and Isolated Practitioners Association (EURIPA) at WONCA Europe, is addressing this task. The UK Department of Health has recently (May 2013) issued a mandate from the Government to Health Education with a focus on delivering high-quality, effective and compassionate care. In this mandate among others, the short-term deliverables and longer-term objectives relevant to NHS values and behaviour as well as working in partnership involving patient voice and local accountability has been clearly presented.

In addition to the above, GPs have a 'front line' role and are ideally placed to offer compassionate care. This is particularly important when they are required to provide comprehensive health care to frail older patients and their families, and to patients approaching end-of-life. Frailty as a state of vulnerability to adverse outcomes is receiving continuous interest in the literature and it is on the epicentre of attention of both geriatricians and GPs. A protocol of a longitudinal qualitative study on needs, appropriateness and utilization of services for end-of-life care for frail older patients in family practice has been recently published by Muller-Mundt *et al.* (2013). Coexisting frailty, multi-morbidity and the high dependence of frail patients on families and caregivers provides a unique place for GPs to test their compassionate capacity to the benefit of patients and families. Certain publications are advising 'sensitivity to the patients' cultural and individual preferences' when physicians are delivering bad news or when they are invited to provide end-of-life services (Ngo-Metzger *et al.* 2008) but compassion seems to be key in facilitating this patient-centred communication in these specific circumstances.

Compassionate care and GP/FM within the economic crisis

Although the World Health Organization (WHO) states that primary care is needed now more than ever (WHO 2008), contemporary Europe faces various challenges as a result of the economic crisis where the focus on primary care has been seriously deregulated in certain countries, including Greece (Tsiligianni *et al.* 2013). Many vulnerable groups have no or limited access to primary care and this presents a challenge for GP. Among these groups are the under privileged populations and migrants with multi-morbidity (O' Donnell *et al.* 2013). GP/FM should test new innovative methods and ideas where either the burden to the health care services or to underprivileged families could be alleviated. GP/FM is challenging to ensure that health equity is not a rhetoric statement and this academic and clinical discipline can be considered as an effective vehicle to guarantee this important component to health policy. The financial crisis is inversely associated with clinical effectiveness. According to Barbara Starfield (2009), effectiveness in clinical practice of primary health care (PHC) can be seen only when PHC is defined on a basis of the first contact, longitudinality, comprehensiveness and coordination. The economic crisis deregulated all those fundamental components and now the question remains as to how compassionate care can be provided in a system where first contact and continuity is not a priority. A primary care-oriented health care system should be responsible for the patient needs and problems as the patient identified. This raises the question as to what extent a system that is predominantly interested in covering its fiscal problems, and GPs who are busy with many other issues are able to recognize the patients' problems? Certainly, GPs as frontline health care professionals under the pressing conditions they meet and severe stress they experience appear to commonly present symptoms of burn-out (Soler *et al.* 2008) and the financial crisis seems to be enhancing this. It remains to be considered and discussed to what extent GPs who offer compassionate and person-centred care are less vulnerable from stress and anxiety within the austerity period. Primary care professionals, and among them GPs, could be an effective vehicle and resource of compassion, while the role of the universities and teaching organizations seems to be pivotal.

The impact of the financial crisis has been studied among various disadvantaged groups, including the elderly, children and migrants (Rechel *et al.* 2013; O'Donnell *et al.* 2013). There are many reports in Greece that the austerity period has led to incidents of hostility, racism and violence against immigrants (Reuters 2012). This period facilitates many voluntary actions that have appeared to alleviate the burden of disadvantaged groups, while voices from scientific consortia, like that of the RESTORE (**RE**search into implementation **ST**rategies to support patients of different **OR**igins and language background in a variety of **E**uropean primary care settings; http://www.fp7restore.eu/) project to protect the right to health care for all persons (O'Donnell *et al.* 2013) independently of the impact of financial crisis.

The role of WONCA and its associated study groups

At an international level, WONCA builds on networks that shape issues of research, education and quality of health care, while it enhances thematic groups that address clinical issues such as diabetes mellitus, cardiovascular and gastroenterology all seen from the perspective of general practice and primary care. Strategic plans for developing further the discipline in Europe is a key issue for that European Association and a new policy strategy is under discussion (Lionis *et al.* 2004, European Academy of Teachers in General Practice and Family Medicine, EURACT 2013), while a new research agenda has been recently published (European General Practice Research Network, EGPRN 2009). Joint efforts to promote the collaboration across the different networks and clinical special interest groups have been recently initiated. To that direction, European Society for Quality and Safety in Family Practice, EQuiP (the network on quality assurance) together with EURIPA (the rural network) have decided to promote patient safety issues in rural settings, while EURIPA jointly with EGPRN (the research network) will meet in Malta this year to discuss a common research agenda in rural areas. Although there is strong involvement of this organization with regard to subjects that affect clinical effectiveness in general practice and primary care, the concept of compassion is still not visible either in the new definition or in the policy statements. However, it is visible that compassion needs to be included in the core competences of the definition of GP/FM which is under revision according to the recent EURACT statement. The concept of compassion could be included in the current agenda of certain European networks including EGPRN, EQuiP and EURACT with the main focus on working together towards a European strategy to promote the concept of compassion. It is important that this concept is incorporated into the European strategy that intends to promote the discipline across the region. The creation of a study group (working party on compassionate care) under the WONCA international umbrella may enhance the forms on that subject and turn the general practice light towards a less clinical definition and measurement within clinical practice. The forthcoming launch of a new journal (*Journal of Compassionate Health Care*) could help to support such an effort.

Conclusion

Although the concept of compassion is frequently referred to within the health care arena and is closely associated with medical performance, it does not yet appear to have received its central role when the definition of GP/FM as discipline of health care services. The inclusion of compassionate care as a key subject in the medical curriculum and the training programmes for residents may have an impact in its global consideration for the incorporation of additional skills in the capacity of GPs. GPs – often being the first point of contact for a number of health related issues – could make a major contribution in terms of delivery, and research into the importance concept of compassionate care.

Care Experiences: through compassion into healing*

Elefteria (Greece)

This is the case of a 47-year-old man followed in the GP ambulatory who was diagnosed with borderline personality disorder for treatment for dependency on illegal drugs in a community detoxification programme. In the first visit when he was asked to talk about his medical history, he was aggressive and suspicious so the interview was interrupted and preceded with a careful physical examination. During that time he slowly started to explain his situation. He referred to chronic symptoms mostly low back pain and muscle cramps after a very severe car accident years ago. He had visited various specialized physicians as orthopaedics and rheumatologists trying to determine a solution to his problem but he complained that nobody could help him. He also described a conflictual relationship between him and the physicians of the detoxification programme.

Through compassion demonstrated by our whole ambulatory team, medical and nurse staff, consisting in the creation of a relationship based on trust, kindness, understanding, availability, privacy, and in communication with other health providers, specialized physicians, psychologist and his family we achieved a better investigation of his needs and adherence to the treatment proposed with a relief of his symptoms. Compassion taught us how it can be a convenient tool to improve physician-patient relationship providing compensatory results not only for the patient but for the health care workers as well.

*Inspired by the book *Through Time in to Healing*, author Dr Brian Weiss, Psychiatrist specialist in regression therapy.

Care Experiences: this amazing doctor changed my life

Patient (New Zealand)

This is a complimentary story about the life-changing help and support I have received from my GP.

I am 46 years old and for probably 30 years have suffered from panic attacks and anxiety. I always believed there was something else wrong with me and that it wasn't stress and anxiety at all. For years I spent hundreds of dollars traipsing around to different specialists for various tests, all of which basically came back okay. I still refused to believe that a panic attack could cause all the symptoms I suffered and continued trotting from one medical centre to another trying to find the answer. I was meanwhile in a dreadful space, still suffering attacks of panic and anxiety, feeling stressed all the time – chasing my tail to find answers and getting nowhere – UNTIL . . .

I decided I needed my own GP. The one I found listened to me and for once in my life I did not feel like an idiot. Fortunately for me, this GP has a particular interest in stress and anxiety. He treated me with respect and a genuine interest in my situation. Although he advised me that certain types of medication would help, I was reluctant to take any pills. Instead of pressuring me to take the medication, he gave me his mobile phone number.

This was to be a safety net for me as I was able to phone him when I had a panic attack. He would talk me through it as he did on numerous occasions and I might add this was at all hours. Not once did he lose his patience with me.

I spent a lot of time at his surgery in various states of panic convinced I was in the middle of a heart attack or something else life-threatening. He and his staff were always amazing and helped me so much.

Eventually I decided that I would try the recommended medication although I was convinced it wouldn't work. Much to my surprise I have never been better in my life. I have always believed I had something far more sinister than panic and anxiety attacks. I have now learned through the patience and understanding of my GP that panic and anxiety is a very serious and nasty disorder and that it can be very hard to treat. I am living proof of that.

I cannot speak highly enough of this dedicated man who has basically saved my life. I am now able to spend more quality time with my daughter and even attended her school camp much to her delight.

I am not sure what else to say, but even if I was to win lotto and gave it to this man, it still wouldn't be enough to show my appreciation and gratitude. He has been amazing in the way he understood and handled my case – giving me back my dignity and my life.

Care Experiences: Jenny's story

Interview between Sue and Jenny (UK)

In the text that follows, we hear of Jenny's experience which captures a key example of lack of care:

(continued)

(continued)

The importance of care, and attention to detail, within a primary care setting

In a recent discussion with Jenny, she told the editors of the following experience which could have potentially led to very serious, and perhaps even life-threatening circumstances.

It had been the period leading up to Christmas, and Jenny was hanging Christmas decorations when a radiator which was not securely fixed to the wall fell onto her leg. Although no serious injury was recognized, and her leg was just grazed, Jenny decided to seek advice from the treatment room of the local Health Care Centre. The staff at the treatment room dressed the wound, and asked her to return for the dressing to be changed. Over the course of the next three weeks, apart from when the Health Centre was closed for Christmas, Jenny returned every day to have the dressing changed. However, the injury did not appear to be healing.

On one occasion, Jenny noticed a strange smell when the dressing was being changed – she questioned the nurse about this, asking if this smell was coming from her wound. The nurse responded that it wasn't, and that it was coming from a man in the next cubicle.

The lack of attention to the fact that Jenny's wound was not healing was eventually picked up on by a different nurse, who asked Jenny when she had last seen a doctor. Jenny replied that she had never seen a doctor regarding her injury. This new nurse then acted immediately by contacting a doctor, and Jenny was sent to the local hospital straight away.

In the hospital ward, Jenny was told that she needed complete rest and that cellulitis had set in. What had started as a graze on her leg was now a large hole. She was informed that if this deterioration of the wound had gone through to her bone, there was risk of amputation. Jenny's husband was keen to take action concerning the lack of care that had led to this situation, but they were told by the surgeon that it was just 'one of those things'.

Fortunately, staff at the hospital were able to treat the injury, thus saving Jenny from amputation.

However, this story reminds us of the importance of good initial care, particularly in primary care settings which are the first port of call for many symptoms and injuries. It appears from this story that the staff who initially treated Jenny simply 'did not care' and thus did not pick up on the developing seriousness of her injury.

Jenny said to the editors 'if it had not have been for that nurse, I could have lost my leg'. Luckily, and eventually, some-one did deliver the attention and care that was needed, but this should have occurred much sooner.

There are several reasons why basic care, attention to detail, and humanity towards the patient are so important in primary health care settings. Not only because good care in these settings can prevent serious outcomes, but also because such care within the community setting can help to reduce hospital admissions.

References

Allen, J., Gay, B., Grebolder, H., Heyrman, J., Svab, I., Ram, P. (2002) The European definition on the key features of the discipline of general practice: The role of the GP and core competencies *British Journal of General Practice* 52, 526–527.

Allen, J., Gay, B., Grebolder, H., Heyrman, J., Svab, I., Ram, P. (2011) *The European Definition of General Practice/Family Medicine.* Short version. WONCA Europe 2011.

Barry, M., Edgman-Levitan, S. (2012) Shared decision making-pinnacle of patient centered care *N Engl J Med* 366, 780–81.

Derksen, F., Jozien, B., Lagro-Janssen, A. (2013) Effectiveness of empathy in general practice: A systematic review *British Journal of General Practice* 63 (606), e76–84.

EGPRN (2009) *Research Agenda for General Practice/ Family Medicine and Primary Health Care in Europe* by Hummers-Pradier, E., Beyer, M., Chevallier, P., Eilat-Tsanani, S., Lionis, C., Peremans, L., Petek, D., Rurik, I., Soler, J.K., Stoffers, H.E., Topsever, P., Ungan, M., Van Royen, P. Maastricht: EGPRN.

Gay, B. (2013) What's new in the updated European definition of general practice/ family medicine? *Journal of General Practice* 1,111.

Gilbert, P. (2010). *Compassion Focused Therapy.* London: Routledge.

Hummers-Pradier, E., Beyer, M., Chevallier, P., Eilat-Tsanani, S., Lionis, C., Peremans, L., *et al.* (2009) The research agenda for general practice/family medicine and primary health care in Europe. Part 1. Background and methodology *European Journal of General Practice* 15 (4), 243–250.

Jani, B.D., Blane, D.N., Mercer, S.W. (2012) The role of empathy in therapy and the physician-patient relationship *Forschende Komplementärmedizin* 19(5), 252–257.

Larorain, S., Sultan, S., Zenasni, F., Catu-Pinault, A. *et al.* (2013) Empathic concern and professional characteristics associated with clinical empathy in French general practitioners *European Journal of General Practice* 19(1), 23–28.

Lionis, C., Shea S., Markaki A. (2011) Introducing and implementing a compassionate care elective for medical students in Crete *Journal of Holistic Health Care* 8, 38–41.

Lionis, C., Shea, S. (2012) Enhancing compassionate care as an integral part of primary care and general practice *Global Journal of Medicine and Public Health* 1(5), 1–2.

Mercer, S.W., Reynols, W.J. (2002) Empathy and quality of care *British Journal of General Practice* 52(suppl), S9–12.

Mercer, S.W., Jani, B.D., Maxwell, M., Wong, S.Y.S., Watt, G.C.M. (2012) Patient enablement requires physician empathy: a cross-sectional study of general practice consultations in areas of high and low socioeconomic deprivation in Scotland *BMC Family Practice* 13, 6.

Muller-Mundt, G., Bleidorn, J., Geiger, K., Klindtworth, K., Pleschberger, S., Hummers-Pradier, E., Schneider, N. (2013) End of life care from frail older patients in family practice (ELFOP)-protocol of a longitudinal qualitative study on needs, appropriateness and utilization of services *BMC Family Practice* 14, 52.

Ngo-Metzger, Q., August, K.J., Srinivasan, M., Liao, S., Meyskens, F.L. (2008) End-of-life: Guidelines for patient-centered communication *Am Fam Physicians* 77(2), 167–174.

NHS 2013. *Review into the quality of care and treatment provided by 14 hospital trusts in England: Overview report*, chaired by Sir Bruce Keogh, London July 2013.

O'Donnell, K., Burns, N., Dowrick, C., Lionis, C., MacFarlane, A. on behalf of the RESTORE team. (2013) Health-care access for migrants in Europe *The Lancet* 382, 393.

Pulse (2013) www.pulsetoday.co.uk (accessed September 2013).

Rakel, R.E. (2000) Compassion and the art of family medicine: From Osler to Oprah *Journal of the American Board of Family Medicine* 13(6).

Richards, T.D. (2003) New GP contract and European definition *British Journal of General Practice* 155.

Peabody, F.W. (1927) The care of the patient *JAMA* 88, 877–882.

Rechel, B., Mladovsky, P., Ingleby, D., Mackenbach, J.P., McKee, M. (2013). Migration and health in an increasingly diverse Europe *Lancet* 381 (9873): 1235–1245.

Science Daily (2012) www.sciencedaily.com/releases/2012/12/121203145952.htm (accessed November 2013).

Soler, J.K., Carelli, F., Lionis, C., Yaman, H. (2007) The wind of change: After the European definition orienting undergraduate medical education towards general practice/family medicine *European Journal of General Practice* 13, 248–251.

Soler, J.K., Yaman, H., Esteva M. *et al.* (2008) Burnout in European family doctors: The EGPRN study *Fam Pract* 25, 245–265.

Starfield, B. (2009) Primary care and equity in health: The importance to effectiveness and equity of responsiveness to people's needs *Humanity and Society* 33, 56–73.

Tarrant, C., Windridge, K., Boulton, M., Baker, R., Freeman, G. (2003) Qualitative study of the meaning of personal care in general practice *BMJ* 326(7402), 1310.

Taylor, M.B. (1997) Compassion: Its neglect and importance *British Journal of General Practice* 47, 521–523.

The Mid Staffordshire NHS Foundation Trust Inquiry (2013) *Independent Inquiry into Care Provided by Mid Staffordshire NHS Foundation Trust January 2005 – March 2009 Volume I and II, Chaired by Robert Francis QC.* London: Stationery Office.

Tsiligianni, I., Anastasiou, F., Antonopoulou, M., Chliveros, K., Dimitrakopoulos, S., Duijker, G., *et al.* on behalf of the Cretan Practice based Primary Care Research Network 'G. Lambrakis' and the Clinic of Social and Family Medicine, School of Medicine, University of Crete (2013) Greek rural GPs' opinions on how financial crisis influences health, quality of care and health equity *Rural Remote Health* 13(2), 2528.

WHO (2008) *The World Health Report 2008: Primary Health Care Now More Than Ever.* World Health Organization, Geneva, Switzerland (available at: www.who.int/whr/2008/whr08_en.pdf).

9 Care, compassion and ideals
Patient and health care providers' experiences[1]

Jill Maben

Introduction

In the past three years in the UK there have been numerous reports highlighting poor quality patient care in hospitals (e.g. Health Service Ombudsman 2011; CQC 2011; Commission on Dignity in Care 2012). None more potent than the Francis Report, which followed the public inquiry into Mid Staffordshire hospital (Francis 2013). Patient testimonies highlighted a 'disturbing lack of compassion' and Robert Francis QC, noted a focus on finance and figures at the expense of patient care, underpinned by a pre-occupation with a narrow set of top down targets (Francis 2010). The second Francis Report (2013) calls for culture change and suggests that we need to select recruits to the profession who evidence the 'possession of the appropriate values, attitudes and behaviours; ability and motivation to enable them to put the welfare of others above their own interests [Recommendation 185]'. No one could deny we want to recruit nurses with the appropriate values, attitudes and behaviours, but the underlying assumption is that to date we haven't been doing so and that this is a key indicator of where things have gone 'wrong' with nursing. But what if largely we haven't been getting recruitment wrong? What if we have recruited nurses with great values and nursing ideals, only for them to be dashed, eroded and crushed in challenging practice environments? What if we have not equipped and supported staff well enough to do the difficult work asked of nurses every day in the NHS? What if nurses start their career very compassionate and caring yet the system in which they work leaves them unable to show this compassion?

We know that 'really relating to patients takes courage, humility and compassion, and requires constant renewal by practitioners and recognition, re-enforcement and support from colleagues and managers. It cannot be taken for granted' (Maben *et al.* 2010). In this chapter I argue that it has been taken for granted that there has been insufficient recognition of the challenging work healthcare staff do each and every day and insufficient support for staff. Research evidence and my own work suggests we haven't necessarily been recruiting the wrong people – but rather we have not been providing sufficiently positive practice environments for their ideals, care and compassion to be realised, to flourish and be sustained. I will draw on my own personal journey as a nurse and my research over 20 years focusing on three key projects, all of which have examined staff experiences of caring work; the experiences of their patients and contextualise this in the wider literature to examine cultural issues and the challenges healthcare staff face in terms of compassionate care delivery, before suggesting potential solutions.

Background

There has long been concern about the demands placed on staff in health-care and the effects of these on the health and well-being of staff (Karasek 1979; Cox and Griffiths 1995). Medical and nursing staff is known to have high levels of stress (Payne and Firth-Cozens 1987; Mimura and Griffiths 2003), burn-out (Maslach and Jackson 1982; Schaufeli *et al.* 1993) and psychological morbidity (Taylor *et al.* 2005; Wall *et al.* 1997; McManus *et al.* 2002). The way in which healthcare staff experience their job impacts on individual performance, patients' experience and healthcare outcomes and the productivity and performance of organisations as a whole (West 2004; 2013). Health care staff work in highly pressurised environments and their work is complex, intense and emotionally challenging. My own and others' work suggests staff well-being impacts directly on patient care affecting staffs' ability to show empathy and compassion to patients and their carers (Taylor *et al.* 2007; Goodrich and Cornwell 2008; Raleigh *et al.* 2009; Maben *et al.* 2012a). My research on staff well-being and its links to patient experience has shown a clear relationship between the well-being of staff and patients' experiences of care; individual employee well-being is an antecedent, rather than a consequence, of patient care performance (Maben *et al.* 2012a). The UK Boorman review of staff health and well-being in the NHS found 80 per cent of staff felt their health and well-being impacted on their care for patients, but only 40 per cent thought that their employer was proactively trying to do something to improve it (Boorman 2009).

We know that the majority of people who enter professional doctor and nurse training are, at least initially, motivated by ideals and a sense of altruism (Lowenstein 2008), but cynicism can develop and these same staff can become less empathetic during their training, and more distant from their patients. Early work in medicine found that medical students develop cynicism in specific situations, but their idealism is not lost and is reasserted as the end of training approaches (Becker and Geer 1958). A recent study in the USA also identified medical students entering the profession with a lot of idealism: 'they want to be of help and service' but 'then something starts to happen when they are exposed to clinical care' when an empathy gap develops (Hojat *et al.* 2009). A study of nursing students suggested that they hold long-term altruistic and professional ideals which they may temporarily abandon in order to meet the requirements of the moment (Melia 1987). My own research shows that ideals and values such as individualised and holistic patient care held dear by graduating students can become abandoned and crushed in a short time, with nurses reporting some degree of burn-out within two years of qualification, leading in some cases to job-hopping or abandonment of nursing altogether (Maben *et al.* 2007). I explore this work in more detail below, but first a personal story.

A personal story . . .

In 1979 I entered nursing with a strong sense of compassion – yet was to leave nursing just two years after qualifying. I thought never to return. In 1983 I moved to London and had my second staff nurse post; 14 months later I had left nursing – I thought for good.

> I was 22 and was working on a busy 32-bedded male medical ward and was often in charge of the whole ward. One evening it was particularly busy. Tom, a man in his fifties, was confused and also very frustrated. As I went to take his blood pressure he grabbed the metal sphygmomanometer (spyhg) (they were heavy metal boxes in those days), got out of bed and threatened to throw it through the window. I therefore got myself between him and the window thinking it may stop him, at which point he said he'd throw it at me. There was only one other member of staff on the ward at the time and they were calling security (who incidentally never came). If it was already a difficult situation it then got much worse when the patient in the next bed who was recovering from a Myocardial Infarction (heart attack) he'd had two days earlier got between me and Tom. At that stage I don't know if I was more worried about the sphyg going through the window, it hitting me, or Jack, my knight in shining armour, having another MI. After a five-minute stand-off with me pleading with Jack to get back into bed, the sphyg eventually went through the window; no one was hurt as such, my blood pressure returned to normal and life on the ward carried on.
>
> Around the same time six patients died in a single week: two unexpectedly from cardiac arrests and another – Eddie after coming in for diagnostic tests only 3 days earlier – seemingly well. I had bonded well with him and with his wife, felt their bewilderment and their distress as he rapidly went downhill and died 3 days after admission from an inoperable cancer. Comforting Eileen his wife was impossible, but I tried. She came back to visit to say thank you. She bought me a begonia and she said I was kind. I didn't feel kind. I felt powerless, useless, bewildered and out of my depth – both as a nurse and as a human being. The senior nurse found me crying in the sluice that week, told me to pull myself together and get back on the ward . . . two months later I left. I had to get away, away from the stress, the distress and the sense of failure.

Keeping in touch with humanity

To deliver compassionate care staff need to keep in touch with their own humanity, which in a demanding busy environment is not always an easy feat. Yet we know that patients value the human touch, care, kindness and compassion. The little things matter to patients and it is the presence or absence of compassion that often marks the lasting and vivid memories patients and family members retain about the overall experience of care in hospital and other settings (Cornwell and Goodrich 2009). A young woman admitted to an acute admission ward after an overdose noted:

> I didn't know where the bathrooms were, I didn't know how to get unhooked from the machine so I could go to the bathroom, I didn't have any toiletries with me, I didn't have anybody coming to see me immediately . . . I was freezing and asked for a blanket, but they didn't bring me one . . . Nobody introduced themselves to me . . . I couldn't tell you anybody's name . . . I was in there for about three days and I didn't eat at all, but nobody noticed.
>
> (Maben *et al.* 2012a)

Conversely in the same environment another patient observed good care of another patient (Maben *et al.* 2012a):

> I did observe a young, auxiliary nurse, and an old lady who couldn't feed herself. Honestly, I was moved to tears. This young auxiliary nurse fed her, and was chatting away to her in such a lovely, lovely way. The old lady wasn't speaking much, but they were having a really nice conversation . . . They seemed to have the time to deal with patients individually, which was wonderful. It was so lovely . . . watching this young woman, just how she dealt so beautifully with this old lady who was in a great deal of pain.

Such care demands that staff empathise, consider the patient and family's perspective and go out of their way to help and be compassionate. Healthcare professionals and patients have long known that caring for patients well is not only the right thing to do, it also aids recovery and makes sense (Hayward 1975; Shuldham 1999; Suchman 1993; Boore 1978).

Patients in today's healthcare settings are almost invariably vulnerable, very sick and in need of support and care at a time of anxiety, discomfort or distress. A patient on an oncology ward reflected on the importance of the little things and relational care:

> The little things seem to me to be some very, very simple things – that you're offered a cup of tea, you're offered a drink of water, you're offered a biscuit, you're offered a snack, you're offered a meal, by the nursing staff and the nursing assistants as well as by volunteers . . . everyone's

always offering you a cup of tea, a drink, and stopping for a bit of rep-
artee. So it's a nice thing; it's just more of a human approach really.

(Maben *et al.* 2012a)

Whilst staff don't go to work to give 'bad care' (Iles 2011), from the patient
perspective sometimes that is what happens, with how staff communicate
with them, one of the issues raised most by patients, their failure often to
see the person in the patient (Goodrich and Cornwell 2008).

Study 1: compassion erosion: the fate of ideals and values, experiences of newly qualified nurses

I believe most nurses enter the profession motivated by ideals of altruism
and a desire to 'make a difference' in the lives of others. However, in some
environments a transformation occurs so that over time these same people
are forced to abandon their ideals and protect themselves against a system
that erodes humanity and caring (Maben *et al.* 2007). My doctoral study
involved asking students at the end of their course in a questionnaire:

> As a qualified nurse what do you anticipate will be your ideals for prac-
> tice? That is if you were able to choose how to practice what would be
> the kind of care you would like to give?

The responses to this question gave me their nursing values and ideals
which I subsequently showed to participants in follow-up interviews, asking
'Can you nurse in this way?', 'If not why not?', 'What gets in the way?' and
'If so what helps?'

From an initial sample of 86 students who responded to the questionnaire, I
followed up 26 of these as they became qualified nurses in a longitudinal study.
There were 22 women and 4 men and I interviewed them when they had been
qualified between 4 and 6 months and again between 11 and 15 months. I analysed the fate of their ideals and values over this period. What was the experience like for them and how this might change over time? Analysis revealed that
at the end of their course, newly qualified nurses emerged with a strong set of
values and ideals and I was able to identify three broad categories:

- patient-centred holistic care
- quality care
- nursing knowledge and research-based care.

For example, one student suggested she would like to:

> See the client as an individual and having time to support them in a
> holistic way. Being able to pick up when they are worried or distressed
> while at the same time ensuring their independence.

I identified three groups in relation to the new nurses' ability to implement these ideals in practice: Sustained idealists, who were able to retain their ideals because they experienced the following in their work environments: support, good role models; sufficient staffing and mix of skills in the team and a philosophy of care that promoted compassionate care, who were able to retain their ideals (just 4 out of the 26 newly qualified nurses). The two other groups identified compromised (14 out of 26) and crushed idealists (8 out of 26) who could not very often implement their ideals of practice and reported the need to compromise their ideals or adjust them on a daily basis (compromised idealist group) or they had buried or lost their ideals and were demotivated (crushed idealists) (See Figure 9.1).

Another story, this time from one of my participants, a newly qualified nurse. Maria one of the crushed idealist group, said after just 14 months in practice:

> I felt that I had really compromised my belief in how (dying) people shouldn't be alone. I am sure I definitely do compromise my ideals like talking to patients rudely, that's one and ideally I would quite like to say *ok rant and rave at me, I can sit here I can take this, I've got half an hour to sit here with you, once you have calmed down we will go through it,* but you just haven't got that time.

She went on to talk about a very busy night shift:

> this woman just started screaming, and screaming at the top of her voice. I still hadn't done my IVs and there was loads to do, I went in there and I just said will you be quiet for five minutes just be quiet . . . I'll shut the door and you can calm down and then I'll come back and as I shut the door, she just really started screaming, really loud, and the sister walked on and started saying what do you think you're doing, and I said ok I know I am wrong, but I am at the end of my tether here.

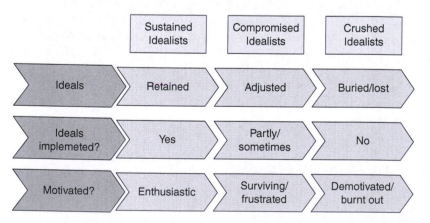

Figure 9.1 Idealism journey

I really felt like I had compromised myself then because I was so rude to this patient, and it was really bad, and I shouldn't have been – that was horrible, I didn't even compromise my ideal, I lost one! I was just so tired, and at the end of my tether. She, like me, received little support and understanding of the demands and complexities of the work.

Nurses were well aware of the fact that their compassion was being eroded and of the impact of this on patients:

> I am slightly less compassionate than I perhaps would be if I was a student, which is not a good thing . . . I feel quite sad that I'm not able to give my all to patient care all the time . . . I still want to. I do feel quite drained when I come in from work, because I am trying to sit down and talk with patients as well as get on with everything else I've got to do. That will probably get less and less as I get more experience . . .
>
> [Anna: interview 1 – admissions ward]

Nurses' ideals were thwarted through structural and organisational con-straints beyond the control of individuals. Key thwarting factors were time pressures, role constraints, staff shortages, work overload and through the organisation of nursing work in which care was task- as opposed to patient-orientated.

Role models were very important and whilst so-called 'negative roles models' could be helpful in showing new nurses what they didn't want to be like, if there were too many of these in practice environments, and not enough good roles models, this could be very detrimental to the newly qual-ified nurses ability to nurse in a way that was consistent with their ideals and values. One new nurse said . . . 'They said that I'd soon settle down and stop being so innovative'.

This doctoral study contributed to the development of a model in terms of what facilitates a positive environment of care (Figure 9.2). It identifies what is needed in practice environments to enable new nurses to retain their ideals and to prevent too much compassion and ideals erosion.

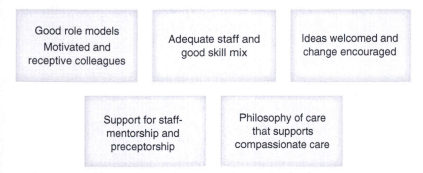

Figure 9.2 Positive environments of care – (i)

Three years after qualification, of the 26 students in the study, two had left nursing for good and two had left for a while at least. These were the so-called crushed idealists who, together with the compromised idealists, were most likely to experience stress and burn-out (see Figure 9.1 above). Even at the first interview (4–6 months after qualifying) Janet said:

> burnout – I can see it happening already (laughs) I think it's just the fact that it's a very stressful environment . . . you can see yourself getting worn out and your energy level depleting and you are dissatisfied . . . when you're tired, I don't think it's that I care any less – sometimes I just haven't got the energy to show it.
>
> [Janet: Interview 1]

The proportion of doctors and other healthcare professionals showing above threshold levels of stress has remained constant at 28 per cent compared to 18 per cent in the general working population (Iverson *et al.* 2009). In a recent European study undertaken at the National Nursing Research Unit, King's College London (RN4cast) UK nurses were second only to recession-hit Greece. Forty-two per cent of English nurses surveyed were assessed as being burned out, while 44 per cent stated that they intended to leave their job in the next year due to dissatisfaction (Aiken *et al.* 2012). The more patients a nurse looks after the higher the emotional exhaustion, job dissatisfaction and patient mortality (Rafferty *et al.* 2007). Emotional exhaustion has increasingly come to be regarded as the core dimension of burn-out (Schaufeli and Bakker 2004; Taris 2006) and refers to the feeling of being overextended and depleted of one's emotional and physical resources (Maslach and Schaufeli 2011). Pines and Aronson (1988) suggest that:

> Burnout strikes precisely those individuals who had once been among the most idealistic and enthusiastic . . . to burnout a person needs to have been on fire at one time.
>
> (Pines and Aronson 1988: 10–11)

Burn-out can cause withdrawal from patients because of the natural human defences we develop in reaction to trauma and this can manifest itself in numbing, a distancing reaction and withdrawal from really connecting with patients (Cornwell and Goodrich 2009).

My doctoral study was undertaken between 1996 and 2000 and in the last decade or so I would argue that the pressures and challenges on nurses have become even greater, with an increasingly ageing population with even greater care needs and health complexity, coupled with the need for cost containment in the English NHS coupled with a reduction in the number of registered nurses (RCN 2012). This is likely to increase pressure on the existing nursing workforce with more patients per registered nurse increasing the likelihood of more stress, burn-out and compromised care delivery.

Doctors, occupational therapists and nurses report staff shortages as being one of their most significant stressors (Leonard and Corr 1998; Rafferty *et al.* 2007; Firth-Cozens 1990). A recent study in Finland found a correlation between overcrowded wards in general hospital (bed occupancy 10 per cent higher than limit for six months) and the use of anti-depressants by doctors and nurses (Virtanen *et al.* 2008); higher patient workload has also been found to predict compassion fatigue in genetic counsellors (Udipi *et al.* 2008). A study of healthcare staff in Sweden (Glasberg *et al.* 2007a) suggested factors such as emotional exhaustion were to do with feelings of troubled conscience, and staff reported 'having to deaden one's conscience', and 'stress of conscience' from lacking the time to provide the care needed, work being so demanding influenced home life, and not being able to live up to others' expectations (Glasberg *et al.* 2007b). NHS staff have been identified as more vulnerable to stress-related behaviours and illnesses than staff in other organisations (Wall *et al.* 1997).

Study 2: employee engagement and retention in the nursing workforce

This second study was a longitudinal study of nurses' experiences in one UK trust undertaken from 2005 to 2007. It had a similar study design to Study 1, but this time the sample was not newly qualified nurses but nurses new to the trust. Participants included some very experienced and many internationally recruited registered nurses from India and the Philippines (Maben 2007). The aim of the study was to examine what keeps nursing staff engaged in an organisation and what influences nursing staff to leave or stay in post? Questionnaires were completed by all new nursing 'starters' over two months (n = 108): of these, 26 nurses were selected to participate in two rounds of in-depth interviews. Staff were asked what makes a good working environment, and adequate staff emerged as an important determinant (see Table 9.1), as in Study 1.

Demotivating factors for nurses differed across the two interviews. At interview 1, the worst experiences described by interviewees tended to focus on issues of support and relationships with colleagues. Issues at interview 2

Table 9.1 What makes a good working environment

Good team, good teamwork; staff help each other, are friendly and offer camaraderie
Good support and feedback
Adequate staff, with good ratios and safe staffing levels
Good staff development and education; feeling stretched, learning, being developed
Good management that is approachable and supportive
Feeling valued and appreciated

focused on the financial savings the hospital was making at the time, and the perceived impact of this on workload and the quality of patient care. In the second round of interviews nurses reported feeling rushed, more stressed and not having sufficient time to give the quality of care they wanted to:

> If you usually, you look after six patients and sometimes we may get ten or 12 . . . So we will not have enough time to give the proper care, to talk with the patient or really, well, to understand the problems.
>
> (ID 059: interview 2)

Overall, participants expressed greater levels of disillusionment and dissatisfaction in the second round of interviews compared to their first interviews. One participant used a powerful metaphor to describe their sense of being overstretched:

> I think a lot of nurses probably lose their focus and lose their faith. I mean, you're on an elastic band: how far can you stretch before it twangs?
>
> (ID 083: interview 2)

These interview results in particular revealed a workforce whose pride in their professionalism was challenged when they saw standards suffer from budgetary pressures, and certainly when they saw patients suffer from their speeded-up workdays. Intrinsic and extrinsic motivators were identified at interview as important to their desire to undertake nursing work, but primarily these focused largely on intrinsic motivators (Table 9.2). These reflected why participants chose to become nurses in the first place and reasons for working at the trust.

Common reoccurring challenges for staff in their practice environments included:

- Lack of time for patients and sense of overwork
- Poor skill mix, the stress of having to support others
- Nurses did not feel 'heard' and the nursing point of view was felt to be dismissed
- Poor leader or manager caused staff to feel unsupported and undervalued, with little feedback and direction.

Table 9.2 Intrinsic motivations

Meaningful work
Feeling valued
Making a difference to patients and their families
Improving practice
Working for a larger good

Staff who feel valued and are satisfied with their responsibilities report lower levels of stress and levels of social support at work can have a protective effect on healthcare professionals mental health (Stansfield *et al.* 2000; Weinberg and Creed 2000; Rada *et al.* 2004). This study provides further data for the positive practice environments model (see Figure 9.3 below).

Study 3: the relationship between patients' experiences of care and the influence of staff motivation, affect and well-being

My most recent research study examined the potential link between staff experiences of work and their psychological well-being and patient experiences of care (Maben *et al.* 2012a). Building on work undertaken outside health care where there is evidence to suggest that happy staff means happy customers this study was one of the first to examine these links in the NHS and to link staff and patients at team and individual levels (Maben *et al.* 2012a). Successful companies outside health – Disney and John Lewis for example – understand well the business case for supporting staff and the John Lewis motto is 'partner's first' – i.e. their staff – knowing that if staff feel well supported, good customer care will follow.

In this study we undertook detailed field work in eight case studies – four in the community (including a rapid response team and adult community nursing) and four in the acute setting (including acute admissions and care of older people). The study involved over 200 hours of direct care observation, over 100 patient interviews and nearly 500 patient surveys, interviews with 55 senior managers, surveys of over 300 staff and 86 staff interviews

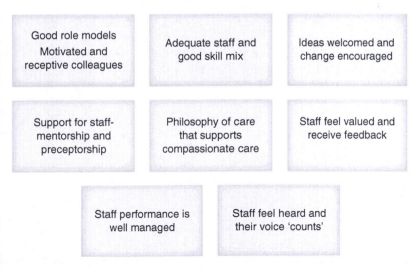

Figure 9.3 Positive environments of care – (ii)

at four different trusts. The majority of our respondents were nurses, with some doctors and allied health professionals. The study found a relationship between staff well-being and patient experience. Staff well-being is an important antecedent of patient care performance and we were able to identify seven staff variables ('wellbeing bundles') which correlated positively with patient-reported experience:

- local/work-group climate
- co-worker support
- job satisfaction
- organisational climate
- perceived organisational support
- low emotional exhaustion, and
- supervisor support.

One of our key finding is that in all settings it was not the wider organisational climate that mattered most to staff (as evidence outside healthcare suggests), but that the local team climate is crucial- what our participants called 'family at work'. Our evidence supports calls for investment in unit level leadership to create well-functioning teams in challenging contexts. We also make the case for staff well-being champions to be embedded in NHS trusts at board level so that staff experience becomes as important as patient experience for the board, because we now have evidence that the two are so closely intertwined – we thus argue that looking after staff is key to creating better experiences for patients. One of the doctors interviewed in this study spoke of the need to be resilient in caring work:

> Everyone will say you need to be good at communicating, you need to be good at basic science, but one of the main things I think you need is resilience, because you work in a job that knocks you down constantly. You've just got to brush yourself off pick yourself up and say, 'That was bad, that was awful, but here we go again.' I think if you take it all home with you, and if you take it all on board, you simply wouldn't be able to come back to work the next day.
>
> (Dr P., Senior House Officer)

In our medicine for older people's setting we observed a work environment where very frail and dependent patients created very high levels of demand on staff who, in turn, felt little control over their day-to-day routines and resources. Leadership and management of staff at ward level was identified as critical for setting expectations of values, attitudes and patient-centred care and for creating a local climate where staff felt valued and appreciated for the difficult work they undertook day in, day out. An unsupportive work environment with bullying and incivility between staff created a difficult place to work and in turn affected patient care delivery. In a paper based on the data from this case study (Maben *et al.* 2012b) we drew on

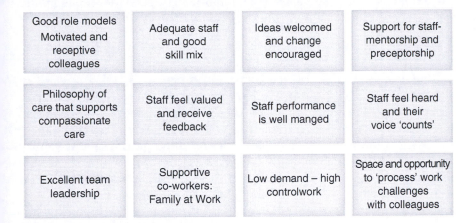

Good role models Motivated and receptive colleagues	Adequate staff and good skill mix	Ideas welcomed and change encouraged	Support for staff-mentorship and preceptorship
Philosophy of care that supports compassionate care	Staff feel valued and receive feedback	Staff performance is well manged	Staff feel heard and their voice 'counts'
Excellent team leadership	Supportive co-workers: Family at Work	Low demand – high controlwork	Space and opportunity to 'process' work challenges with colleagues

Figure 9.4 Positive environments of care – (iii)

the unpopular patient literature to highlight how in poor ward and patient care climates staff seek job satisfaction through caring for the 'poppets', the patients staff found most endearing, leaving less favoured – and often more complex patients – to receive less personalized care. These patients felt like 'Parcels'. Thus we found that in poor work environments staff try hard to make work satisfying by selectively giving compassionate care to the rewarding poppets. This study has provided further data to develop the positive environments model (Figure 9.4).

Thus the practice environment is crucial in supporting nurses to deliver the high quality compassionate care. Returning to the issues raised at the beginning of this chapter, we know that it 'takes courage, humility and compassion to really relate to patients. We also know this requires investment and constant renewal by practitioners with recognition, re-enforcement and support from colleagues and managers' (Maben *et al.* 2010). Promoting meaningful connections with patients in which practitioners see each patient 'as a person to be *engaged with* rather than a body to *do things to*' (Nicholson *et al.* 2010) takes resilience and courage, and staff need support and renewal.

There are a number of initiatives that provide support for staff and opportunities for reflection on practice and renewal. For example, restorative supervision (Wallbank and Woods 2012), a pilot in the NHS of 'Samaritans' type buddying scheme to support staff (Sawbridge and Hewison 2011) and methods of providing reflective space such as After Action Reviews (Walker *et al.* 2012), Balint Groups in Primary care (Balint *et al.* 1993), resilience training/workshops (Antonovsky 1987) and Action learning sets (Pedler 1997) as well as Schwartz Center Rounds (Lown and Manning 2010; Goodrich 2011; 2012). Drawing on the theoretical literature, reflective spaces may be expected to produce benefit through the mechanisms of self-disclosure and a potential rise in self-compassion, an important aspect of developing positive affect and compassion for others (Gilbert 2010; Derlega *et al.* 1993).

Conclusions

So what does all this research tell us? What light does it shed on the issues at Stafford hospital? I suggest the work environment at Staffordshire hospital was the living embodiment of a poor work environment with crushed ideals and covert rules; with poor role models, poor mentorship and preceptorship, and a philosophy of care that did not support compassionate care. We know in many wards staff did not feel valued, were not performance-managed well and did not get good feedback; the staff voice was not able to be heard and there was poor team leadership with a bullying culture where staff did not feel well supported by colleagues in some work settings. With a high demand and low control work environment there was little opportunity to process the difficult emotionally demanding work staff were undertaking and we know that staffing and skill mix were inadequate. It was system wide failure that left nurses unable to do the job they came into nursing to do:

> I have never met a nurse who comes to work to do a bad job. The nurses were so under-resourced . . . to give adequate care to patients. If you are in that environment for long enough, what happens is you become immune to the sound of pain . . . or you walk away. You cannot feel people's pain, you cannot continue to want to do the best you possibly can when the system says no to you, you can't do the best you can.
> (Dr in A and E, Mid staffs Inquiry 1 2010)

Austin Thomas, lead nurse for Paralympics GB, suggested nurses are suffering from care fatigue and their morale has been eroded:

> If you send a soldier into battle without what they need they'll get battle fatigue – well we as the nursing profession have got care fatigue . . . not enough of us, not enough kit . . . 80 per cent of nurses are so overwhelmed they haven't got enough left in them to smile.
> (Austin Thomas, RCN Congress 2013)

Creating a good work environment, really supporting, listening to and acting upon staff experiences is key to compassionate care for patients. It also is morally the right thing to do for a staff group who are asked to go the extra mile at work every day. So if we want to support healthcare staff better so that they are not overwhelmed and do not become indifferent we need to fix the job:

> If the job is making doctors sick, why not fix the job rather than the doctors?
> (Chambers and Maxwell 1996)

Summary box

Students enter the profession to give good care – yet ideals, compassion and empathy erode and can become crushed in poor practice environments.

Lack of staff, no role models, little support and preceptorship contribute to this erosion.

Covert rules socialise new nurses into the culture of the ward.

Nursing staff are intrinsically motivated and an inability to provide good care saps motivation – indeed, when they cannot give good care moral distress ensues.

Nurses need to feel valued, listened to and get timely and accurate feedback to feel engaged.

There is a link between staff experiences of work and patient experiences of care.

Staff well-being is an important antecedent of patient care performance.

Important for good practice environment is supportive leadership and local team climate – 'family at work'.

Care Experiences: the importance of kindness

Andrew (UK)

In June 2003 I went to my local G.P. with what I thought was just an ulcer in my mouth – he immediately made an appointment for me at the Facial Clinic in our local hospital.

I met the consultant on the following Monday, who did a biopsy and a week later he diagnosed Carcinoma of the floor of my mouth – there and then he made a bed available for the following Monday and Tuesday. The next day I underwent a 15-hour operation to remove the tumor and replace under the tongue with a graft of skin and bone taken from my left forearm.

After 14 days I was discharged! Treatment by my consultant, doctors, nurses and everybody concerned was exemplary. About a month later I was given 5 weeks of daily radio therapy – again superb effective and very professional treatment.

Since then I have had restorative dentistry and after 10 years still have a six-monthly appointment with my consultant to check that all is well – and thanks to the wonderful treatment by all concerned, all is well! Beyond technical expertise, what made this experience so positive for me was the general kindness, care, politeness, consistency, reassurance and trust.

Care Experiences: compassionate care and the patient and carer views

Jean (UK)

These are my mother's comments about her stays in hospital recently and four years ago for a lower leg amputation. At that time, she did have good care overall, and the surgery was faultless but in the post-operative period she had a nasty experience with a young surgical houseman who ripped off her dressing, causing her much pain and agony during a ward round. This episode was followed up with the hospital but no one was willing either to believe this had happened or take responsibility for the incident. The team leader of the surgical team told me that my mother has 'probably imagined it, as she was on a medicine that had CNS effects'. As my mother is neither over-imaginative nor demented, this was adding insult to the injury. There was no resolution then or since. At the hospital where she was transferred, there was a lack of care due to staff shortages and use of agency nurses who kept to a defined protocol and so people were left without water, without turning to relieve pressure sores, and made to feel objects rather than patients. As the following shows, both hospitals have made great progress in patient management and are applying the best traditions of nursing care and compassionate management on the wards.

This is my mother's statement:

My name is Marjorie Moran (known in hospital as my first name, Bessie). I have been in hospital twice, four years ago to have my lower right leg amputated and this year just recently, to have to have my big toe amputated due to an ulcer which had formed on the side of my foot (all due to a lack of circulation). I can only say from my own experiences that I could not have had better care and attention and particularly the second operation. This from the wonderful surgeons, nurses and staff at A and St. P the physio girls and chaps at R Hospital. Wonderful care all round. The hospitals were wonderfully clean, the food was great and such varied menus! This is, as I say from my own experience and my family will join me in this, especially my younger son who is also my carer and my best friend.

Notes from my brother Brendan who cares for my mother when she is home, and is her main contact and escort when she has to go to hospital for treatment. Brendan has spent a LOT of time on hospital wards as a result, and this is his response on the issues of ward management, patient contacts and caring:

From my perspective all contact with both hospitals (St P and A Hospital) has been friendly and helpful. What I saw of my Mum's care was impressive and noticeably improved since she was in the first time at St P. Mum says she particularly noted the understanding, calm and caring that the nurses and staff showed anyone that was hard of hearing or distressed.

I witnessed myself the lady with dementia being treated with respect and care when I visited Mum. She would call out and a nurse would arrive within seconds and if it was just a random shout for no reason, she wasn't berated or dismissed. There was an understanding/caring voice making sure she was OK.

There is a particularly wonderful Nurse 'Annie' at St P on H Ward who took so much trouble even to call me on Mum's behalf to remind me to bring something over or that she had been moved to another ward, etc. When Mum had a particularly bad night her bubbly reassuring personality alone was a tonic that made Mum feel better. I don't think that the effect of this can be underestimated when it comes to a patient's recovery.

I have noticed a change since Mum was in the first time. Within a week I wasn't as worried about leaving Mum at hospital after witnessing the quality all round. The culture seems to have changed big time at St P, for the better.

Care Experiences: Jenny's story

(interview between Sue and Jenny (UK))

In the text that follows, we hear of Jenny's experience which captures an inspirational example of kindness and compassionate care:

Following a routine mammogram, Jenny was diagnosed with breast cancer. Although the cancer was small, it was of a very aggressive form. There were surrounding cells that were also identified as cancerous and these were removed immediately. After the cancerous cells were removed, Jenny underwent a series of chemotherapy and radiotherapy. Chemotherapy can of course be a very unpleasant experience, but this was alleviated by the kindness of the healthcare team by which Jenny was treated:

'The girls are lovely, they ask you what you want to be called . . . I've seen that they've written 'Jenny' on my notes . . . very, very caring people – some are still learning but there is always a sister who sits with them . . . cleanliness – the ward is spotless, they are always putting plastic aprons on, cleaning their hands, and so on. Very very nice people.'

'They make you feel at ease – during the whole procedure I always felt that they had my best interests at heart. They don't talk down to you . . . even the surgeon.'

(continued)

(continued)

Jenny also told the editors that the ward where she had been treated dealt with all different types of cancer. Recently, during a chance encounter with the oncologist who had been treating Jenny; the oncologist had remembered her name and her personal condition, and had greeted her with warmth and humanity – even personally arranging another appointment for her.

The editors asked Jenny whether this kindness was applicable to the entire health care team and she told the editors:

'They were all so lovely . . . the radiotherapy team – there was a bond . . . they tell you things, they open up, and this makes you open up too. Even the chap with the tea trolley would say "Would you like a cup of tea or some soup?" with such kindness . . . everyone was on Christian name terms . . . they were very nice people.'

'They are never aggressive, they come and check on you . . . they cross check the notes on drugs . . . the cancer people are second to none – very very caring people – they put you at ease because they are so caring.'

Jenny's story is heart-warming and uplifting, demonstrating how kindness can have a positive effect on even the most traumatic conditions and procedures. Hearing such stories is an inspiration to us all.

Note

1   This chapter is based upon an inaugural lecture delivered orally 1 May 2013 at King's College London by Professor Jill Maben RN; BA (Hons) MSc; PhD. Director, National Nursing Research Unit, Florence Nightingale School of Nursing and Midwifery, King's College London and Trustee Point of Care Foundation. Project 3 was funded by the National Institute for Health Research Service Delivery and Organisation programme (project number SDO/213/2008).The views and opinions expressed therein are those of the authors and do not necessarily reflect those of the NIHR SDO programme or the Department of Health.

References

Aiken, L.H., Sermeus, W., Van den Heede, K., Sloane, D.M., Busse, R., McKee, M., *et al.* (2012) Patient safety, satisfaction, and quality of hospital care: Cross sectional surveys of nurses and patients in 12 countries in Europe and the United States *BMJ* 344, e1717.

Antonovsky, A. (1987) *Unravelling the Mystery of Health: How People Manage Stress and Stay Well.* San Francisco, CA: Jossey-Bass.

Balint, E., Courtenay, M., Elder, A., Hull, S., Paul, J. (1993) *The Doctor, the Patient and the Group: Balint Revisited.* London: Routledge.

Becker, H.S., Geer, B. (1958) The fate of idealism in medical school *Journal of Health and Social Behavior* 23(1), 50–56.

Boore, J. (1978) *Prescription for Recovery.* London: Royal College of Nursing.

Boorman, S. (2009) *NHS Health and Well-Being Review: Interim Report and Final Report.* London: Department of Health.

Care Quality Commission: CQC (2011) *Review of Compliance: Winterbourne View.*

Chambers, R., Maxwell, R. (1996) Helping sick doctors *BMJ* 312(7033), 722–723.

Commission on Dignity in Care (Age UK, NHS Confederation and Local Government Group) (2012) *Delivering Dignity: Securing Dignity in Care for Older People in Hospitals and Care Homes. A Report for Consultation.*

Cornwell, J., Goodrich, J. (2009) Exploring how to enable compassionate care in hospital to improve patient experience *Nursing Times* 105, 15.

Cox, T., Griffiths, A. (1995) The nature and measurement of work stress: Theory and practice. In: Wilson, J.R., Corlett, E.N. (eds), *Evaluation of Human Work: A Practical Ergonomics Methodology.* London: Taylor & Francis.

Derlega, V.J., Metts, S., Petronio, S., Margulis, S.T. (1993) *Self-Disclosure.* Thousand Oaks, CA: Sage Publications.

Firth-Cozens, J. (1990) Sources of stress in women junior house officers *BMJ* 301, 89–91.

Francis, R. QC (January 2005 – March 2009) *Independent Inquiry into Care Provided by Mid Staffordshire NHS Foundation Trust.* London: The Stationery Office (Vols 1 and 2).

Francis, R. QC (2013) *Report of the Mid Staffordshire NHS Foundation Trust Public Inquiry.* House of Commons: Stationery Office (Vols 1–3).

Gilbert, P. (2010) *The Compassionate Mind.* London: Constable.

Glasberg, A.L., Eriksson, S., Norberg, A. (2007a) Burnout and 'stress of conscience' among healthcare personnel *Journal of Advanced Nursing* 57(4), 392–403.

Glasberg, A.L., Norberg, A., Soderberg, A. (2007b) Sources of burn-out among healthcare employees as percieved by managers *Journal of Advanced Nursing* 60(11), 10–19.

Goodrich, J. (2011) *Schwartz Centre Rounds®: Evaluation of the UK Pilots.* London: The King's Fund.

Goodrich, J. (2012) Supporting hospital staff to provide compassionate care: Do Schwartz Center rounds work in English hospitals? *Journal of the Royal Society of Medicine* 105, 117–122.

Goodrich, J., Cornwell, J. (2008) *Seeing the Person in the Patient: The Point of Care Review Paper.* London: The King's Fund.

Hayward, J. (1975) *Information – A Prescription against Pain.* London: Royal College of Nursing Contract No. 5.

Health Service Ombudsman (2011) *Care and Compassion? Report of the Health Service Ombudsman on Ten Investigations into NHS Care of Older People.* London: Department of Health.

Hojat, M., Vergare, M.J, Maxwell, K., Brainard, G., Herrine, S.K., Isenberg, G.A., *et al.* (2009) The Devil is in the Third Year: A Longitudinal Study of Erosion of Empathy in Medical School. *Academic Medicine* 84(9), 1182–1191.

Iles, V. (2011) Why reforming the NHS doesn't work. The importance of understanding how good people offer bad care. Available at: www.reallylearning.com (accessed 30 September 2013).

Iversen, A. Rushforth, B. Forrest, K. (2009) How to handle stress and look after your mental health *BMJ* 338, b1368.

Karasek, R.A. (1979) Job demands, job decision latitude, and mental strain: Implications for job redesign *Administrative Science Quarterly* 24(2), 285–308.

Leonard, C., Corr, S. (1998) Sources of stress and coping strategies in basic grade occupational therapists *British Journal of Occupational Therapy* 61(6), 257–262.

Lowenstein, J. (2008) *The Midnight Meal and Other Essays about Doctors, Patients, and Medicine.* New Haven, CT: Yale University Press.

Lown, B.A., Manning, M.A. (2010) The Schwartz Center Rounds®: Evaluation of an interdisciplinary approach to enhancing patient-centered communication, teamwork, and provider support *Academic Medicine* 85, 1073–1081.

Maben, J. (2008) A critical analysis of employee engagement, turnover and retention in the nursing workforce: A case study of an inner London acute trust. Funded by a post-doctoral fellowship by the Health Foundation. Available at: www.kcl.ac.uk/nursing/research/nnru/publications/Reports/NursingRetention finalreport-2008.pdf.

Maben, J., Latter, S., Macleod C. (2007) The challenges of maintaining ideals and standards in professional practice: Evidence from a longitudinal qualitative study *Nursing Inquiry* 14(2), 99–113.

Maben, J., Cornwell, J., Sweeney, K. (2010) In praise of compassion in nursing *Journal of Research in Nursing* 15(1), 9–13.

Maben, J., Peccei, R., Adams, M., Robert, G., Richardson, A., Murrells, T., Morrow E. (2012a) *Patients' experiences of care and the influence of staff motivation, affect and well-being.* Final report NIHR Service Delivery and Organisation programme. Available at: www.netscc.ac.uk/hsdr/projdetails.php?ref=08-1819-1213).

Maben, J., Adams, M., Robert, G., Peccei, R., Murrells, T. (2012b) Poppets and parcels: The links between staff experience of work and acutely ill older peoples' experience of hospital care *International Journal of Older People Nursing: Special Issue: Acute Care* 7(2), 83–94.

Mackintosh, C. (2007) Protecting the self: A descriptive qualitative exploration of how registered nurses cope with working in surgical areas *International Journal of Nursing Studies* 44(6), 982–990.

McManus, I., Winder, B., Gordon, D. (2002) The causal links between stress and burnout in a longitudinal study of UK doctors *The Lancet* 359, 2089–2090.

Maslach, C., Jackson, S.E. (1982) Burnout in health professionals: A social psychological analysis. In: Sanders, G.S., Suls, J. (eds), *Social Psychology of Health and Illness.* Hillsdale, NJ: Lawrence Erlbaum Associates.

Maslach, C., Schaufeli, W.B., Leiter, M.P. (2001) Job burnout *Annual Review of Psychology* 57, 397–422.

Melia, K. (1987) *Learning and Working: The Occupational Socialization of Nurses* London: Tavistock.

Mimura, C. Griffiths P. (2003) The effectiveness of current approaches to workplace stress management in the nursing profession: An evidence based literature review *Occupational and Environmental Medicine* 60(1), 10–15.

Nicholson, C., Flatley, M., Wilkinson, C., Meyer, J., Dale, P., Wessel, L. (2010) Everybody matters 2: Promoting dignity in acute care through effective communication *Nursing Times* 106(21), 12–14.

Payne, R., Firth-Cozens J. (1987) *Stress in Health Professionals.* Chichester: John Wiley & Sons.

Pedler, M. (1997) *Action Learning in Practice.* Aldershot: Gower.

Pines, A., Aronson E. (1988) *Career Burnout: Causes and Cures.* New York: Free Press.

Rada, R., Johnson, C. (2004) Stress, burnout, anxiety and depression among dentists *Journal of American Dental Association* 135(6), 788–794.

Rafferty, A.M., Clarke, S., Coles, J., Ball, J., James, P., McKee, M., Aiken, L.H. (2007) Outcomes of variation in hospital nurse staffing in English hospitals: Cross-sectional analysis of survey data and discharge records *International Journal of Nursing Studies* 44(2), 175–182.

Raleigh, V., Hussey, D., Seccombe, I. (2009) Do associations between staff and inpatient feedback have the potential for improving patient experience? An analysis of surveys in NHS acute trusts in England *Quality and Safety in Health Care* 18, 347–354.

Stansfield, S., Head, J., Marmot, M. (2000) *Work Related Factors and Ill Health. The Whitehall II Study.* Suffolk: HSE.

RCN (2012) Frontline First: Analysis of NHS Information Centre Data. London: RCN.

Sawbridge, Y., Hewison A. (2011) *Time to Care? Responding to Concerns about Poor Nursing Care.* Birmingham: Health Services Management Centre, University of Birmingham.

Schaufeli, W., Maslach, C., Marek T. (1993) *Professional Burnout: Recent Developments in Theory and Research.* Washington, DC: Taylor & Francis.

Schaufeli, W.B., Bakker, A.B. (2004) Job demands, job resources, and their relationship with burnout and engagement: A multi-sample study *Journal of Organizational Behavior* 25, 293–315.

Shuldham, C. (1999) A review of the pre-operative education on recovery from surgery *International Journal of Nursing Studies* 36, 121–177.

Suchman, A. (1993) *Partnerships in Healthcare Transforming Relational Processes.* Rochester, NY: University of Rochester Press.

Taris, T.W. (2006) Is there a relationship between burnout and objective performance? A critical review of 16 studies *Work and Stress* 20, 316–334.

Taylor, C., Graham, J., Potts, H., Candy, J., Richards, M., Ramirez, A. (2005) Changes in mental health of UK hospital consultants since the mid-1990s *The Lancet* 366, 742–744.

Taylor, C., Graham, J., Potts, H., Candy, J., Richards, M., Ramirez, A. (2007) Impact of hospital consultants' poor mental health on patient care *British Journal of Psychiatry* 190, 268–269.

Thomas, A. (2013) Against the odds. Royal College of Nursing Congress and Exhibition 21–25 April 2013. Liverpool. Available at: www.rcn.org.uk/newsevents/congress/2013/tuesday/austin_thomas_-_against_the_odds (accessed 30 September 2013).

Udipi, S., Veach, P.M., Kao, J., LeRoy, B. (2008) The psychic costs of empathic engagement: Personal and demographic predictors of genetic counsellor compassion fatigue *Journal of Genetic Counseling* 17, 459–471.

Virtanen, M., Pentti, J., Vahtera, J., Ferrie, J., Stansfeld, S., Helenius, *et al.* (2008) Overcrowding in hospital wards as a predictor of antidepressant treatment among hospital staff *American Journal of Psychiatry* 165, 1482–1486.

Walker, J., Andrews, S., Grewcock, D., Halligan, A. (2012) Life in the slow lane: Making hospitals safer slowly but surely *Journal of the Royal Society of Medicine* 105, 283–287.

Wall, T.D., Bolton, R.I., Borrill, C.S., Carter, A.J., Golya, D.A., Hardy, *et al.* (1997) Minor psychiatric disorders in NHS Trust employees: Occupational and gender differences *British Journal of Psychiatry* 171, 519–523.

Wallbank, S., Woods, G. (2012) A healthier health visiting workforce: Findings from the restorative supervision programme *Community Practitioner* 85(11), 20–23.

Weinberg, A., Creed, F. (2000) Stress and psychiatric disorder in healthcare professionals and hospital staff *The Lancet* 355(9203), 533–537.

West, M. (2004) *Effective Teamwork: Practical Lessons from Organisational Research* Oxford: Blackwell.

West, M. (2013) Quality and Safety in the NHS. Available at: http://www.lums.lancs.ac.uk/files/quality-safety-nhs-f.pdf.

10 Compassionate Clowning: improving the quality of life of people with dementia

A playful compassionate approach from the Hearts & Minds 'Elderflowers'

Magdalena Schamberger

Introduction

This chapter will explore Hearts & Minds' use of Compassionate Clowning specifically in relation to our Elderflowers performing arts programme for people with dementia. However, before focusing on the subject of Compassionate Clowning and playful compassion, an exploration on why compassion in dementia care is of the utmost importance, appears necessary.

The Royal College of Psychiatrists states, that 'Dementia often starts off with just memory problems' (Royal College of Psychiatrists 2013). However the condition, which affects a large part of the brain, can lead to a wide range of challenges, which will get increasingly worse over time. These may include: 'difficulty managing day-to-day tasks; difficulty communicating; changes in mood, judgement or personality . . . people with dementia become increasingly dependent on others to help them as the illness progresses'. It seems that, it is this increasing dependency of people who previously have been in control of their lives, as well as their bodily functions, combined with the element of confusion, which can increase challenging behaviour, frustration and depression. The most successful remedies, in my experience, are empathy and compassion shown towards the individual and their situation. Not pushing the individual towards being the person they no longer are, but kindly supporting them in who they have become at that particular moment in time.

Alzheimer Scotland states that 'Dementia can affect every area of human thinking, feeling and behaviour, but each person with dementia is different – how the illness affects someone depends on which area of their brain is damaged'.

Imagine feeling vulnerable, confused and upset, and imagine the possible needs associated with these feelings. Using a playful compassionate approach, enables a carer to engage with the personality behind the dementia and focus on the person's feelings and human needs.

The NHS dementia guide explains, that:

> when a person with dementia finds that their mental abilities are declining, they're likely to feel anxious, stressed and scared. They may be aware of their increasing clumsiness and inability to remember things, and this can be very frustrating and upsetting for them.

In addition the guide suggests that to sensitively offer support and to avoid being critical is central in supporting people with dementia. It explicitly mentions the importance of being understanding as well as retaining a sense of humour. This is where the importance of playful compassion and the Hearts & Minds approach come into play.

Hearts & Minds is an arts-in-health organisation based in Edinburgh, Scotland. Our mission is to support the improvement of the health care environment by using the performing arts with playful compassion to build meaningful and lasting relationships with children, young people, elderly people with dementia and their families as well as health care staff in a variety of care settings.

Our unique Clowndoctors and Elderflowers programmes use clowning, humour and playful compassion to provide sensitive, safe and individually tailored quality interactions for our participants, delivered by professionally trained and experienced arts-in-health practitioners. Hearts & Minds practitioners use their creative skills to engage with the individual person to encourage and enable communication. Within the Elderflowers programme, it is specifically the notion of the Elderflowers family unit that appears to improve levels of interaction and enhances the relationships between participants, practitioners, fellow residents and family members as well as care staff.

Trust and respect are the basis of our programmes. Creating authentic connections, engagement and communication with the individual are at the heart of our interactions. Hope, laughter and increased resilience are often the most noticeable byproducts. Our philosophy is always to look beyond the illness or special needs of the person and instead look at their individual psychological and emotional needs, thereby helping to overcome challenges such as stress, pain, frustration, loss of control and grief. We know from feedback that our work supports the promotion of dignity and respect, as our skills and activities help to connect with the whole person: the person beyond the symptoms of their illness.

The Hearts & Minds Elderflowers programme specifically uses the performing arts to engage with people in the mid to advanced stages of dementia in a health care environment, aiming to positively contribute to their quality of life. This chapter on Compassionate Clowning will explore how playful compassion can be implemented within assessment and long-term care by means of the Elderflowers family approach and the unexpected use of European style theatre clowning in this environment. It aims to highlight the positive impact this can have on residents, staff and relatives. The chapter also attempts to generalise some of its learning in regards to its concept and communication techniques, which may be considered useful for medical and nursing students, practicing health care professionals as well as artists working in a health care environment.

Background

Following the success of the Hearts & Minds Clowndoctors programme for children in hospital and hospice care (established in 1999), we recognised quite quickly that we had found an approach which seemed especially effective in communicating and engaging with particularly vulnerable children, terminally ill children and children with special communication needs. By using artistic engagement and highly visual and often non-verbal communication approaches/methods we were able to create choices and possibilities, which appeared to engage many children who otherwise were considered beyond reach.

We were very keen on building on this concept and experiences and were looking to extend our activities to reach a different age range in 2001 and develop a programme for elderly people.

With the encouragement of the Dementia Services Development Centre at the University of Stirling we started to look at how Hearts & Minds could specialise in the creation and delivery of 'engaging' activities tailored for people with dementia.

As Artistic Director I was put in charge of this development. The lack of personal experience in this area created a feeling of apprehension and curiosity toward the subject, prior to my initial research visits in two dementia units in the Scottish Borders. However, during the visits valuable insights on both a personal and artistic level were gained:

> **First**, I understood instantly that to be able to establish connections and communication with the residents I needed to be relaxed and interested; to have no agenda; to offer a friendly and approachable face, soft and welcoming eyes and to have a presence without any apprehension, judgement or fear. I also needed lots of time.

> **Second**, I noticed that residents seemed to find it difficult to remember their own names as well as those of other resident's and staff and therefore frequently called each other 'hen', 'darling' or 'dear'. An immediate artistic decision was taken to use similar memorable endearments such as Blossom, Bonnie, Buddy, Handsome, Honeybunch, Petal, Pickle, Sweetie-Pie, Toots, etc. for all the Elderflowers characters. The unexpected use of pet names and diminutives now often forms the basis of a first interaction with the Elderflowers.

> **Third**, I was struck by the residents' need and determination to try and communicate. The less others appeared to understand the content of their conversation, the stronger the determination seemed to grow. Even the slightest sign or acknowledgement of understanding or

agreement seemed to be greeted by an immediate feeling of 'lighting up', relaxation and well-being. A connection was made and appreciated.

Finally, I left with the feeling that most residents were looking for something: looking to go home, looking for familiarity, their family, their names, their dogs, their belongings or even for something they no longer knew they were looking for. However, I was also touched by the immediate celebration and feeling of success they showed when finding 'something' and sharing this with me, creating a little community of two.

We therefore tailored our Elderflowers Programme in response to all of these insights. Our aim was to create a programme, which would respond to the needs, challenges and abilities of this particular client group.

Why it works

The following principles underpin the Hearts & Minds Elderflower programme.

Our ethos is the respect for people, their lives, their history, their challenges and their personal circumstances. The basis of our work is our belief that in spite of the diagnosis of dementia and the deterioration of cognitive function, the personality of an individual remains and can be reached. Therefore the Elderflowers' approach focuses on the abilities and communication preferences of the individuals and always aims to connect with the 'essence' of the person beyond the illness.

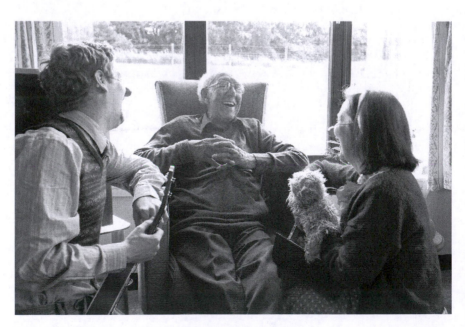

Figure 10.1 Photograph of Elderflowers interaction (1)

A starting point and guiding light for each interaction is the genuine 'sharing of a moment': the Elderflowers are always in the present, not concerned about the past or the future. The Elderflowers interaction does not reflect anything about the participants' illness and the present moment is where they meet and have the opportunity to enjoy themselves.

The Elderflowers believe that people with dementia are still experts in their own lives, and always consider their life experiences. Even though they may no longer be intellectually aware of their former professions, likes and dislikes, their physical expression and rhythm is still often a manifestation of their lives and habits. For example: a gentlemen we have worked with regularly uses a repetitive gesture in a rhythm, which appears abstract and does not apparently make sense to us for his current living circumstances. However, when we found out that during his lifetime he had been a keen cyclist we realised that his gesture was connected to checking his bicycle tyres.

People with dementia are still trying to communicate but often no longer have words available that make sense to us as listeners. The Elderflowers practitioners are able to suspend their need to comprehend the logic of a conversation, but instead connect with the person and their abilities, for example by using their names, their verbal or physical rhythm or personal history.

The importance of giving and receiving: rather than performing 'at' or 'for' the participants, the Elderflowers encourage participation and interaction, enabling participants to give as well as receive. Often, due to circumstances of care, people with dementia are frequently in the position of having to accept/receive what is presented to them, such as medication, food, clothing, personal care. Feeling themselves in a position to 'give' something valuable to someone else: aide, advice, sympathy, information, is an extremely important part of the Elderflowers engagement.

Elderflowers encounters often start with a relevant theme, a problem that needs to be solved, a choice to be made. Every suggestion will be accepted and playfully developed. For example the Elderflowers may seek advice on how to behave at a special event (such as a wedding), give a choice of what props to use or which hats to wear; help with a decision on which colour to paint the walls. Input will be sought according to the abilities of the participants and can be given verbally or non-verbally.

A charge nurse at Clackmannan Community Hospital shared the following observation with us about an Elderflowers interaction:

> they create scenarios, for example at one session they appeared as brother and sister, when talking to a patient they told him they were having a disagreement about what they wanted for lunch and as they did not know the area they asked if he knew of anywhere. The patient then became engaged in a conversation about different eating places in the area. This was giving this gentleman the opportunity to share his knowledge and give his opinion. These sessions give patients the opportunity to escape from the hospital environment and routine, and offer a way for them to express themselves, therefore feeling valued.

Even small interactions that transform a situation from one of being 'cared for' to one of being able to 'give to' are extremely valuable in restoring a sense of purpose, dignity and humanity to people with dementia.

The nurse continues:

> Resources for Occupational Therapists and Nursing staff time are limited. Staff do not always have time for activities in the ward due to a busy schedule or heavy workload. The Elderflower Project contributes greatly to maintaining a person-centred approach within this health care setting.

The Elderflowers offer a 'menu' of different performing arts activities and different art forms as tools. Clowning forms the basis of their approach; however, in addition they use a menu of live music, singing, dancing, poetry, storytelling, improvisation, puppetry and multi-sensory tools, etc. to tailor activities to the needs, tastes and preferences of the individual participants.

Case study

Over the last 18 months the Elderflowers have been working regularly with Mary (name changed) who has Alzheimer's disease. The deterioration in her condition has been less marked than that of other members in her group and the challenge has been for the Elderflowers to find ways to keep developing activities with her, to boost her self-confidence and to encourage her to stay connected to the group.

Throughout her life, Mary has had an interest in the arts, particularly in the area of music. She has a good sense of rhythm and is always tuneful when playing a harmonica or, more recently, a small electric piano, which she plays using the black keys only. She can also pick up a rhythm with the group with clapping, and sometimes conduct a little. It is at these times that she is in most contact with her group.

Mary also enjoys colours and beautiful objects. But it is her rhythmic sensibility in particular that the Elderflowers plan to keep nurturing. As her condition changes this is likely to be the way in which the practitioners can keep her focused. She responds well to one-to-one visits, and the Elderflowers plan to see how she might respond to more challenging requests, for example if she 'conducts', the Elderflowers will dance.

Hearts & Minds practitioners follow a referral system. They plan their activities and tailor them according to the location, needs and abilities of the individual participants. We have individuals with dementia referred to us by health care staff. In addition we gather as much information as possible about the participants' life history from carers as well as observations during our interactions. The aim is to connect, engage, relax and create a sense of well-being in the participants. Smiles and laughter are often a byproduct although they are not the immediate focus. The practitioners know that they may be seeing participants for many years to come. At the end of each programme day the practitioners write a report back and in some of the units they are asked to contribute to the medical notes of the participants.

In addition to the participant's life history and personal information we receive from staff or relatives, the Elderflowers take great pride and care to research further into the 'time', culture and social history of the towns, places and regions we visit. This also includes looking at local jobs and industry as well as music and poetry and traditions. Often this knowledge becomes the starting point for interactions between practitioners and participants and often contributes to opening up further channels of communication, giving an opportunity for others to join in as part of a joint social and cultural network.

The participants themselves are always our starting point. The Elderflowers begin their encounters without any preconceptions. Practitioners are prepared to respond to the participants' age, rhythm and notion of time. The creative exchange is signified by simplicity and clarity to avoid further confusion. Pauses are an invitation to respond. Although the presence of the Elderflowers family has a purpose, the interactions are relaxed and without any pressure. The only goal is the attempt to create a meaningful connection and possibly invite a response, whatever

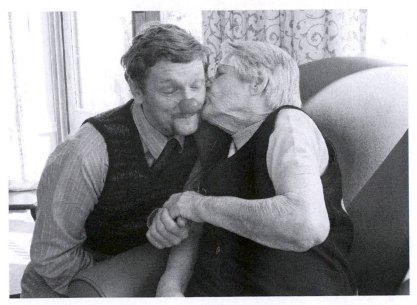

Figure 10.2 Photograph of Elderflower interaction (2)

this response may look like. Within the arts, there is no right or wrong. Everything goes.

Visual stimulation: the Elderflowers are dressed up for a special occasion and their costumes hark back to an era that participants may remember. Rather than focusing on verbal engagement the Elderflowers use a range of visual stimuli: from the red nose, the costumes, hats, juggling scarves, colourful musical instruments, suitcases full of props (ranging from abstract props, to gloves, fans, old telephones, old watches bicycle parts in need of repair, post cards, perfumes, etc.) as well as an Elderflowers family album and photographs.

Why clowning?

When we first proposed the use of 'clowning' to engage with people with advanced dementia in assessment and long-term care, we were met with a few sceptical opinions and raised eyebrows – to say the least. We were lucky enough to find some open minds, who gave us permission to run pilot programmes on their wards. Over time we seem to have proven our value and although sometimes staff or relatives may find that we are not to their taste, most will be able to look beyond their own preconceptions and focus on the needs of their patients and family members.

> Elderflowers is bringing out a response from clients who normally have no or little response. Clients are starting to recognize practitioners and are showing stimulation of short-term memory.
>
> Nurse, Findlay House, Edinburgh

Over time I have noticed and marked the following unexpected connections and similarities between Compassionate Clowns and people with dementia.

The Elderflowers use European style theatre clowning to engage with participants, instead of colourful wigs, big shoes or theatrical make up, they simply use the red nose as their trademark and point of recognition for participants.

The red nose is our calling card, our identity, our focus, our surprise, our signifier, our transformer, our sign of recognition; a sign of our playfulness, openness and vulnerability. It aids the performer to transform into their other self/alter egos – the Elderflowers.

For the performers, the red nose is widely considered the smallest mask in the world. It connects them with their own vulnerability, openness and playfulness. For the residents it is first, a visual focus and signifier, clearly drawing attention to the eyes and therefore establishing immediate connection.

It is this shared vulnerability and positive outlook on life that people with dementia recognise and are drawn to. Within their daily routine people with dementia are often – due to necessity – surrounded by staff members in control, needing to give medication, perform personal care duties, etc. People with dementia are no longer in the 'know' – that is what they have in common with clowns: they share their vulnerabilities, insecurities and humanity of making mistakes without the ability of being able to hide them. Clowns never learn from their mistakes and, try as they might, they fail over and over again – a reality for many people with dementia. However the positivity of celebrating mistakes and never giving up creates a positive experience and aids their well-being.

In addition, red is often seen as a colour which can be differentiated by the ageing eye for a very long time. Furthermore, the reflection of the plastic nose seems to attract particular interest and attention from people with dementia. The shape of the clown nose is round. It softens the outline of the face and draws you to the eyes, immediately evoking a non-confrontational, non-judgemental and ultimately friendly character. The red nose is a visual signifier, invites engagement and assists memory of engagement. A lady with dementia expressed the following sentiment after an interaction with the Elderflowers: 'Someone said: "You've missed your breakfast" – I said, "Well, I don't mind – but have I missed the red noses?"'

What makes Compassionate Clowns attractive to people with dementia

- Clowns have a friendly and eternally optimistic outlook. They believe 100 per cent in what they are doing. They are therefore able to fully engage with and surrender to the participants' reality.
- Clowns, not unlike people with dementia, act 'in the present moment', without any social pressure or judgement.
- They are always happy to be 'there', wherever they are.
- Clowns appear 'different' and out of the norm – this is something people with dementia seem to relate to. Rather than hiding their differences they point to them.
- Clowns are used to highlighting failure and making mistakes. They regularly pick themselves up, dust themselves off, retry and fail over and over again. Within this optimism and naiveté they enjoy the freedom of celebrating their mistakes rather than hiding them, hence sharing their 'humanity'.
- They also forget their failure (and successes) very quickly and repeat them over and over again. They share this apparent lack of short-term memory with people with dementia.
- They are highly visual.
- They encourage verbal and non-verbal communication.
- They are looking for beauty and are able to find it in any situation, environment and within anybody they encounter.

Compassionate Clowning principles relevant for the Elderflowers work

- A starting point for the clowns is the present moment in space and time, where nothing much happens. This is offered as an invitation to the participants, in which they have time to respond.
- They have a curious outlook on life and are always searching and looking for love, encouragement and validation by others.
- The first idea is the best idea. Clowns will try anything and stick with it to the end.
- Simplicity – one thing at a time.
- They use creativity, rhythm and humour to facilitate an interaction.
- 'When you get old, you don't get to experience music informally, it's always played at you. What you've just done is wonderful, thank you, it was lovely and special' – Female participant, Queen Margaret Hospital, Dunfermline.
- Failure, success and repetition – clowns never give up, repeat their successes and mistakes. Therefore the participants have many chances to join in and be affected.
- The individual clown characters have strong and clear personal rhythm.
- They share the element of 'being confused'; of not knowing the answer and the vulnerability that accompanies this feeling.
- They don't solve the problems and don't fill in the blanks.
- They adapt their approach, making it up as they go along.
- They take things seriously and never give up.
- They have a respect for authority – everybody knows more than they do.
- They are 'different' and therefore often considered outsiders.
- They can be outrageous.
- They don't take anything personally.
- They are unexpected in a health care environment and signify a break from the norm and daily routine.
- David Sheard describes the experience of dementia as 'crossing a bridge moving from one reality to another.' As performers and artists it is easier for us to suspend 'our' reality and accompany people with dementia across this bridge rather than calling them back into the 'current' reality.

The 'Elderflower family' concept

Although people with dementia often no longer remember their own families or their position within their own family unit, they appear to have an innate understanding of what family bond and sibling rivalry mean. The family approach gives a degree of safety, identity, community and reference. The Elderflowers present themselves as a family unit of brothers, sisters and cousins. They have a made-up family history and family tree as well

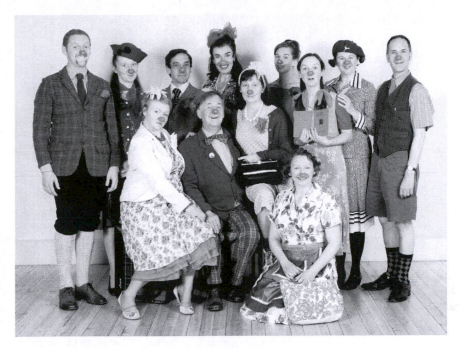

Figure 10.3 Photograph of Elderflowers family

as pictures and stories they can share. It also opens up creative play using sibling rivalry. As members of this family they have an identity and a purpose – the visit. In addition they also introduce a sense of excitement and adventure.

The Elderflowers also often act as a substitute family or family friends for those who don't get visitors very often. One gentleman with dementia expressed his feelings towards the Elderflowers with the following words: 'You are from the heart and genuine friends, truly genuine.'

Sometimes the Elderflowers even become substitute family members for the relatives. The daughter of a participant passed on the following message: 'I just want to take the opportunity to tell you what you are doing here means a lot to me and the whole family. My mother loves you. Bless you.'

The Elderflowers wear costumes that are inspired by and hark back to the times of Cary Grant, Audrey Hepburn, Doris Day and so forth. They are dressed up for a special occasion. Participants may still remember more distant times in their past. As their short-term memory deteriorates, their long-term memory often continues to function or is more easily accessible, and the clothing of the Elderflowers can help stir those memories, help create a connection with, or just bring a sense of comfort to the participants.

Case study

When Rose (name changed) first met the Elderflowers she was intrigued but a little hesitant about joining in. However, over a number of visits she began to welcome them with open arms. She remembered them from week to week and was curious when new Elderflower siblings turned up.

When Rose moved to another ward, visits became tailor-made for her needs. She was very happy when she found out that the Elderflowers also visited her new home. She showed them around and introduced them to the staff as her friends. She treated them as close friends who were always welcome in her room, even on days when the staff had difficulty getting permission to enter.

Rose loves to watch and play with the Elderflowers. She has a red nose, which she keeps in her bag. She sings with the Elderflowers with her nose on and gives good advice on everything from dancing and acrobatics to cooking and arranging a party. In May, Rose had her 80th birthday, which happened to be on a day the Elderflowers were visiting. The staff asked the Elderflowers if they could persuade her to come into to the living room for coffee and cake to celebrate with the other ladies and gentlemen. She had refused but was more than happy to do it with the Elderflowers. They gave her a photo of the Elderflowers family and together they put it up on the wall in her room.

The Elderflowers also love working with Rose. They feel that she really likes them and together they have found a level of play where fantasy and reality have a place. Sweetie-Pie Elderflower comments: 'I don't think she ever confuses us with family but she accepts us as we are and seems to enjoy every visit. A wonderful lady.'

The Elderflowers always work in a duo providing undivided two-to-one interactions. Some participants respond better to male, some to female practitioners. In any case – working in a duo enables an indirect approach and play (working between the partners for the benefit of the participant), which can be useful during a first encounter with more anxious or worried participants.

Compassionate Clowning for person-centred care

Listen with an open mind.

Suspend logic and the need to understand.

Listen with eyes as well as ears, to understand beyond spoken words.

Summary

The Hearts & Minds Elderflowers programme uses *Compassionate Clowning* to focus on individuals, their personality and the positive aspects of behaviour rather than any element of their illness. In my experience a sense of fun, positivity and playful compassion help to minimize frustration, distress and anxiety levels as well as challenging behaviour.

The Scottish Government appears to concur and officially states their commitment to:

> always exploring therapeutic approaches as the first alternative in intervening in such circumstances; always regarding the use of psychoactive medications as the last treatment option.
>
> (Scotland's National Dementia Strategy (2011))

In addition the Scottish Government describes in their Common Standards of Care for Dementia that 'the standards explicitly assert that people have the right to be treated as a unique individual and to be treated with dignity and respect'.

I could not agree more. It is important to remember that people with dementia will have spent their lives contributing to our society. They deserve our respect and should be treated as a person with feelings, wants and needs, in spite of their diagnosis.

They remain experts of their own lives and history.

They have names we need to remember, even if they no longer can.

They have feelings, which need attention.

They have likes, dislikes and preferences, which they are entitled to.

They may have different communication needs, which require patience, time and listening.

They may have a family who are no longer able to visit the person they have known all their lives.

Treat them like you would like your own family members to be treated.

Treat them like family.

Care Experiences: presentation delivered during interview for job as Mental Health Advocate

Chris (UK)

Passions change and mature as the individual does. Circumstances dictate how and where one can channel their energies therefore when unforeseen events enter and alter your life irreparably; your whole mind set, passions and interests undergo a seismic shift and are rarely ever the same again.

(continued)

(continued)

Therefore I would like to talk about the diagnosis and treatment of my mother's illness and how it has affected both my mother and my family as a whole.

My mother contracted *HSE* (*Herpes Simplex Encephalitis*) following her release from hospital after having undergone a routine biopsy to determine why she was intermittently losing the sight in her left eye. Having received a diagnosis of *Giant Cell Arteris* she was placed on a course of *prednisolone* steroids; a drug that's effect is to wipe out the body's own immune system, and discharged home.

Although we had been told to avoid contact with young children with chicken pox and presented with a small blue card that my mother was to carry at all times notifying any health care professionals that she was on steroids, that was the sum total of the information we were furnished with. Therefore who would have thought that something as seemingly innocuous as a cold sore could have such a devastating effect upon a person?

One just has to read the newspapers regarding the High Court case involving the family of a woman known as 'M' to see the devastating suddenness of this viral infection. Here the family of 'M'; who's minimally conscious state which is one stage up from a persistent vegetative state, has secured the courts judgement allowing the withdrawal of life supporting treatment.

'It's not about us at all,' her former partner, identified as S, said. 'We can only speak up for her, nothing more. We are her voice. We have no ulterior motive. We just know who she was and her opinions.'

Herpes Simplex Encephalitis affects at least 1 in 500,000 therefore it is little wonder that information relating to this devastating condition is so sparse. However, given that the latent cold-sore virus is so prevalent amongst adults (as much as 90 per cent of adults carry the virus) why is information so lacking as to the infections potentially devastating consequences?

How is anyone ever meant to protect themselves adequately from just such an infection whilst on a course of immunosuppressant medication, if they are not being furnished with all or even adequate information? Surely the potential risks involved if and when a person becomes infected with *HSE* would result in a greater level of information and education being relayed to the individual, their family and the public at large, but at no time where we made aware of these risks.

Even when I was informed of her diagnosis and the word '*encephalitis*' was mentioned my ignorance led me to think she had contracted *CJD* (*Creutzfeldt–Jakob disease*) as a result of eating meat contaminated with *BSE* (*Bovine Spongiform Encephalitis*) and that her condition would be fatal.

Although we were eventually given an Internet print-out pertaining to the *HSE* infection after my mother's condition was diagnosed and treatment was underway with the administration of the anti-biotic *Aciclovir*, I feel that had we been better informed of the potential risks then we as a family could have taken the appropriate steps to ensure minimal contact with the outside world until such a time as the treatment of steroidal medication had ceased and my mother's immune system had returned to normal.

Despite recovering from her illness my mother is by far a very different person now than to what she was before. Once so independent and mentally alert, she is now in need of constant care and supervision. However, we do feel fortunate that her disposition is one of eternal sunshine or blissful ignorance as my father would say, always smiling and rarely unhappy she still to this day brings joy and laughter to all she meets.

It was in part due to the treatment I felt my mother received at the hands of the health care professionals that I decided to return to university and complete my Law degree as is evident in the choice of modules studied from tort law, medical law and human rights law, all highly important matters that would one way or another affect my mother's situation.

I strongly believe that my mother's illness could have been prevented had we been fully informed of the risks associated with a potential infection resulting from an eradicated immune system; the length of time it took with which to diagnose her *HSE* infection and, due to the rarity of the condition itself, the apparent lack of education exhibited by certain members of the health care staff in terms of treatment and understanding.

So in conclusion, whereas once my passions were orientated around my own interests and desires, due to the massive impact my mother's illness has had on all our family I believe I have become less self-centred and more compassionate as a person and it is for that reason that I welcomed the opportunity to channel and focus this compassionate side of myself into the role of Independent Mental Capacity Advocate.

References

Alzheimer Scotland, Information & Resources, about dementia (available at: www.alzscot.org/information_and_resources/about_dementia) (accessed 30 July 2013).

David Sheard, Dementia Care Matters (available at: www.dementiacarematters.com/pdf/howbridge.pdf) (accessed 26 June 2013).

Dementia Services Development Centre (available at: http://dementia.stir.ac.uk/) (accessed 26 June 2013).

Hearts & Minds Business Plan (available at: www.heartsminds.org.uk/) (accessed 26 June 2013).

Hearts & Minds, Home of Clowndoctors and Elderflowers (available at: www.hearts minds.org.uk/) (accessed 26 June 2013).

NHS Choices: Looking after someone with dementia – Dementia guide (available at: www.nhs.uk/conditions/dementia-guide/pages/dementia-carers.aspx) (accessed 30 July 2013).

Red Nose Coming DVD: clowning and dementia in Care Homes; Dementia Services Development Centre 2009 (available at: www.dementiashop.co.uk/products/red-nose-coming-dvd-clowning-and-communication-care-homes) (accessed 26 June 2013).

Scotland's National Dementia Strategy (2011) One Year on Report page 2 The Scottish Government, Edinburgh (available at: www.nationalarchives.gov.uk/doc/open-government-licence/version/1/open-government-licence.htm) (accessed 30 July 2013).

The Royal College of Psychiatrists (2013) Memory problems, Alzheimer and dementia (available at: www.rcpsych.ac.uk/expertadvice/problemsdisorders/memory-problemsanddementia.aspx) (accessed 26 June 2013).

Photographs of Elderflowers interactions: courtesy of Colin Dickson, Lasswade Scotland.

Photograph of the Elderflowers family: courtesy of Susan Burrell, Susan Burrell Photography, Dalkeith, Scotland.

11 Compassionate care of patients with diabetes mellitus

A personal account

Stathis Papavasiliou

Brief introduction by Sue Shea

Long-term conditions require a number of efforts in daily self-management. In particular, people with diabetes face many challenges, as the condition involves a number of emotional issues, in addition to physical factors. As such it is important for people with diabetes to maintain a positive proactive response and to engage with a supportive health care provider (Shea and Wynyard 2009). Diabetes requires a number of lifestyle changes, and in many cases, as the literature suggests, people with diabetes may view such changes as threatening and may overestimate their ability to control the condition, while underestimating the seriousness of it (Coelho *et al.* 2003; Thoolen *et al.* 2009).

Patient-centred care is a term frequently used in relation to long-term conditions, and a recent thematic analysis conducted by Hudon *et al.* (2012) emphasized new dimensions of such care in relation to chronic disease management, including acknowledging patient expertise, offering hope and providing advocacy. In addition, the Diabetes Attitudes Wishes and Needs 2 (DAWN2) study Peyrot *et al.* (2013), has adopted a multinational focus on psychosocial issues and patient-centred care, aiming to identify new avenues for improving diabetes care.

Compassion, empathy and support towards patients with diabetes are of great importance in assisting the patients in coming to terms with their illness, and thus improving physiological and psychological outcomes. However, until recently the term 'compassion' has not been greatly utilized in connection with diabetes, although a study by Pace *et al.* (2009) suggests that engagement in 'compassion meditation' may reduce stress-induced immune and behavioural responses.

Britneff *et al.* (2013) remind us that mental health issues are common amongst people with diabetes and are associated with poor glycaemic control and self-management. Thus it would seem logical that a compassionate approach to people with diabetes is essential in alleviating the burden and helping patients to understand and cope with their condition.

(continued)

(continued)

Furthermore, in a study by Hojat *et al.* (2011), the hypothesis that physician empathy is associated with positive health outcomes for patients with diabetes was confirmed, in that empathy was shown to be an important factor associated with clinical competence and patient outcomes.

An interesting perspective on diabetes care and education is put forward by Anderson and Funnell (2008), who point to the fact that 'effective diabetes education involves a combination of art and science' and that ' . . . establishing a therapeutic alliance with patients is an art . . . '. These authors remind us of the importance of interpersonal skills and values that diabetes educators should adopt, and that they should be able to feel and express compassion, empathy and warmth.

In the following chapter, endocrinologist Stathis Papavasiliou offers a moving and informative personal account of working and caring for people with diabetes. Using a military analogy, Papavasiliou speaks of 'war against the disease', and the importance of support of patients and their families and education in self-care, thus providing an interesting and insightful learning tool.

Compassion is defined as 'sympathetic consciousness of others' distress together with a desire to alleviate it' (www.merriam-webster.com/dictionary/compassion). Therefore, it would seem to me, that compassionate patient care is the sum total of all medical decisions and actions. These decisions and actions should take into conscious account the distress and discomfort a patient experiences by the illness itself, compounded by the discomfort caused by diagnostic and therapeutic actions. It is a necessary addendum that the caregiver explains and delivers all of the above, in a climate of active emotional supportive participation toward the patient and his/her family and makes every effort to alleviate the discomfort.

This is not an easy path to follow.

To begin with, compassion it is not a subject that is systematically taught in medical schools and there are no well-defined quantitative scientific standards. No one knows for sure that it can be taught. The attitude toward compassionate care is transferred by example from generation to generation of physicians, either in the positive direction of creating in the trainee the desire to meet and if possible exceed the standards of the teacher or occasionally in the negative direction of avoidance of the behaviour of his/her technically and scientifically advanced, morally impeccable but emotionally dry and less than considerate superiors.

Following the path also depends on the personality of the caregiver, the value system he/she grew up with, the ethnic background, religious and socioeconomic factors, and sometimes physical and psychological stamina. It is very difficult to be compassionate at the end of a long and arduous sleepless call, with an inordinately heavy patient load and very little time to spend per patient.

Then there are other difficulties and errors either on the side of excess or deficiency. A show of pretentious compassion may serve as a cover for inadequate knowledge and skills on the part of the caregiver. It may be an effort to avoid confronting difficult diagnostic and therapeutic decisions; competition with colleagues; a whole host of other reasons that belong to the category of unacceptable ethical and professional behaviour.

Lack or withdrawal of compassion may be the result of aversion toward the beliefs and behaviour of a patient, the fears and inhibitions of the caregiver, covert or overt anger toward the patient, while the loss of the ability and skill to be compassionate is, among other things, a sign of the so-called 'burn-out' syndrome in health care professionals and a clear sign they must withdraw from the front lines. All of the above relate to sub-standard care and require thorough discussion, clear lines of communication and appropriate corrective action.

Excessive emotional involvement in the suffering of patients on the part of the caregivers is a well-known and recognized reason for rendering them incapable of appropriate and timely action and results in partial or some-times permanent incapacitation of physicians and other health care profes-sionals. There is a clear warning by Osler in 'Aequanimitas' against such a contingency that remains valid to this day.

However, it is the opposite attitude of aloofness, indifference, arrogance and distance that go hand in hand with apparent or real disregard for the patient's suffering and fears which has caused a worldwide wave of protest by patients and their advocates and a call for change in the attitudes and behaviour of health professionals. More so, if the patients we are called to care for suffer from a chronic disorder with serious long-term complica-tions, such as diabetes mellitus.

On the right side wall of the office of Dr F. Whitehouse MD, Clinical Professor of Medicine at 'Henry Ford' Hospital in Detroit, Michigan, where I received my basic training in internal medicine and diabetes mellitus under his wise tutelage, there was a shield-shaped plaque with an entrenchment tool, a shovel, attached to it. Under the plaque there was an inscription: 'For leading his men into battle'. For years I thought that it was a war memento dedicated to him, by grateful comrades in arms. His overall bearing, his even temper during crises, his crew cut and self-discipline, leadership by example without a trace of arrogance or self-importance, bore all the marks of a mili-tary leader. He was also the archetypal compassionate physician, a moral and professional leader and above all an exemplary teacher. I had the privilege to observe him in his daily interaction with diabetic patients and their families for three years and take in all the lessons he offered.

It was his wife, Iris Whitehouse RN, a diabetes nursing educator and training expert of rare abilities and kindness, who told me during her visit with us in Crete at our request, for the purpose of educating the nursing staff at the University Hospital of Crete and in rural outposts of the Greek NHS in Crete, that it was a gift by his residents at 'Henry Ford'. It was F. Whitehouse that instilled in me the dual approach to diabetes mellitus.

War against the disease; support for and mobilization through education in self-care, of the patients and their families.

1. The enemy

Diabetes mellitus is a generalized disorder of metabolism, including the metabolism of carbohydrates, proteins and lipids characterized by hyperglycaemia and caused by relative or absolute insulin deficiency. The disease has been known for millennia and there are many causes. Autoimmune destruction of insulin-producing β-cells in the pancreas is the most common cause of type 1 diabetes that affects young people, has an acute onset and is characterized by absolute insulin deficiency. Type 2 diabetes mellitus affects primarily adults who are usually overweight or obese; they commonly have relatives with the disease and it is accompanied by insulin resistance. Insulin resistance means that for the same quantity of insulin, the biological effect of the hormone is less than that observed in a normal person. Thus, in most patients with type 2 diabetes although there is insulin in the bloodstream and sometimes in excess compared to normal people, it is not enough to hold the blood glucose in the normal range because of endogenous factors, mostly related to excessive weight, that prevent the hormone from exercising its full biological effect. Hence, the term 'relative insulin deficiency' in the definition of diabetes mellitus, stated above.

As the years go by, the secretory capacity of the beta islet cells may diminish and varying degrees of true insulin deficiency may result, in addition to insulin resistance. Diabetes mellitus manifests with polydipsia, meaning excessive thirst, polyuria, meaning excessive urine output, and polyphagia meaning excessive hunger and food intake. Cramps, blurred vision, unwanted and unplanned weight loss and other less commonly encountered symptoms complete the presentation symptomatology.

A third common type of diabetes mellitus is the diabetes of pregnancy that requires special awareness and care for the mother and the foetus. Collaboration with the obstetricians is mandatory and ideally joint meetings between the two teams to discuss progress and problems of pregnant women with diabetes of pregnancy are very productive. Diabetic women in their reproductive years should plan with their diabetes team the timing of getting pregnant and subsequent care that is far more intensive and complex than the usual care of other categories of diabetics.

Acute complications of diabetes mellitus include diabetic ketoacidosis, and hyperosmolar coma.

Diabetic ketoacidosis is the result of acute insulin deficiency, usually precipitated by an intercurrent illness and is commonly the end result of autoimmune destruction of the insulin-producing beta-cells of the pancreatic islets. It is a serious deregulation of the acidity of the internal environment of the patient caused by the overproduction of an organic acid called beta-hydroxy-butyric acid and ketones, accompanied by dehydration and electrolyte imbalances, because of polyuria caused by the ensuing hyperglycaemia. If left untreated, it becomes life-threatening and leads to coma and death. Today this is a rare occurrence in the developed world. In patients with known type 1 diabetes, the usual causes are omission of insulin doses or an acute illness that raises their insulin needs or prevents them from following their prescribed therapeutic programme.

Hyperosmolar coma is an elevation of the osmotic pressure of the plasma because of very high glucose levels that may cause profound dehydration. The result is malfunction of the central nervous system manifesting as stupor and coma. It usually occurs in adult elderly patients. In these patients, even small amounts of circulating insulin are sufficient to keep ketone and β-OH-butyric acid production in check and ketoacidosis does not develop. As in the case of diabetic ketoacidosis this complication may become life-threatening and lead to coma and death if left untreated, but this is a rare occurrence today.

Diabetes mellitus is also accompanied by chronic complications that take years to develop but may result in early loss of life and chronic disability.

These include macrovascular complications, microvascular complications and diabetic neuropathy.

The macrovascular complications arise from accelerated atherosclerosis affecting large arteries such as the carotids, the coronary arteries, the arteries supplying the lower limbs, the bifurcation of the aorta and the pelvic arteries and other large vessels.

The result is ischaemia of the areas of the body that are receive their nutrients and oxygen via these large vessels and may result in cerebrovascular accidents, angina and myocardial infarction, ischaemia and sometimes gangrene of the legs and feet requiring amputation, impotence and erectile dysfunction in men, etc.

Microvascular complications are the result of a complex process that eventually causes occlusion of the small vessels supplying vital organs such as the kidneys, the vessels of the retina, the small vessels of the myocardium, the small vessels of the feet, etc.

The end result is ischaemia of the affected tissues with loss of function or in the case of the lower extremities, ulcers of the feet.

The most widely known microvascular complications are diabetic retinopathy and nephropathy. In retinopathy vision is threatened and in nephropathy the end result may be end-stage renal failure requiring dialysis.

Diabetic neuropathy affects both myelinated and non-myelinated nerves and causes loss of tactile, pain and temperature sensation, most commonly in the lower extremities where neuropathic foot ulcers may develop. Loss of deep sensation may result in damage of the ankle and knee joints. Paraesthesias such as pinprick sensation or causalgia, meaning burning pain usually in the lower extremities or frank pain, may degrade the quality of life of patients.

Autonomic neuropathy may result in diabetic gastropathy, neurogenic bladder, orthostatic hypotension, impotence and erectile dysfunction in men.

Susceptibility to a whole host of infections, ranging from dermal mycoses to serious vital organ infections, such as for example pneumonia, further increase the morbidity and mortality due to diabetes mellitus.

2. The battleground

The battleground is the pre-existing pathology of the patient, along with all the extraneous factors that may influence the outcome, such as the social environment, health care system and administrative machinery governing the rules and regulations of benefits, medications and consumables related to the care of diabetes.

3. The troops

The troops are the health care professionals, organized in a team that includes one or more physicians, a diabetes teaching nurse, a dietician, a psychologist and secretarial support. However, in most settings in my country this is way beyond realistic, and usually the physician along with the diabetes teaching nurse and other nursing staff bear the weight of patient care, with some help from the dietetics department in public hospitals. Psychological expert support is usually on request to the psychiatry department and is utilized sparingly and if serious psychiatric problems arise. I have never had the luxury of a personal secretary.

The patient becomes part of the troops; so are the family and friends who are able and willing to offer support.

The first contact with the newly diagnosed patient is extremely important. After a thorough history and physical examination, the first objective is to make sure that the fear and sense of loneliness of the patient are alleviated and reassure him/her that a lot has changed in their lives but nothing is lost with the diagnosis of diabetes. Using language that is as simple as possible, but not simplistic, we usually explain what diabetes is and what we are going to do about it in broad terms.

We direct the discussion to the immediate priorities of getting the blood sugar under control and treating the acute complications if present. We explain that from now on we are a team.

If we detect denial, or a casual approach to diabetes we make a note and defer stressing differences of opinion and approach for a later time when we know more about the patient and his/her circumstances.

We explain the plan of education and training in diabetes self-care and try to establish a positive attitude toward the process, stressing that although we will always be there if the patient wishes us, the purpose is to make him/her self-sufficient. It is also explained that the burden of their self-care is theirs; not their mother's; not their wife's or husband's. Of course this approach does not apply to patients with disabilities, such as vision problems, problems with joints and elderly patients requiring care, or children.

Initial instructions regarding diet, exercise and medications are given and we make ourselves available at all times via telephone, email, etc. 24/7 and appointments are made with the teaching nurse, and the dietetics department. The patient is in boot camp.

Extra time is devoted to the families of teenagers and young people in general who are newly diagnosed with type 1 diabetes, to make sure that the guilt, the fear, the sense of doom that accompanies the announcement that insulin injections are unavoidable, are contained and the integrity of the family is not threatened.

Rarely, it is imperative to intervene dynamically in favour of the patient on first sight to protect him/her from their social environment. On one occasion, we had to literally drag a young peasant woman who was pregnant and had type 1 diabetes, from the clutches of her mother-in-law, who had brought her to the hospital to have an abortion right then and there, because she wouldn't have 'the cripple's child" for a grandchild. We admitted her in our ward where she stayed until she had a healthy baby girl, who recently got married. She learned to count to 20 while with us, during her hands-on instruction of the use of an insulin pen.

4. Training to battle diabetes

Following the initial contact, the patient's skills are built up through education with either a physician or a teaching nurse and follows a programme similar to other centres. Education means teaching the theoretical background that is necessary to understand the disease and its complications and training means application of theoretical knowledge. Education is carried out individually or in small groups during a visit. Training includes hands-on experience with equipment, such as insulin pens and blood sugar measuring devices, the supervised planning and decision-making related to diabetes over the telephone, email, or other means of communication. It includes handling situations that arise in daily life, such as going out to dinner with friends, going to a trip, response to a hypoglycaemic episode, adjustment of insulin dose, treating a minor illness, knowing when to get to the hospital in a hurry, etc.

Praise is in order for correct decisions and a brief reminder of what they have been taught and eliciting the correct modified response otherwise. At every stage, the purpose of the knowledge or skill that is taught is clearly and simply stated and it is emphasized that repetition and questions make perfect. Reinforcement of a positive attitude toward insulin shots is particularly important.

In my environment, insulin injections continue to be viewed as invasive and are frequently equated to shots taken by drug addicts. Explaining the difference between addiction and necessity is done frequently and in the most positive possible terms until the negative attitude associated with insulin administration weakens and disappears.

Knowledge of the long-term complications of diabetes is introduced in advancing stages of sophistication, making sure that the patients are not scared out of their minds, starting to feeling hopeless, and getting the impression that the whole effort of fighting the disease is futile. Balancing encouragement with criticism is an art that we health care providers learn over time. The end result of the process of education and training is hopefully an independent patient who can take care of his/her needs and make appropriate use of the resources available. The patient is now a diabetes warrior.

5. The battle

Diabetes is a chronic disease that demands vigilance, motivation, knowledge, discipline, perseverance and patience on the part of both patients and caregivers.

Maintaining a good quality of life and attaining important professional and social goals without developing complications is a major victory for both the patients and the health care team. In some cases the trials and tribulations of the daily care of diabetes fade and become necessary daily habits. Attaining a particular goal becomes all important and is enjoyed for its sake.

The case of a master vine grower from a village just outside Heraklion comes to memory. He loved his family and what he was doing so much, that for over 30 years he took outstanding care of himself just to be able to work in his vineyard and enjoy being with his family. His job involves daily exercise in a sunny healthy environment; his family, and especially his wife who took care of his diet and corrected the rare deviations from his programme, made sure he kept every appointment throughout this period and took care of logistics, which contributed to his working in his eighties and facing the prospect of retirement with horror. He has become a valued personal friend and it is I who draws strength from his success.

Another patient was a young man of 12 when he was first diagnosed with type 1 diabetes, who with rare discipline and determination grew over 2 metres and played professional basketball.

However, these are inspiring exceptions.

As in any conflict, sooner or later problems develop.

The usual points of friction with patients are weight and diet management across all age groups, denial and a continued nonchalant attitude toward diabetes, pseudodefiance of the disease, unnecessary dependence on others for self-care, blatant non-compliance with therapy, using diabetes to manipulate the social environment.

Disagreements arise and the temperature of personal relationships may and does rise.

As long as the caregiver is aware that it is not a conflict of egos, we believe that this is part of any meaningful and caring human interaction.

The patient is given the option of continuing his care with another physician or making an effort to adhere to the programme and the rules of our relationship.

The usual outcome is that for some time patients may go elsewhere, but they usually return to us.

A case in point is a young lady brought to us at the age of 14 by her mother.

She had been diagnosed with diabetes type 1 four years prior to her visit to us and although initially she was a model patient, during the turbulent times of adolescence she revolted. We established a good relation with both the family and the patient and contained the revolt for a few years.

As time went by, she started 'missing' shots of insulin, adopted a totally inappropriate dietary regime, her blood sugars became erratic and she gained weight. We had several visits where tension started building up and eventually it was impossible for any member of the team to get through to her about the dangers of such blatant non-compliance with her programme. Complications started developing, including retinopathy and mild nephropathy. Suddenly, she stopped seeing us altogether.

About three years later she came back because she 'missed us'. In the meantime she had married and had two boys. A few months after her return, her younger son also developed diabetes type 1 and she went through a serious episode of depression because although she was taking her son's illness in stride, someone in the environment said that it was the 'vengeance of God'. This was the straw that broke her overburdened back.

The whole team pulled together with her and slowly but steadily she came out of the depression and is now taking much better care of herself. Unfortunately, we will have a rocky road ahead because of the complications. Hopefully, we will manage.

I wish I had got to that part of her soul that made her snap out of the depression earlier, but I didn't know how. She has never left since.

Handling defeat is difficult for both patients and caregivers, but it is a reality.

The prospect of blindness, the amputation of a limb because of ischaemia, advancing renal failure requiring dialysis, a massive myocardial infarction with resulting heart failure are situations that try the fighting spirit of both patients and caregivers to the extreme. Of course the physician has to present the facts and the options and let the patient and the family participate in the decision-making process, guiding firmly but gently. The involvement of other specialties becomes central to patient care. He/she must be there to absorb some of the shock of the impact of such situations.

This is not the time to remind the patient of the countless warnings and admonitions issued by the team over the years. The comfort and easing of the daily life of the patient takes precedence.

At this stage, one of our concerns is to make sure that the flow of information is smooth, there are no conflicting messages from various sources that increase the anxiety of the family and the patient, giving the impression that one team does not know what the other is doing. We also go to great pains to inform the patient and the family who is leading the effort to solve a particular problem and what our role is in this setting.

In the narrowing defensive perimeter, spirits must be maintained and choices, however small, must be presented, thus negating as far as possible the loss of independence and lightening the weight of increasing disability.

Parting with a patient forever is always taxing to the team and it takes some time before we regroup. Contact with the patient's family is maintained during the mourning period and we make sure that we solve administrative problems that may arise. However, the loss also serves as a new starting point, steeling our determination to do better.

Epilogue

The scientific strides in the research of all aspects of diabetes mellitus have resulted in marked improvement of the daily life of millions of patients around the world. However, diabetes mellitus and its kin disease, obesity, continue to affect growing numbers of patients.

In a global environment dominated by economic efficiency, limited resources and the information revolution, patients feel that they are 'processed', rather than cared for and they are reacting to this trend in health care delivery. This wave of protest is particularly relevant in patients with chronic diseases such as diabetes mellitus and highlights the necessity to reevaluate concepts and practices such as 'compassionate care' that were taken for granted so far, and devise ways to maintain the deeply personal nature of health care on one hand while meeting the necessities of the new economic environment on the other.

In the personal account presented in this report we presented the 'traditional' model as applied in our environment. It is an open question whether it is viable and optimal and what additional research and education of health care providers needs to be implemented to make it so.

Care Experiences: the importance of a compassionate approach following diagnosis of diabetes

Robin (UK)

Nothing quite prepares you for the shock of hearing that you have dangerously high blood sugar levels and that there is imminent danger of you having a stroke or heart attack. This was the case with me the day before an essential trip to Greece with my partner Sue. After an emergency visit to my local surgery and a visit to a late night pharmacy, we set off for Greece the next day. I had a large bag with me containing test strips, lancets, glucose monitor, ketone testing kit, blood glucose and cholesterol lowering medications.

Prior to this revelation I had been aware that something was not quite right with me or my body. I was suffering from intense fatigue, exacerbated anxiety and carelessness when driving or crossing roads. I was also having problems with my eyes and starting to experience extreme depression. The depression was exacerbated by the fact that I didn't have a clue what the contents of my bag of medical 'goodies' was for or even how to use them.

Fortunately for us we have a close friend in Greece, Stathis, who is an endocrinologist. The calming process started as soon as we went to see him, and I realized that I was in the hands of a compassionate and caring doctor. He spent ages with me explaining everything in the minutest detail, even drawing a diagramme showing times when to eat regularly throughout the day. He thought long and hard about the medication that I had been prescribed by my local GP surgery in the UK. Although this was the correct medication he wanted to prescribe something else that would immediately start to bring my astronomically high blood sugar levels down. To do this he sent out to a local pharmacy for the appropriate medication. He then tackled my eye problem arranging a consultation with an ophthalmologist.

I can never thank this man enough, nor will I ever forget the kindness and compassion shown to me. He treated me as an individual, listened to my worries, yet never once did I feel that I was being treated as a case book diabetic. What sticks in my mind most of all, and I always smile when I think of it, was the phrase '*taming the beast*' that he used when helping me to tackle my diabetes.

References

Anderson, R. M., Funnell, M. M. (2008). The art and science of diabetes education: A culture out of balance, *The Diabetes Educator* 34 (1): 109–117.

Britneff, E., Winkley, K. (2013) The role of psychological interventions for people with diabetes and mental health issues. *Journal of Diabetes Nursing* 17: 305–310.

Coelho, R., Amorim, R. N., Prata, J. (2003). Coping styles and quality of life in patients with non-insulin dependent diabetes mellitus. *Psychosomatics* 44: 312–318.

Hojat, M., Louis, D. Z., Markham, F. W., Wender, R., Rabinowitz, C., Gonnella, J. S. (2011). Physicians' empathy and clinical outcomes for diabetic patients. *Acad Med.* 86 (3): 359–364.

Hudon, C., Fortin, M., Haggerty, J., Loignon, C., Lambert, M., Poitras, M. (2012). Patient-centered care in chronic disease management: A thematic analysis of the literature in family medicine, *Patient Education and Counseling* 88 (2): 170–176.

Pace, T. W. W., Negi, L. T., Adame, D. D., Cole, S. P., Sivilli, T. I., Brown, T. D., Issa, M. J., Raison, C. L. (2009). Effect of compassion meditation on neuroendocrine, innate immune and behavioral responses to psychosocial stress, *Psychoneuroendocrinology* 34 (1): 87–98.

Peyrot, M., Burns, K. K., Davies, M., Forbes, A., Hermanns, N., Holt, R., *et al.* (2013). Diabetes Attitudes Wishes and Needs 2 (DAWN2): A multinational, multi-stakeholder study of psychosocial issues in diabetes and person-centred diabetes care, *Diabetes Research and Clinical Practice* 99 (2): 174–184.

Thoolen, B. J., de Ridder, D., Bensing, J. *et al.* (2008). Beyond good intentions: The role of proactive coping in achieving sustained behavioural change in the context of diabetes management. *Psychology and Health* 23: 52–56.

Shea, S., Wynyard, R. (2009). The importance of a proactive response to a diagnosis to type 2 diabetes, Diabetes Voice 54 (1): 17–19.

12 The health impact of financial crisis

Omens of a Greek tragedy

Alexander Kentikelenis, Marina Karanikolos, Irene Papanicolas, Sanjay Basu, Martin McKee and David Stuckler

Brief introduction by Robin Wynard

David Stuckler, Alex Kentikelenis and their research colleagues have conducted groundbreaking research into the nature of austerity and recession, and the impact of these on the health of people and health-care systems around the world. In a recently published book Stuckler and Basu reach the staggering conclusion that '… austerity involves the deadliest social policies. Recessions can hurt but austerity kills' (Stuckler and Basu 2013: xx).

The so-called *Troika* of the International Monetary Fund, the European Union and the European Central Bank have decided massive bailouts to countries such as Greece, Portugal, the Irish Republic and Cyprus. Greece alone, a country very familiar to the editors of this book, has been awarded an €110bn bailout by the Troika. Of course such debts have to be repaid eventually, and austerity has been seen as a measure to cut down demand for consumer goods and luxuries. This it has undoubtedly done but it has brought in its wake all kinds of social ills.

It has to be remembered that it is not only members of the Euro zone like Greece that have been dealt harsh austerity measures and have had to suffer sweeping social problems as a result of these. In the UK the Trussell Trust, the UK's biggest provider of food banks said more than 350,000 people required help from its food banks during 2012:

> up to half of all people turning to food banks are doing so as a direct result of having benefit payments delayed, reduced or withdrawn altogether and changes to the benefit system are the most common reasons for people using food banks.
>
> (BBC News 30 May 2013)

As a boy growing up in the East End of London near to the City in the 1950s, I was aware of the nature of austerity, shortages were everywhere and we were all in need. I was also aware that being in a similar situation, people helped each other with something akin to what might be called compassion. The UK and Europe were rebuilding after a devastating war. Most items of food, clothing, petrol, etc. were rationed by a scheme of ration books and coupons, a scheme which did not end until 1954. There was, care of the *Utility Furniture Scheme*, the so-called *austerity furniture* of which my parents were inordinately proud. Playing on bomb sites for me seemed to be a way of life which was casually accepted because they just happened to be there.

But there is a massive difference between this austerity and the world of austerity that Kentikelenis *et al.* have poignantly and thoroughly researched. For me and many others the war was over and there seemed to be some hope for a better future world.

The following article reprinted from *The Lancet* by permission, together with the addition of a postscript by Kentikelenis cogently explores the austerity measures imposed on Greece by the Troika and their impact on the health and well-being of the nation and obvious implications of the need for compassion.

Greece has been affected more by the financial turmoil beginning in 2007 than any other European country. Fifteen years of consecutive growth in the Greek economy have reversed. Unemployment has risen from 6.6 per cent in May 2008 to 16.6 per cent in May 2011 among adults (youth unemployment rose from 18.6 per cent to 40.1 per cent) (Hellenic Statistical Authority 2011), as debt grew between 2007 and 2010 from 105.4 per cent to 142.8 per cent of GDP (€239.4 to €328.6 billion) compared to the EU-15 average change from 66.2 per cent to 85.1 per cent of GDP in this same period (€6.0 to €7.8 trillion) (Eurostat 2011). Greece's options were limited, as its government ruled out leaving the euro, precluding them from one of the most common solutions in such circumstances: devaluation. To finance its debts, Greece had to borrow €110bn from the IMF and Eurozone partners, under strict conditions that included drastically curtailing government spending. While other countries in Europe (e.g. France, Germany) now show signs of economic recovery, the crisis continues to evolve in Greece; industrial production fell by 8 per cent in 2010 (Hellenic Statistical Authority 2011).

The Lancet's editor has asked whether anyone is looking at the effect of the economic crisis on health and healthcare in Greece (Horton 2011), in light of the adverse health effects of previous recessions (Stuckler *et al.* 2009). Here, we describe changes in health and healthcare in Greece based on our analysis of European Union Statistics on Income and Living Conditions (EU-SILC) data (Eurostat 2007; 2009), which provide comparable cross-sectional and longitudinal information on social and economic characteristics and living conditions throughout the European Union. In Greece, representative samples of 12,346 and 15,045 respondents were recruited in 2007 and 2009 respectively, using consistent methodology, of which a total of 26,489 had complete socio-demographic data (see Web Appendix Table 12.1

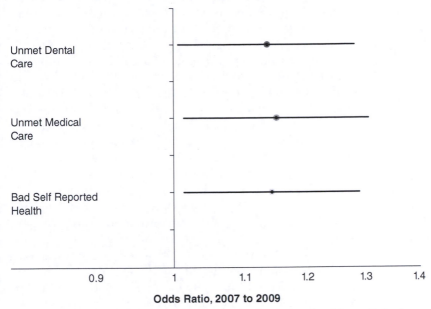

Figure 12.1 Changes in self-reported health and access to healthcare linked to financial crisis, population representative surveys of Greece, 2007 compared with 2009, adjusted estimates

Notes: 95 per cent confidence intervals presented. X-axis on log-scale. Data are from the Greece EU Survey on Income and Living Conditions, 2007 and 2009 survey waves. Models correct for potentially confounding differences of survey respondents, including age, a dummy for age over 65, sex, marital status, the degree of urbanization (from 1 to 3), and educational attainment; similar patterns found when including measures of household income. See Web Appendix Table 12.2 for more details.

for more details). We also drew on reports collected from medical research institutes, health prefectures and non-governmental organizations. These include epidemiological indicators, data on hospitalisations, and reports on mental health problems and the status of vulnerable groups.

As shown in Figure 12.1, compared with 2007, the pre-crisis baseline, there was a statistically significant increase in people reporting that they did not go to a doctor or dentist despite feeling it was necessary in 2009 ($OR_{doctor} = 1.15$, 95 per cent CI: 1.02 to 1.30; $OR_{dentist} = 1.14$, 95 per cent CI: 1.01 to 1.28, see Figure 12.1 and Web Appendix Table 12.2), after correcting for differences in survey respondents including age, sex, marital status, educational attainment, and urban/rural residence. The main reasons for not seeking medical care did not appear significantly linked to an inability to afford care (OR = 0.87, 95 per cent CI: 0.74 to 1.02), but to long waiting times (OR = 1.83, 95 per cent CI: 1.26 to 2.64), travel distance to care (OR = 2.50, 95 per cent CI: 1.35 to 4.63), waiting to feel better (OR = 1.93, 95 per cent CI: 1.26 to 2.96), and other reasons not captured by the survey tool (OR = 1.54, 95 per cent CI: 1.05 to 2.27); (Web Appendix

Table 12.3). As Greece's universal public health care system entitles citizens and those with social insurance to visit GPs free of charge and attend outpatient clinics of hospitals for between zero and 5 euros, these observed reductions in access likely reflect supply side problems: there were about 40 per cent cuts in hospital budgets (Telloglou 2011), understaffing and reported occasional shortages of medical supplies as well as bribes given to medical staff to jump queues in already-overstretched hospitals (Telloglou *et al.* 2011). Although people were less likely to visit general practitioners and outpatient facilities, there was a rise in public hospital inpatient admissions of 24 per cent in 2010 compared to 2009 (Liakopoulou 2011), and 8 per cent in the first half of 2011 compared to the same period of 2010 (Polyzos 2011). Major private health providers, although comprising a smaller fraction of care delivery than public providers, were also hit by pressure on personal budgets and registered losses after the onset of the crisis. A 2010 study reported a 25–30 per cent decline in admissions to private hospitals (Hellastat 2010).

There are signs that health outcomes have worsened, especially among vulnerable groups. We observed a significant rise in the prevalence of people reporting their health was 'bad' or 'very bad' (OR = 1.14, 95 per cent CI: 1.02 to 1.28; Figure 12.1). Suicides rose by 17 per cent in 2009 from 2007 and unofficial 2010 data quoted in parliament mentions a 25 per cent rise (Avgenakis 2011). The Minister of Health reported a 40 per cent rise in the first half of 2011 compared to the same period in 2010 (Loverdos 2011). The national suicide helpline reported 25 per cent of callers faced financial difficulties in 2010 (Katsadoros *et al.* 2011) and recent reports in the media indicate that the inability to repay high levels of personal debt may be a key factor in the increase in suicides (Tsimas 2011). Violence also has risen; homicide and theft rates also nearly doubled between 2007 and 2009 (Carassava 2011; Krug *et al.* 2002; Sundquist *et al.* (2006). The numbers of people able to obtain sickness benefits has declined (OR = 0.61, 95 per cent CI: 0.38 to 0.98) between 2007 and 2009, likely due to budget cuts, with further reductions to access and the level of benefits anticipated once austerity measures are fully implemented (Web Appendix Table 12.4; EU-SILC 2009).

A significant increase in HIV infections occurred in late 2010. The latest data suggest that new infections will rise by 52 per cent in 2011 compared with 2010 (922 new cases versus 605), with half of the currently observed increases attributable to infections among intravenous drug users (Paraskevis *et al.* 2011). Data for the first seven months of 2011 show more than a 10-fold rise in new infections among these drug users compared with the same period in 2010 (Paraskevis *et al.* 2011). The prevalence of heroin use reportedly rose by 20 per cent in 2009, from 20,200 to 24,100 according to estimates from the Greek Documentation and Monitoring Centre for Drugs. Budget cuts in 2009 and 2010 have resulted to the loss of a third of the country's street-work programmes (EKTEPN 2010); one survey of

275 drug users in Athens in October 2010 found 85 per cent were not on a drug-rehabilitation programme (EKTEPN 2010). Many new HIV infections are also linked to an increase in prostitution (and associated unsafe sex) (EKTEPN 2011). An authoritative report described accounts of deliberate self-infection by a few individuals to obtain access to benefits of €700 per month and faster admission into drug substitution programmes (EKTEPN 2011). The latter offer access to synthetic opioids and can have waiting lists of three or more years in urban areas.

Another indicator of the effects of the crisis on vulnerable groups is increased use of street clinics run by NGOs. Until recently, these primarily catered to immigrants, but the Greek chapter of Medicins du Monde (Doctors of the World) estimates that Greeks seeking medical attention from their street clinics rose from 3 to 4 per cent of the total pre-crisis to about 30 per cent (Karatziou 2011).

Despite many adverse signs, there are some indications of improvement. There have been marked reductions in alcohol consumption (Hellastat 2010) and, according to police data, drink-driving has decreased (EKTEPN 2010). These trends were not artefacts of reduced detection due to police force budget cuts, as police checks remained the same and more drivers were screened in 2009 than 2008.

Overall, the picture of health in Greece is concerning. It reminds us that, in an effort to finance debts, ordinary people are paying the ultimate price: losing access to care and preventive services, facing higher risks of HIV and STDs, and in the worst cases losing their lives. Greater attention to health and healthcare access is needed to ensure that the Greek crisis does not undermine the ultimate source of the country's wealth – its people.

Care Experiences: experiences from a Greek Primary Care Unit

Christos (Greece)

Last Thursday, I attended to a 46-year-old lady who had visited our Primary Care Unit. I noticed that she had lost weight since the last time I had seen her.

When I asked how I could help she asked me for a prescription for an anti-depressant drug. As I dislike prescribing such medicines without first listening to the patient and asking him/her to communicate their personal story, I invited the lady to tell me why she felt she needed such drugs.

The lady explained that her husband had owned a small enterprise in the town centre, wherein the eldest son had also worked. However, financial restraints had caused the business to close, and shortly

(continued)

(continued)

afterwards her husband had had a heart attack and was currently still unwell. The lady's two younger sons were having trouble at school, and were encountering learning difficulties.

I asked the lady how she spent her daily life, and she replied 'trying to find something to cook'. She told me that twice a week she visited rural areas looking for 'snails', in order to obtain food for two days. She said she also visited the local market for fruit and vegetables, and that she had a small garden where she was currently cultivating wild vegetables just to have something to eat.

I identified that this lady had potential thoughts of self-harm and suicide and I wanted to help her beyond my normal responsibilities as a medical doctor. I gave her my mobile number and my card, and I tried to communicate various coping styles to her. Suddenly the lady burst into tears, to the shock of myself and the nurses who were present at the time.

I told her that I would try to find her a small job, even if only a small cleaning job, and even if it would only provide 100 euros per month. This seemed to provide some hope to the lady, and she started to breathe again.

The experience allowed me to reflect on the fact that at these times of crisis my role needs to go beyond the usual responsibilities of prescribing and offering advice as a medical doctor. Such situations are not only about dealing with starvation, they are about offering kind words, networking, and providing compassion and hope.

I did of course prescribe the lady the anti-depressant tablets that she was seeking, but I explained that this was not the only therapy, and that alternatives such as Cognitive Behavioural Therapy which might help her to think differently was also an option . . . '

A new gateway to the world – (*Written outside the Church of* Panagia *Greece*)

Christos (Greece)

It was a warm day in June
The atmosphere was heavy with uncertainty
Visitors stood in silent grief

The cloudy and sad eyes of the young lady,

the usual dress of the patients in current time

The drug was over, the result of poverty, poverty is everywhere in this country.

The search for a permanent ray of light is a continuous expectation,

The tears that fell from the eyes of the young visitor radiated power assembled from years.

One world crystallized years collected throughout my academic life.

Hundreds of images of my childhood life, forgotten souls, memories, stories passing in front of me,

Images of immigrants, from Asia Minor, Armenians, sacrifices and falls of Greece

This is my new book.

Happiness or pain?

Joy's distillation or scar tissue in my soul?

It's my new world, my new life.

Outside the church of Panagia

The leaves of the trees give life to the sound and movement of the wind

The soul of my father, the souls of my ancestors and those who had not time to offer them.

Postscript to 'Omens of a Greek tragedy'

When we first wrote in *The Lancet* in October 2011, we called attention to the health consequences of the economic crisis in Greece. The then Minister of Health promptly responded in a World Health Organization conference:

> all vulnerable groups have access to health care, even if they have no health insurance at all, even if they are jobless, homeless, refugees or illegal immigrants . . . It is not the case [that the financial crisis deprives the Greeks of access to health care services].
>
> (Loverdos 2011)

To our dismay, the leadership did not take the mounting evidence of Greece's health crisis into consideration when designing health reforms and introducing additional austerity measures in the subsequent months (Economou *et al.* 2014). Instead, some Greek politicians and officials adopted techniques established previously by vested commercial interests to discredit evidence on the causes of ill health (Diethelm and McKee 2009, 2010). Denialism substituted for the lack of urgent policy action to address the health needs of the population (Kentikelenis *et al.* 2013).

Since then, a growing number of studies have linked the economic crisis and associated economic adjustment policies to adverse effects on public health (Economou *et al.* 2014). Mental health status has significantly worsened since the onset of the crisis: suicides (Kondilis *et al.* 2013), suicidality (Economou *et al.* 2011), and major depression (Economou *et al.* 2012) have markedly increased. Infectious diseases have also been affected (Bonovas and Nikolopoulos 2012). In particular, a rapid rise in HIV infections has been observed, driven largely by infections among injecting drug users; the number of new cases among this population rose from 14 in 2010 to 522 in 2012 (KEELPNO 2013). This coincided with a scaling back of resources available for HIV prevention services (ECDC 2012). Access to healthcare services and medicines has also declined following budget cuts. There has been a 40 per cent increase in unmet medical need between 2007 and 2011, mainly attributed to treatment being too expensive and long waiting lists (Eurostat 2013). The human stories behind these statistics have been conveyed in shocking detail by excellent investigative journalism (Kelland 2012; Daley 2012; Badawi 2013).

At the time of writing, several European countries are experiencing unprecedented welfare state cutbacks and reorganization of public health services (Karanikolos *et al.* 2013; Stuckler and Basu 2013). In these cases, health expenditure reduction is commonly the key consideration behind reforms. How should such changes be studied? Linking different levels of analysis is necessary to elaborate on the links between macro-level socioeconomic change (economic crisis, unemployment, welfare state retrenchment) to meso-level mechanisms (specific policy change, alternative care structures) to micro-level responses to adversity by individuals, families and communities. In the case of Greece, patients' experience of 'crisis' is the experience of long waiting lines, discontinued treatments, unobtainable medicines, high and hidden healthcare costs, and a demotivated health personnel. Further research is urgently needed to disentangle how rapid economic change affects the lives and health of individuals, socioeconomic groups, and communities.

Alexander E. Kentikelenis
King's College, Cambridge
November 2013

References

Avgenakis, E. (2011) Question: Dramatic increase in the number of suicides due to the economic crisis and rumors on the operation of networks of usurers and blackmailers; Reference number: 16171 Athens: Hellenic Parliament.

Badawi, Z. (2013) Greece – In Sickness and in Debt. BBC World Service [available at: www.bbc.co.uk/programmes/p01bn6m8, accessed on 16 July 2013].

Bonovas, S., Nikolopoulos, G. (2012) High-burden epidemics in Greece in the era of economic crisis. Early signs of a public health tragedy *Journal of Preventive Medicine and Hygiene* 53, 169V171.

Carassava, A. (2011) Crime casts Long Shadow over Athens *Los Angeles Times* (accessed on 31 May 2011).

Daley, S. (2012) Greeks Reeling From Health Care Cutbacks. *New York Times.* [available at: www.nytimes.com/2011/12/27/world/europe/greeks-reeling-from-health-care-cutbacks.html, accessed on 24 March 2012].

Diethelm, P., McKee, M. (2009) Denialism: What is it and how should scientists respond? *The European Journal of Public Health* 19, 2–4.

ECDC (2012) *Risk assessment on HIV in Greece.* Stockholm: European Centre for Disease Prevention and Control.

Economou, C., Kaitelidou, D., Kentikelenis, A., Sissouras, A., Maresso, A. (2013) The impact of the financial crisis on health and the health system in Greece. In: Thomson, S., Jowett, M., Evetovitis, T., Mladovsky, P., Maresso, A., Figueras, J. (eds), *The Impact of the Financial Crisis on Health and Health Systems in Europe* Copenhagen: European Observatory on Health Systems and Policies.

Economou, M., Madianos, M., Peppou, L.E., Patelakis, A., Stefanis, C.N. (2012) Major depression in the era of economic crisis: A replication of a cross-sectional study across Greece *Journal of Affective Disorders* 145, 308–314.

Economou, M., Madianos, M., Theleritis, C., Peppou, L.E., Stefanis, C.N. (2011) Increased suicidality amid economic crisis in Greece *The Lancet* 378, 1459.

EKTEPN (2010) Annual Report on the State of the Drugs and Alcohol Problem. Athens: Greek Documentation and Monitoring Centre for Drugs – EKTEPN.

EKTEPN (2011) Report of the Ad Hoc Expert Group of the Greek Focal Point on the Outbreak of HIV/AIDS in 2011. Athens: Greek Documentation and Monitoring Centre for Drugs – EKTEPN.

Eurostat (2011) News Release: Euro area and EU27 government deficit at 6.0% and 6.4% of GDP respectively. Luxembourg: Eurostat.

Eurostat (2013) EU-SILC Survey Data.

Eurostat. Cross-sectional European Union Statistics on Income and Living Conditions (EU-SILC), 2007 and 2009 users' database. Luxembourg: European Commission, Eurostat; released March 2011. Disclaimer: Eurostat has no responsibility for the results and conclusions which are those of the authors.

Hellastat (2010) Sector Study: Alcoholic Beverages. Athens: Hellastat.

Hellenic Statistical Authority (2011) Press Release: The Production Index in Industry recorded a decline of 8.0% in March 2011 compared with March 2010. Piraeus: Hellenic Statistical Authority.

Hellenic Statistical Authority (2011) Press Release: Unemployment rate at 16.6% in May 2011. Piraeus: Hellenic Statistical Authority.

Horton, R. (2011) Offline: Looking forward to some surprises *The Lancet* 377, 2164.

Karanikolos, M., Mladovsky, P., Cylus, J., Thomson, S., Basu, S., Stuckler, D., Mackenbach, J.P., McKee,M. (2013) Financial crisis, austerity, and health in Europe *The Lancet* 381(9874), 1323–1331.

Karatziou, D. (2011) Society in Humanitarian Crisis. *Kyriakatiki Eleftherotypia,* 24 July 2011.

Katsadoros, D., Bekiari, E., Karydi, K., Liakopoulou, E., Violatzis, A., Lytra, M., *et al.* (2011) Suicide Help Line 1018: Characteristics of callers for January–December 2010. 21st Panhellenic Conference of Psychiatry, Athens.

KEELPNO (2013) HIV/AIDS Surveillance in Greece, 31 12 2012. Athens: Center for Disease Control and Prevention.

Kelland, K. (2012) *Basic Hygiene at Risk in Debt-Stricken Greek Hospitals* Reuters. [available at: http://uk.reuters.com/article/2012/12/04/us-greece-austerity-disease-idUSBRE8B30NR20121204, accessed on 27 March 2012].

Kentikelenis, A., Karanikolos, M., Reeves, A., McKee, M., Stuckler, D. (2013) Greece's health crisis: From austerity to denialism *The Lancet*: in press.

Kondilis, E., Ierodiakonou, I., Gavana, M., Giannakopoulos, S., Benos, A. (2013) Suicide mortality and economic crisis in Greece: Men's Achilles' heel *Journal of Epidemiology & Community Health* 67(6), e1.

Krug, E.G., Mercy, J.A., Dahlberg, L.L., Zwi, A.B. (2002) The world report on violence and health *The Lancet* 360 (9339), 1083–1088.

Liakopoulou, T. (2011) Since last year private hospitals are in touble while NHS is doing better *Kathimerini* (accessed on 12 June 2011).

Loverdos, A. (2011) Response to Question by Member of Parliament, Reference number: 56885. Athens: Ministry of Health and Social Solidarity.

Loverdos, A. (2011) Social Determinants of Health and Development. Presentation at the WHO World Conference on Social Determinants of Health, Rio de Janeiro [available at: http://loverdos.gr/gr/index.php?Mid=68&art=2244, accessed on 24 March 2011).

McKee, M., Diethelm, P. (2010) How the growth of denialism undermines public health *BMJ* 341, c6950.

Paraskevis, D., Hatzakis, A. (2011) An Ongoing HIV Outbreak among Intravenous Drug Users in Greece: Preliminary Summary of Surveillance and Molecular Epidemiology Data. EMCDDA Early Warning System.

Paraskevis, D., Nikolopoulos, G., Tsiara, C., Paraskeva, D., Antoniadou, A., Lazanas, M., *et al.* (2011) HIV-1 outbreak among injecting drug users in Greece, 2011: A preliminary report *Euro Surveill* 16 (36), 19962.

Polyzos, N. (2011) ESY.net: Presentation of the Secretary General of the Ministry of Health and Social Solidarity. Athens: Ministry of Health and Social Solidarity.

Stuckler, D., Basu, S. (2013) *The Body Economic: Why Austerity Kills* New York: Basic Books.

Stuckler, D., Basu, S., Suhrcke, M., Coutts, A., McKee, M. (2009) The public health effect of economic crises and alternative policy responses in Europe: An empirical analysis *The Lancet* 374, 315–323.

Sundquist, K., Theobald, H., Yang, M., Li, X., Johansson, S.E., Sundquist, J. (2006) Neighborhood violent crime and unemployment increase the risk of coronary heart disease: A multilevel study in an urban setting *Social Science and Medicine* 62(8), 2061–2071.

Telloglou, T. (2011) Interview with Minister of Health Andreas Loverdos. In: Papahelas, A., Telloglou, T., Papaioannou, S. (eds), *Folders*. Greece: Skai TV.

Telloglou, T., Kakaounaki, M. (2011) Three weeks and one night on duty. In: Papahelas, A., Telloglou, T., Papaioannou, S. (eds), *Folders*. Greece: Skai TV.

Tsimas, P. (2011) *Erevna*. Greece: Mega TV.

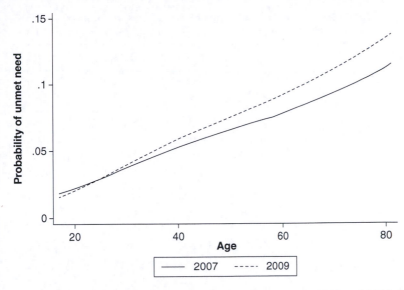

Figure 12.2 Probability of unmet medical need and age in 2007 and 2009 (lowess regression)

Web Appendix Table 12.1 Comparison of EU-SILC Greece survey socio-demographics, 2007 and 2009 waves

Variable	2007		2009		T-test	p-value
	n	Mean (Std. Dev)	n	Mean (Std. Dev)		
Age (17–81)	12346	49.78 (18.83)	15045	50.39 (18.82)	−2.6716	0.0076
Sex (male =1)	12346	0.48 (0.50)	15045	0.48 (0.50)	0.3814	0.7029
Family status (married =1)	12346	0.63 (0.48)	15045	0.63 (0.48)	−0.1258	0.8999
Degree of urbanisation (1-high, 3-low)	12346	2.16 (0.93)	15045	2.14 (0.93)	2.1398	0.0324
Education (1-lowest, 4-highest)	11899	1.97 (1.04)	14590	2.08 (1.07)	−8.0697	<0.0001

Web Appendix Table 12.2 Change in prevalence of key health indicators between 2007 and 2009, ages 17–81 (Odds ratios), weighted

Covariate	Bad self-reported health (bad or very bad=1)	Chronic illness	Health limitation	Unmet medical need	Unmet dental need
Financial crisis dummy	1.141*	1.02	1.064	1.150*	1.135*
	[1.015 to 1.283]	[0.934 to 1.113]	[0.970 to 1.167]	[1.015 to 1.303]	[1.006 to 1.281]
	(0.028)	(0.663)	(0.186)	(0.029)	(0.040)
Age	1.078***	1.086***	1.081***	1.030***	1.020***
	[1.069 to 1.087]	[1.081 to 1.092]	[1.075 to 1.087]	[1.024 to 1.037]	[1.014 to 1.025]
	(0.000)	(0.000)	(0.000)	(0.000)	(0.000)
Age 65 or older	0.709**	0.827*	0.98	0.686***	0.459***
	[0.569 to 0.884]	[0.714 to 0.957]	[0.835 to 1.149]	[0.551 to 0.853]	[0.368 to 0.573]
	(0.002)	(0.011)	(0.800)	(0.001)	(0.000)
Male	1.096	0.955	0.934	0.799***	0.993
	[0.964 to 1.245]	[0.872 to 1.045]	[0.848 to 1.029]	[0.704 to 0.908]	[0.880 to 1.121]
	(0.162)	(0.315)	(0.166)	(0.001)	(0.913)
Married	0.558***	0.648***	0.684***	0.874	0.915
	[0.487 to 0.639]	[0.584 to 0.718]	[0.614 to 0.762]	[0.756 to 1.010]	[0.792 to 1.058]
	(0.000)	(0.000)	(0.000)	(0.068)	(0.232)
Degree of urbanisation (1-high, 3-low)	1.008	0.909***	0.972	0.811***	0.832***
	[0.944 to 1.076]	[0.866 to 0.954]	[0.923 to 1.023]	[0.759 to 0.868]	[0.781 to 0.887]
	(0.817)	(0.000)	(0.280)	(0.000)	(0.000)
Education level (1-lowest, 4-highest)	0.645***	0.702***	0.671***	0.776***	0.773***
	[0.595 to 0.702]	[0.668 to 0.738]	[0.636 to 0.709]	[0.721 to 0.835]	[0.720 to 0.829]
	(0.000)	(0.000)	(0.000)	(0.000)	(0.000)

Notes: Odd ratios presented with 95% confidence intervals; p-values in parentheses. Number of individuals is 26,489.*p < 0.05, **p < 0.01, ***p < 0.001.

Web Appendix Table 12.3 Change in prevalence of unmet need for medical examination or treatment between 2007 and 2009, by reason for unmet need (weighted)

Covariate	Cannot afford care (1)	Waiting list (2)	Lack of time (3)	Too far to travel (4)	Wait to get better (5)	Other reasons (6)
Financial crisis dummy	0.867	1.828**	1.329	2.497**	1.931**	1.540*
	(0.082)	(0.001)	(0.174)	(0.004)	(0.003)	(0.029)
Age	1.030***	1.018*	1.002	1.034	1.036***	1.047***
	(0.000)	(0.047)	(0.818)	(0.108)	(0.001)	(0.000)
Age 65 or older	0.597***	1.624	0.309**	1.377	0.939	0.424*
	(0.001)	(0.126)	(0.008)	(0.526)	(0.851)	(0.012)
Male	0.744***	0.758	0.814	1.002	1.399	1.077
	(0.000)	(0.131)	(0.348)	(0.996)	(0.100)	(0.711)
Married	0.713***	1.199	5.562***	0.648	1.1	0.668
	(0.000)	(0.329)	(0.000)	(0.272)	(0.689)	(0.052)
Degree of urbanisation (1-high, 3-low)	0.801***	0.467***	0.884	2.898***	0.864	1.071
	(0.000)	(0.000)	(0.267)	(0.000)	(0.220)	(0.559)
Education level (1-lowest, 4-highest)	0.660***	0.864	1.169	0.685**	0.894	0.998
	(0.000)	(0.117)	(0.107)	(0.006)	(0.356)	(0.988)
Pseudo R-squared	0.0492	0.0726	0.0523	0.129	0.044	0.026
Sample size	26489	26489	26489	26489	26489	26489

Notes: Odd ratios presented; p-values in parentheses. Sample size is 26,489

1 Could not afford to (too expensive, not covered by insurance).
2 Waiting list (on actual waiting list, perception of the long waiting list or 'applied' and still waiting to see a medical specialist).
3 Could not take time because of work, care for children or for others.
4 Too far to travel/no means of transportation.
5 Wanted to wait and see if problem got better on its own.
6 Other reasons include fear of doctor/hospitals/examination/treatment, respondent didn't know any good doctor or specialist, refusal, other).

Web Appendix Table 12.4 Change in prevalence of access to social benefits between 2007 and 2009 (weighted)

Covariate	All benefits	Unemployment	Old age	Survivors	Sickness	Disability	Education
Financial crisis dummy	0.961	1.111	0.925	0.904	0.608*	1.025	0.988
	(0.421)	(0.257)	(0.188)	(0.305)	(0.040)	(0.840)	(0.972)
Age	1.103***	0.989**	1.174***	1.092***	1.019*	1.067***	0.903***
	(0.000)	(0.004)	(0.000)	(0.000)	(0.031)	(0.000)	(0.000)
Age 65 or older	3.492***	0.0645***	2.338***	0.521***	0.577	0.0470***	n/a
	(0.000)	(0.000)	(0.000)	(0.000)	(0.149)	(0.000)	
Male	1.752***	1.221*	3.618***	0.0634***	1.465	1.261	1.39
	(0.000)	(0.036)	(0.000)	(0.000)	(0.110)	(0.071)	(0.322)
Married	0.313***	1.325*	1.775***	0.00209***	0.824	0.407***	0.31
	(0.000)	(0.035)	(0.000)	(0.000)	(0.477)	(0.000)	(0.063)
Degree of urbanisation (1-high, 3 - low)	1.135***	1.276***	1.249***	0.713***	0.918	1.170*	0.580*
	(0.000)	(0.000)	(0.000)	(0.000)	(0.543)	(0.029)	(0.010)
Education level (1-lowest, 4-highest)	0.897***	0.886*	1.089**	0.705***	0.610**	0.500***	2.084***
	(0.000)	(0.014)	(0.009)	(0.000)	(0.002)	(0.000)	(0.000)

Notes: Odd ratios presented; p-values in parentheses. Sample size is 26,489 except for education with 19,891.

Part IV

Organizational issues

When considering the benefits of delivering care which is compassionate in nature, it is important to take into account organizational and structural elements which can affect both patients and healthcare providers. This section investigates organizational issues, current initiatives for addressing organizational issues, and the importance of avoiding 'compassion fatigue' within the organization. This section provides important links between the individual and the organization.

13 How good people can offer bad care

Understanding the wider factors in society that encourage non-compassionate care

Valerie Iles

Synopsis

That health care has changed from being a covenant of care between care giver and care receiver to a set of auditable transactions, performance managed by scrutiny of data dashboards, is largely a result, not of particular governments or managers, but of macro technological and societal changes.

These changes are themselves the results of some of our universal human longings and we cannot hope to influence the nature of care within our society unless we name and explore these factors and these longings.

If our care processes are to encompass human-to-human relating (and not all care does require this) we need to become aware of how our individual behaviours as citizens contribute to the diminishing of care. Only then can we approach NHS reform in ways that help rather than hinder.

Introduction

Blaming is very easy. When we hear descriptions of poor care, worse, scandalous care, it is a very human response. When we think about poor care across a system then there is even more. Health care professionals blame managers. Economists and policy makers blame the 'vested interests of the professions'. Everyone blames the short-termism of politicians. But this isn't helpful and distracts us from where our attention is needed.

Where is it helpful to direct our attention instead? To the technological and societal forces that form the environment within which health care is offered today, to the impact they have on the nature of care, and to the universal human longings that underlie those forces. Until we have named and explored these we will not be able to ensure our care systems offer care givers and receivers the space in which compassion can be practised, protected and valued.

In this chapter I explore some of the most significant of these forces, how we respond to them, and the kind of care that results. I then suggest ways in which we can respond differently and in so doing allow the practice of compassion to be nurtured and protected.

Background

Three years ago a group of thoughtful and experienced contributors to the NHS came together to form a Learning Set and explore how it is that good people can offer bad care. We set out explicitly to look beyond the economic and managerial literature to the fields of anthropology, sociology, political philosophy, psychology, moral philosophy and history, to explore in greater breadth and depth three significant issues: the dynamics of the patient-professional interaction; the allocation of resources in a liberal democracy; and the nature of professionalism.

We did so because we believed that when the economic/managerial paradigm was introduced to the NHS (and to British industry more widely) 30 years ago it was a hugely valuable addition to our ways of thinking, but that since it has swept aside those other ways and become the only game in town, its explanations and remedies are not wrong but impoverished, and are leading to the situation in which we find ourselves.

When we looked at these other schools of thinking we found descriptions that explained the world differently from the prevailing views of economists and policymakers, and also from those of healthcare professionals. We believe it is important to bring together into a coherent argument about how we are where we are and how we could, if we chose, be somewhere different. This chapter draws on the work of that Learning Set.

The technological and societal forces that form today's health care environment

Imagine a large blank sheet of paper. In each of the four corners we are going to write a factor that contributes to the circumstances in which healthcare finds itself today.

In the top left-hand corner let's put the public health measures and technological advances of the last 150 years. These have led to an increase in longevity, so let's write that down too, near that corner. That means there are a larger number of fit and healthy pensioners than in previous generations; and also a larger number of older people with multiple co-morbidities, who need ongoing treatment for their 'long term conditions'. These need to be written down too. So the pattern of disease has changed, and with it an expectation of longer life, and perhaps even a sense of entitlement to that. Perhaps too an assumption on the part of health professionals that this is wanted by everyone – and at whatever cost? Shall we write in some of that too?

In the top right-hand corner let's put the domination of the ideology of neo-liberalism, the marketisation agenda and globalisation. This has, in turn, led to a change in the nature of politics, from the role of reconciling different interests, to that of rationally administering the market place.

This growth in markets has led to many benefits, including increasing food supplies across the world so that our food budget is now only 10 per cent of our income whereas 100 years ago it was closer to 70 per cent. Over the last 30 years too millions of people in developing countries have been lifted out of poverty. However, it has also led to market concentration with many mighty global companies beyond the reach of national governments, and some of these, for example the food and leisure industries, arguably contributing to damage to public health.

In the bottom right-hand corner let's add the digital revolution – our ability to compare and contrast anything at all that can be represented by a code with anything else that can. This has had a huge impact on our lives, and a lot of beneficial consequences including for example a reduction in variation in the performance of individuals and organisations, as well as massive shifts in communication and entertainment. It has also led to a culture of audit across the West which has resulted in the following, which we may think are not so benign:

- A reduction in creativity, largely as a result of performance being measured against predefined objectives which are then given priority over addressing emerging issues innovatively.
- Valuing only the activities than can be codified, because only activities that can be measured are measured this privileges the use of explicit knowledge over tacit knowledge, and activity at the expense of thinking. Thus 'hyperactivity and discourse are privileged over wisdom and silence'.
- Not measuring what is happening, only how we are managing what is happening. Because of the difficulties in capturing the nature of 'first order activities' (the interactions between professionals and patients) it is not these that are monitored but second order processes or 'proxy measures' (things like boxes being ticked).
- Litigation increases because public understanding of professional decision-making processes becomes distorted by league tables and other forms of public dissemination of 'performance' data, and the lowest risk option is privileged in any decision even where there are sound arguments for other options.
- Evidence Based Medicine (EBM) rules the day – and its epistemological foundations are unchallenged: EBM has led to many improvements in care, but it has also led to a perceived hierarchy of evidence in which the RCT [Randomised Control Trial] trumps all others. This makes assumptions about the nature of medical knowledge that are left unsaid and untested. It leaves out of sight questions raised about different epistemologies in which, for example, considerations of complexity may be more valuable.
- Financial aspects become the key factor in clinical decision-making: information about costs and activity can be linked much more easily

than in the past and financial performance becomes a major criterion of organisational support for an activity. This runs counter to the whole concept of a national health service in which risks are pooled across the UK population.

• Policy makers set targets for easily measurable aspects of care and local leaders deliver on those narrow targets rather than achieving them by improving the system.

• Uncomfortable political decisions are moved sideways, so they are 'taken out of the political arena and recast in the neutral language of science'.

You will have noticed that the factors in the four corners don't exist in isolation, they all interact with each other, so, for example, we can see that the digital revolution combines with marketisation so that many more services are available 24/7, and that then leads to increased expectations for service delivery across all sectors including health care. This is sometimes characterised as 'the rise of the demanding consumer'. That's you and me!

Something else has happened too. I mentioned neo-liberalism as one of major factors taking a place in one of the four corners of our page. Neo-liberalism is a set of ideas that gained ground in the United States in the 1970s and has swept the Western (and increasingly Eastern) worlds. It is a politico-economic theory favouring free trade, privatisation, minimal government intervention in business, reduced public expenditure on social services, etc. and is just that – a theory. It was developed entirely rationally with little empirical evidence to support it. It has resulted in the world now being viewed through the lens of economists, instead of through that of sociologists, anthropologists, psychologists, historians or of real people operating in a real world. Economics itself is rooted in theory, and around the theoretical 'rational, self interested man'. These other schools of thinking (and we ourselves) focus on actual experiences, and real, complex, whole people. So this is a manifestation of a phenomenon (described by John Ralston Saul, in *Voltaire's Bastards: The Dictatorship of Reason in the West*) in which logic and reason trump practical experience (Saul 1993).

Another example of this also arises from the interaction of top and bottom right-hand corners (politics dominated by economics + the digital revolution). It is the move away from managing *people* to managing *performance*, from engaging person to person (one multifaceted, idiosyncratic, wonderful, flawed, irritating, emotional person interacting with another), to managing by checking nice clean, tidy, objective data, often in seductively compiled 'dashboards'.

So somewhere near the middle of our page we need to write MANAGERIALISM. The block capitals are those of Henry Mintzberg, the world's most cited management academic, who vividly describes how managers now focus on spurring on the performance of the people in their team, rather than engaging actively with them as people, talking with them about how to do things, supporting them when they are behaving in ways that are likely to be successful and challenging them when their behaviour is likely to be unproductive. 'All too often', (he says) 'when managers don't know what to do, they drive their subordinates to "perform"' (Mintzberg 2011). He suggests that experience, authenticity and intuition are much more important than logical analysis.

This preference for logic and reason over experience seems to arise from our desire to understand, our desire to know how something works, rather than being content that it does. From there it is not very far to speculating/reasoning/theorising about how things might work, what results ought to follow from an intervention, and so on. These are very interesting and our ability to do so has led to great technological advances, but they can also take on a greater persuasive ability than is borne out by facts and direct experience, especially when the systems we are dealing with are complex and not simple. Eugenics is one example. Macro economics another! We should always be careful when theories are not backed by evidence and experience, and we should not be afraid to rely on experience even when we do not understand the causal mechanisms involved.

We could also characterise this desire to understand, to KNOW, for certainty, as a manifestation of our inherent, existential anxiety, our anxiety to survive and thrive – both physically and socially. So let's think of the page we are writing on as representing our anxiety, our own and others.

In the bottom left-hand corner we now need to write the 2008 banking crisis. As we now know, banks across Europe had chosen to over-lend to the Eurozone periphery countries (exploiting the fact that their perceived risk was reduced as a member of the Eurozone) and effectively transferred their risk, and then their debts to their (our) national governments(Blyth 2013). Most of those governments, encouraged by the IMF, have imposed austerity programmes on their public spending, in a doomed but politically expedient attempt to reduce the debts transferred to them by the banks. The consequences of the austerity programmes will impact unevenly, and hit the most vulnerable the hardest ('recession hurts, its austerity that kills' (Stuckler *et al.* 2013)), so we can expect large increases in pressure on public services at a time when they are being squeezed. So the overall cap on spending and the increased need for services must be included on our paper too.

We have already seen that each of these corners interacts with all of the others and with the anxiety that is represented by the paper underlying them. You might like to note down other results you can think, of these interactions between them. You could also add ways in which they impinge upon you personally in your work or home lives. You may find that Figure 13.1 prompts some ideas.

The shaded boxes here look very neat and rather attractive on paper but in real life these are forces and factors that swirl around us like winds, acting and interacting with each other and with us. And if the piece of paper that we are writing on does represent our existential human anxiety – anxiety about mortality, morbidity, social and work relationships, our place in the world, and about everything else –then we need to think again about that swirl! I call it a swirl because it feels to us like a swirl of winds buffeting us. And just like real winds, we cannot ignore them or make them go away, but we can respond to them in ways that are helpful and do not fan the winds or we can add to the force of the winds by our own behaviours.

We must remember that the swirl isn't anybody's fault. And it isn't all bad. Nevertheless there is always a danger that in that swirl, and in our responses to it, something of value will go out of the world. So it is important that we fight for the things we see as important – of value to the world – and that other people do too. Most of all though, we will all be struggling to survive and thrive, to keep our place in the world, and in our struggle we may jeopardise things that other people value, and they will do so too.

Notice that I have used the phrase 'things of value go out of the world' and have not talked of 'trade-offs'. This is an example of where managerial language, sorry MANAGERIAL language, can so easily rob decisions of emotions that have an important part to play. Indeed MANAGERIAL language (remember this is different from managerial language) is always logical and reasonable, and its users talk of the importance of emotional intelligence, by which they usually mean that everyone should agree with them because they are being logical and reasonable. There are two quotes I like to keep in mind when dealing with MANAGERS, or when working with clinicians who are dealing with them and who have in desperation fallen into behaviours of blame and unproductive resistance. John Ralston Saul says 'the expression of any unstructured doubt is automatically categorized as naïve or idealistic . . . Bad for the economy or for jobs' and that is certainly what I see happening, and if you think of your own experiences you might recognise it too.

The other quote is from M. McDonald's chapter in the wonderful book edited by Marilyn Strathern, *Audit Cultures* (Strathern 2000): 'For anthropologists resistance to reforms is not to do with complacency, backwardness, laziness, inefficiency etc. Opposition is encapsulated in a whole symbolic complex through which people can feel their realities traduced'.

I try to keep in mind, too, the Buddhist concept that emotions are energy with a story attached, and that the energy is always a good and wonderful thing even if the story to which it's attached is unhelpful. If we can keep in mind that we are all responding to the swirl, then instead of wasting time and energy blaming individuals or groups and fighting *against* them, we can fight constructively *for* things that matter to us, forming coalitions to do so.

One of the results of this swirl is that health care is becoming diminished, the culture of audit, of MANAGERIALSIM, of marketisation, have led to care being envisaged as a set of auditable transactions in a market economy, instead of as a covenant of are between care giver and care receiver with an element of gift economy in both directions. The difference between these two kinds of care are summarised in Figure 13.2.

As you look at it please try to keep in mind that the transactions that comprise the left-hand column (caring *for* people) are also part of the right-hand (caring *about* them), after all it would be impossible to care about someone and not also care for them. And also that there are many occasions on which the left-hand column is all that is needed. So it is not that transactional care is wrong (or poor) and covenantal (or relational) care is right (or good), but that good care will involve deciding which of these is needed where, or perhaps here – in this situation in front of you.

The trouble is that only the transactional aspects of care are measurable, i.e. codifiable. The relational aspects of care do not lend themselves to being coded or counted; they are much richer than can be represented in such a limited way.

If we care about the UK having an NHS that can offer care as a covenant (when that is needed) we have to find ways of convincing funders, and their/our representatives – governments – and patients, that we are using resources wisely and compassionately. We must therefore find ways of describing and discussing care as a covenant, and ways that are sufficiently independent and hard edged to withstand the suspicion that health care professions are merely protecting their own interests.

Often, in a discussion about this, professionals, especially doctors, will point out that doctors are one of the most trusted groups in society and politicians the least. There is often an air of self-satisfaction and blame about this (!) and that is not at all helpful. The history of reform after reform of the NHS has largely been prompted by frustration on the part of policy makers at the lack of preparedness on the part of professionals to reflect on and redesign services to meet the needs of patients rather than their own convenience and ambitions, and to take a full part in difficult decisions about how to use resources wisely and well. We could almost see this as professionals not using their professional expertise and judgement to play a proper part in the 'swirl', choosing instead to almost take it 'personally' as 'doctor bashing' instead of as a set of forces that impinge upon everyone, and the weakest and most vulnerable the most.

Let's reflect for a moment on these levels of trust. If we do we can see that politicians have given doctors the most fantastic privilege of being able to dispense back to us our own generously, collectively, donated largesse. Naturally then doctors are trusted more than politicians whose role is the inherently unpopular one of reconciling different interests, and who have to subject themselves to re-election by an electorate who don't have the patience to explore the complexities of an issue and instead make their choice based on sound bites.

This is something for doctors to celebrate and enjoy, not use as a weapon against those (or an excuse to avoid) doing a job they themselves could and should participate in – making difficult decisions, with no right or wrong answers, about how best to use resources.

The reason I have laboured this point is that we (all of us) are ourselves an integral part of the swirl. Our own anxiety leads us to make responses to what is going on around us that make the situation worse. We contribute to the dangers facing care just as much as anyone else does. Indeed one way of thinking about the factors is that they are winds that are made up of the breaths of each and every one of us – and while we will not, on our own, be able to halt them we can and should stop adding our breath to them.

We breathe with them largely as a result of our own anxiety, an emotion we find uncomfortable, despite it being very valuable. If we were prepared to accept our anxiety, accept that it is inherent in the health care task and even the most experienced of practitioners will be anxious on occasion, we might even welcome it as a reminder that this is an occasion when we need to take extra care, then we might be able to respond very healthily to it. A healthy response to anxiety includes some or all of the following:

- noticing an unpleasant feeling of anxiety
- bringing it into awareness
- reflecting on the source of it
- seeking support where we need it
- thinking carefully through the needs and wishes of the other
- reminding ourselves of our sense of purpose
- bringing together our own concerns with those of the person who has prompted our anxiety
- deciding to embark on a course of 'aware altruism'
- or of meaningful dialogue with the other the outcome of which cannot be anticipated
- seeking support from someone more experienced in a particular procedure or situation.

This is something we can address as individuals, but we can and must support the ability of *all* our health staff to respond to anxiety in these healthy ways. We must draw on what we know from evolutionary psychology (described in other chapters in this book) and help individuals and teams to ensure that their three major emotional systems (fight/flight; seeking and finding; and soothing and contentment (Gilbert 2009)) are in balance. This will mean a change in our routine organisational processes so that they are no longer primarily risk based but allow elements such as celebration and mourning, connection with others, and the setting of wholesome care ambitions rather than ruthlessly monitored targets. (Think of the routine ward handover processes as you read this list and you may find you see what I mean).

So, I want to leave you with these thoughts.

In the next 48 hours you will be confronted by many of the factors you have drawn on your sheet of paper, and you can respond in an aware manner and healthily to them and contribute to nurturing the ability of the system to offer care that is a covenant, when what is covenant is wanted and needed. Or you can respond in ways that push us closer towards care a set of transactions. What you do will make the system more or less compassionate. Whether the kind of care we have read about on a few wards in Mid Staffs continues or not depends on you as much as it depends on anyone else.

Because although these forces swirl around us like winds, they are made up of billions or trillions of breaths. And you can either add your breaths to them, or you can breathe against them. You won't make them go away but you can stop making them stronger.

Indeed as you think more deeply about this over time you will find that everything in life can be approached as a transaction or as a covenant – and there will be times when each is more appropriate. But you may also find that as you bring these choices into awareness you choose more and more the covenant in whatever you are doing.

But choosing, choosing wisely and being aware is the important thing. For all of us – including and especially me and you.

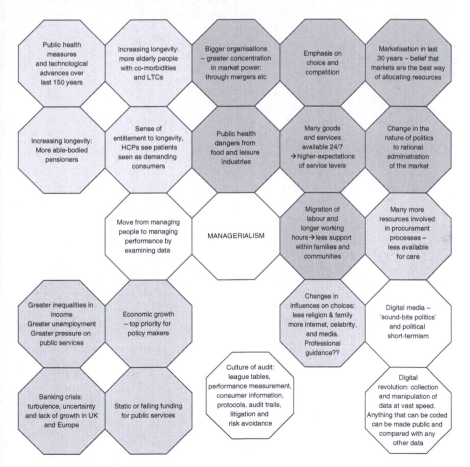

Figure 13.1 Representation of 'swirl'

Transactional care	Covenantal care
Health care as a set of auditable transactions: patient as consumer, professional as provider	*Health care patient and professional are in covenantal relationship*
Patient is cared for	Patient is cared about as well as for
Professionals are seen as givers (or suppliers) of services	Professionals recognise that in their encounters with patients they give *and* receive
Focus on calculation and counting – this can be seen as objective	Focus on thoughtful, purposeful judgement – this is necessarily subjective but incorporates objective measures and evidence
Predetermined protocols	Emergent creativity which can include the use of protocols
Discourse and hyperactivity	Wisdom and silence in addition to discourse and action
Explicit knowledge	Tacit knowledge as well as explicit knowledge
Reflection on facts and figures	Reflection on feelings and ethics as well
Focus on efficiency and effectiveness	Focus on the quality of the moment as well
Dealing with the presenting problem	Keeping in mind the meaning of the encounter – for both parties - while addressing the presenting problem
Competence is what is called for on the part of the professional	The humanity of the professional is also called upon
Individuals have a relationship with the state and with the market	Individuals have a relationship with the community and with wider society
Good policy ideas MUST degenerate as they are translated at every level of the system into a series of measurable, performance manageable actions and objectives. The focus here is on being able to demonstrate the policy has been implemented.	Policy ideas can stay rich and be added to creatively, so that solutions are responsive, humane, practical, flexible, and adaptable. Here the focus is on implementing the spirit and intent of the policy.

Figure 13.2 Differences between transactional and covenantal care

Care Experiences: a Saturday night in the ER . . .

Kathi (Greece)

It was Saturday night and we had arranged with a couple of friends to go out for dinner. We were a little late and as we had invited these friends, it would be nice to be there to welcome them . . .

I was delaying . . . I had a lot still to do . . . the next morning I was leaving for a conference for which I had the responsibility and had not even prepared my address . . . My husband called me for the third time . . . before going down the stairs I remembered that my netbook was not charged, I picked in a hurry the power cable and went down the staircase. Midway, I made a false step, I couldn't regain equilibrium, the cable fell off my hands, my feet get tangled in it, and oops, I fell against the wall, while I leaned with my hand against the wall to reduced the impact of the fall . . .

That was it!! I got immediately that gut feeling that something went terribly wrong . . . and it did! The sudden acute pain did not less much guess work . . . I sat on the staircase holding my wrist. I mumbled something like it's broken.

A few minutes later we were at the ER of the nearby Accidents Hospital. It was almost 10.00 p.m. The hand was already swollen, very painful. The number of wounded people waiting their turn diluted any hopes of quick relief. When I managed to get to the triage desk where a nurse and a doctor were busy giving instructions, writing notes about previous patients, I still had to wait. The doctor without looking at me asked what brought me there. I told him that most probably I had a complete fracture of the wrist. He looked up at my wrist said: 'looks like one' and he gave me a referral for an X-ray.

In my haste and disarray to go to the hospital, I did all the dumb things: I didn't take an analgesic, I didn't take with me something like a stretcher e.g. a ruler, a towel to rest the hand and most important an icepack. Thus, while waiting for more than two hours my turn for an X-ray the pain became unbearable, and made me scream when the radiologist tried to put it in place. When I asked her 'can you please handle it with care? it's uttely painful', the answer was an indifferent 'I need to put in the right angle, let me do my job' . . .

I came out in tears from the pain, not able to find a position that made it less painful. I had to wait an hour more for the X-ray results and when I got it was tell-tale: comminuted fracture of the wrist. I went back with my X-ray to the orthopaedic surgeon, but I was told I had to wait as other patients and new serious accidents had come in.

(continued)

(continued)

I returned back to my seat sweating and trembling from the unbearable pain . . . the night had advanced, it was past 1.00 a.m. and I had no indication when a doctor could see me. In the examination hall with ten beds separated by curtains, reigned chaos with patients coming and going, only two doctors and a nurse for more than twenty patients, with broken arms, legs, car and bike accidents, falls and more. As for cleaning, basic housekeeping, it seems these were forgotten under the steady flow of patients. Doctors and nurses did not bother about patients' modesty, they asked patients to undress without drawing the curtains; no care was taken to change the disposable bed sheet for the next patient, nor to explain what they were going to do to them . . .

I pulled up my courage and went again into the examination room determined to ask for a strong analgesic and learn when a doctor would see me. No doctor or nurse was at sight but I caught one nurse in the corridor:

'Could you please help me, I need a strong analgesic as my hand aches terribly.'

'We don't dispense medicines here, but you may go to the pharmacy outside the hospital and buy one', and she went away.

I looked at her incredibly, how could she be so cruel? She should know from experience what it is like to have a broken arm and that the pharmacy was closed, as it was not on duty that night . . . It appalled me that the hospital had a complete lack of compassion and interest for the crowds of seriously and not so seriously wounded that arrive continuously . . . there was not the slightest sign of compassion or comfort while waiting to be examined from the triage nurse, the admissions desk clerk, the radiologist . . . but the worst was still to come . . .

I pulled myself up and looked for another nurse. I found one and went to her and asked decisively for an analgesic. She answered she didn't have but that she would find an injection that would do the job. She asked me to wait . . . It was 2.00 a.m. and I was a wreck both physically and psychologically as I feared the verdict of the orthopaedic surgeon. After half an hour I spotted her again and asked for the injection. OK she said, wait for me here. So, I waited for her in an empty cubicle that a patient had just left. She came back and asked me to take down my pants. I looked at the dirty examination bed. No need to lay down, she said, just pull down your pants.

Of course, I couldn't as I was holding my broken arm. I asked her to help me . . . and if she didn't mind to pull the curtain. No need she said, no one is going to see whatsoever, I just need your upper thigh . . . I was exhausted, I surrendered . . .

Around 2.30 a.m. I got hold of a doctor, what is the case with me? What can you do for my hand? She said something, 'will try to put in place, I wait for another doctor . . . ' while she was already looking at the cubicle in front of her with the old lady who had fallen from the bed and broken her arm . . . I insisted 'can you please explain to me what kind of a fracture is it? what you will do?'. No answer, only an evasive: 'Return to the waiting room, you will be called.'

At 3.00 a.m. I had lost all remnants of patience from unbearable pain and the five hours waiting. I enquired about the doctor and found her in an argument with an intern. I asked her if she could see me now, she threw me a 'Yes, wait for me in the plaster room'. The nurse that was applying the plaster cast to patients, however, had gone an hour ago, saying he would be back in 20 minutes.

I thought that the doctor would give instructions to the plaster cast nurse on how to apply the cast. I had made the wrong guess as I realised in a few minutes. She came in the plaster room together with the intern while continuing to argue over whether she had to take also more serious cases that night. I was sitting on the bed. Lie, she ordered while continuing her argument . . . I did as well as I could . . . She pulled my hand. I screamed: what are you doing? it aches . . . it's broken.

She didn't pay attention, and continued talking to her colleague who was getting hold of my elbow. At that time I got really angry and shouted at her: 'What are you doing? you are supposed to take care of my hand and instead you are shouting to the intern and pull my hand, as it were an inanimate object. Stop arguing and tell me what is all this fuss!'

At that moment, the intern understood the awkward of the situation: instead of examining the fracture and discussing what were the best movements for putting it back in place, explain to the patient the procedure, they continued their discussion without paying any attention to the patient, they didn't even look at me, they were handling the broken hand as if it were a piece of wood. In fact, the patient was 'interrupting' their discussion . . . He asked her to calm down and told me they would try to put the fracture in place. I still did not know what that meant . . .

At that moment, the plaster nurse arrived and the three of them without further set at the job, the doctor holding and pulling the hand, the intern pulling in opposite direction above the wrist and the nurse puling the elbow. I screamed from the unbearable pain as I have not screamed in my whole life, I had almost fainted when the nurse told me the plaster was ready but that I needed to wait till it hardened before going for another X-ray . . .

(continued)

(continued)

I felt weak, humiliated by the behaviour of these doctors, who left after they washed their hands without a single word to the patient, without informing me at least of the next steps. For them, I was not a person, I was just another 'object of care' to which it was enough to perform the mechanistic movements of care . . .

New wait, new unbearable handling in the X-ray room, new wait to see the doctor: Final verdict: 'comminuted fracture, the replacement is considered satisfactory for the kind of fracture but not perfect, meaning that it may leave some kind of ankylosis that you may improve with physiotherapy . . . '

I did not want to hear more from her . . . I left the hospital and hope never to have to go back again . . . the story does not finish here, but the rest of it is another story: a story of compassion to be told another time.

References

Blyth, M. (2013) *Austerity: The History of a Dangerous Idea.* New York: Oxford University Press.

Gilbert, P. (2009) *The Compassionate Mind: A New Approach to the Challenge of Life.* London: Constable & Robinson.

Mintzberg, H. (2011) *Managing.* Harlow: Prentice Hall.

Saul, J.R. (1993) *Voltaire's Bastards: The Dictatorship of Reason in the West.* New York: Vintage Books; London: Penguin Books.

Saul, J.R. (2009) *The Collapse of Globalism.* London: Atlantic Books.

Strathern, M. (ed.) (2000) Audit Cultures: Anthropological Studies, In: *Accountability, Ethics and Academy.* London: Routledge.

Stuckler, D., Basu, S. (2013) *The Body Economic: Why Austerity Kills.* London: Allen Lane.

14 Current initiatives for transforming organizational cultures and improving the patient experience

Susan Frampton and Joanna Goodrich

Introduction

Many of us have been patients at some point in our lives. Most of us have loved ones who have been in hospitals or nursing homes. These personal experiences teach us a great deal about what is most important to people when they are ill and in need of care. Sometimes the care experience is not optimal and can leave a person feeling that they have been robbed of their dignity and humanity, and determined that the system must change. Changing the entrenched culture found in hospitals and health systems, widely considered to be the most complex organizations existing today (IOM 2001), is particularly challenging. Inherent in this challenge is the significant power differential that traditionally exists between those highly trained professionals delivering care, and people who are often at their most vulnerable when in the role of "patient." Planetree has dedicated itself to addressing this imbalance and the work of the Point of Care programme at The Kings Fund, which is based in England, has focused on the role of staff in creating person-centered environments. Both organizations have pioneered unique ways of integrating the patient perspective into organizational change efforts This chapter presents insights into this transformational work with patients and staff. Planetree is a non-profit patient advocacy organization that was established in the U.S. originally, and now has partner offices in Europe, South America, and Canada, as well as affiliated providers in several additional countries.

Planetree model of patient-centered care (Frampton)

Creating organizational cultures that support and encourage patient involvement in their own care and true partnerships between patients, families and clinicians, begins with a willingness to listen to and value all perspectives. Successful healthcare culture change models must be grounded in the patient's perception of the care experience, and often the experiences that galvanize a patient to agitate for change are not positive ones.

One such patient was Angelica Thieriot, who established Planetree as a non-profit organization in 1978. Angie, a native of Argentina, found herself admitted to a typical U.S. hospital in the late 1970s with a life-threatening illness. The setting was incredibly institutional and alien, and the care largely impersonal and mysterious. Being hospitalized was more traumatic than coming close to death, and the experience motivated her to do whatever she could to change the system.

While Angie felt she had received appropriate clinical care in what appeared to be a clean and efficient environment, the impersonal quality of care and lack of access to meaningful information about her condition and treatment rendered it a very poor healing experience. From her point of view as a patient, she experienced many aspects of the environment of care that were obstacles to healing. She described a setting not unlike a prison, with bare white walls, excessive noise and disturbances to sleep throughout the night including bright overhead lights being turned on multiple times, limitations placed on visitation by her loved ones, and inadequate access to her own medical information:

> As a patient I rebelled against being denied my humanity and that rebellion led to the beginnings of Planetree. We should all demand to be treated as competent adults, and take an active part in our healing. And we should insist on hospitals meeting our human need for respect, control, warm and supportive care, a harmonious environment and good, healthy food. A truly healing environment.
>
> (Thieriot 2010)

Angie believed that she survived her hospital experience in large part due to compassion – in particular the compassion of two nurses who came into her room after she had been hospitalized for several days and was close to death, and called her by name. This was the first time staff had called her by name, and encouraged her to work with them and help with her own healing process. The recognition that she was a unique individual with a name and not just another "case" helped Angie to re-engage in her own recovery process.

Angie came away from this experience with a vision of what a truly healing hospital could be. She envisioned a place where the whole person would be supported – body, mind and spirit. A place where caring, kindness and respect were as highly valued as a good clinical or technical outcome, and where the patient's perspectives would be listened to and used to change the way care was delivered. She founded Planetree and dedicated it to the "personalization, humanization and demystification" of healthcare. She chose as a name the type of tree that Hippocrates, father of modern medicine, sat under to teach the very first medical students, symbolizing the need to recognize the holistic approach at the roots of modern medicine.

Her own experience had clarified for her the powerful potential for a holistic approach to profoundly affect the behavior of care providers and the health outcomes of their patients. She continued to explore various elements of a patient-centered model of healthcare, and this led eventually to the establishment of the very first Planetree model site, a 13-bed medical/surgical unit that opened in 1985 at a large medical center in San Francisco. The unit was supported by several grants from local philanthropic foundations. The success of this unit and several other experimental sites eventually led to expanded adoption of the model and its related implementation methodologies for sustainable culture change. (Martin *et al.* 1998) Currently, the model is being used in hundreds of settings throughout the United States, Canada, and at many sites in Europe and Latin America. This widespread adoption has been aided by the global movement toward patient and person-centric care, and the growing evidence-base supporting core components of the Planetree model (Stone 2008). The Planetree organization currently is organized as a membership and consultation services provider, and its operations are supported primarily through dues, consultation fees, government contracts and foundation grants. Partner offices have been established in several countries through licensing agreements between Planetree International and local entities committed to developing vibrant patient-centered networks in their region. These partners bring a deep understanding of the local healthcare system and cultural context to the work, and contribute to the ongoing growth and development of a global Planetree advocacy network.

In addition to partner offices, Planetree's model has been adapted for use in healthcare settings in many other countries of the world, including in hospitals and health systems in Asia and Africa. The model is flexible, and emphasizes what is most important to the people serving and being served in a wide variety of care settings, from hospitals and health centers, to nursing homes and home care settings. The elements of high-quality, patient-centered care, as well as effective implementation approaches, are similar despite significant differences in the way healthcare systems may be organized and financed.

The model itself comprises ten core components defined by patients as essential to a quality experience. Using these components as a framework to first assess an organization's culture and then identify opportunities for improvement provides a comprehensive framework for patient-centered culture change. These key areas include elements such as compassionate human interactions, involvement of family and friends, access to information, creation of a healing environment, and spiritual support.

Essentials of organiational culture change

Although Planetree's beginning was a very grass-roots effort, in most healthcare organizations a sustainable patient-centered culture starts with capable, visionary leadership. Termed, "transformational leadership" for its ability to truly alter an organization, compassionate human interactions must be evidenced from the board room to the patient's bedside. Specific relationship-building strategies such as leadership rounds, consistent face-to-face meetings with staff at all levels of the organization, transparent communication and the ability to consistently inspire staff to exemplify the organization's mission builds organizational capacity for compassion. (Stevenson 2002).

While the patient experience remains at the center of change initiatives, much of the initial focus is on the employees – both their role and ideas for enhancing the environment of care.

It is well recognized that staff morale impacts patient satisfaction. Research shows when healthcare staff are satisfied with their workplace, this positively influences the care they provide their patients (McHugh 2011). A recent Gallup Education Poll study found only 30 percent of American employees are engaged at work. Engaged employees were defined as those who, are "involved and enthusiastic about their work." Non-engaged employees were shown to be satisfied with their workplace but were "not emotionally connected to them" (Marklein 2013). Organizational change efforts therefore must focus on staff to both sensitize them to the patient experience and gather their thoughts and ideas for improving the environment in which they work and deliver care. Listening to staff and acting upon their ideas and solutions often results in improvements not only in the patient experience, but improved workplace satisfaction and retention of valuable employees (Spence Laschinger *et al.* 2009).

The roles of staff and management in these change efforts were examined in a recent study focused on the Planetree model implementation process (Béliveau 2013). The research sought to identify elements essential to successful knowledge transfer in a variety of clinical settings, in order to facilitate effective and efficient spread of the model. Four phases were identified as critical to successful and sustainable organizational culture change: launching, securing, anchoring, and monitoring. During the initiation of change efforts, a description of the model and the approach to be used in the change efforts was communicated to all employees. The commitment of the leadership team was explicitly demonstrated, and initiation of the implementation process according to the context of the individual setting ensued. Common difficulties to overcome at this stage included employee skepticism of the approach, sensitivity around the potential misperception by staff that they weren't compassionate enough and therefore needed to change, and a lack of understanding of the Planetree model and its foundations. Being attentive to the need for information, affirming and recognizing what is already in place and working well in the organization, and focusing on the new approach as a way to improve the patient experience facilitated a successful launch.

Following this was a phase in which the model and related approaches were translated and adapted in ways that made sense for the specific organizational setting, including connecting improvement strategies back to activities already in place or underway. Strengthening these activities by incorporating recommendations gathered from patients, families and direct care givers, and communicating this widely, ensured employee engagement and commitment.

This engagement then led to a phase in which stakeholder commitment supported implementation of the approach through attitudes and behaviors, as well as in processes and practices. Staff concerns that were found to impact change adoption at this stage included the perception that the approach required more work, that some but not all managers were truly committed to the approach, and that there were relatively few visible results for staff members and/or patients. Ensuring that all staff had a concrete understanding of expectations for organizational results, and that all achieved improvements were well publicized internally and their added value clearly communicated, were important facilitators at this stage. Once the model and related approaches were securely anchored within the organization, the final monitoring phase ensued. At this stage, assessing progress of the strategies employed and making ongoing adjustments and improvements became the focus. Recognizing that organizational culture change is an ongoing process, and that periodic adjustments and innovations are an integral part of the process, is essential to long-term success and sustainability.

The need for continued innovation to sustain a vibrant organizational culture is one that can be supported by participation in a global learning community. The network of Planetree member hospitals, clinics and long-term care communities continues to contribute to the evolution of patient-directed policies, procedures and designs, serving as living laboratories for development of more compassionate organizational cultures. The members share the understanding that the majority of healthcare environments have been designed primarily for the convenience of providers and their tools and technology. They share a desire to modify this so that the basic needs of the human beings receiving care are supported in a kind and caring way. They acknowledge that many in healthcare leadership have lost sight of an essential component of the healing partnership – that of a caring human relationship. Increasingly our hospitals have moved nursing staff away from the bedside, into centralized areas where they can do their work undisturbed by the patients and their families. As the technological sophistication of medical care has increased exponentially, our ability to provide meaningful information and education to patients in ways they can understand has been challenged. The role of the family and community to assist in the care and support of the patient has been minimized over time, as reflected in organizational policies that limit family presence and involvement and in the lack of adequate space available for families in many healthcare settings.

One of the most significant remaining challenges to creating truly patient-centered cultures is to operationalize the concepts into defined practices, and measure the results of implementation efforts. Many health systems around the world today support the concepts of humanization of care and person or patient-centered philosophies of care (Frampton *et al.* 2013) and yet relatively few healthcare organizations are successfully *doing* it. In 2005, Planetree initiated a project to identify a set of common practices found at our most successful member hospitals and health centers. Success was defined as having achieved some of the highest levels of patient and staff satisfaction following implementation of the Planetree model, along with the highest quality of clinical care, as defined by sets of standardized care process and outcome measures (Williams *et al.* 2005). These common organizational structures and practices were then developed into a set of patient-centered designation criteria and a process to encourage, assist, measure and recognize those organizations able to meet the criteria. During the test phase of the patient-centered designation project, data comparing the scores of the six participating hospitals to national benchmarks revealed an encouraging relationship between adoption of these common practices and better performance on patient experience scores and clinical process of care measures (Frampton *et al.* 2009). This correlation has continued to be demonstrated in the more than 40 acute and long-term care settings that have since achieved designation in the U.S., Canada, the Netherlands and Brazil (Planetree Contributes to National Priorities Partnership Report 2011). One of the very unique features of this designation process is the integral role of patients, their families and their direct care givers. Each organization applying for recognition at the gold level must be able to validate, through focus groups and interviews with patients and staff members, that each of the 55 criteria are indeed in place and a part of the lived experience of care. These criteria include such practices as patient-directed visitation, open access to

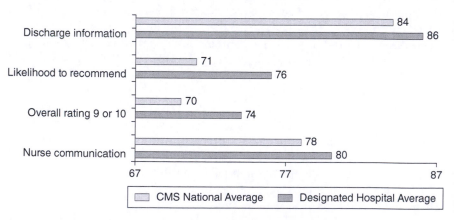

Figure 14.1 Comparison of U.S. Planetree Designated Hospital Patient Satisfaction Measures Average Scores and CMS National Average Reporting Time Period: 1 July 2011 – 30 March 2012

medical records, patient and family involvement in developing treatment and care plans, establishment of patient and family advisory councils, and provision of compassionate communications training for staff.

Patient-centered, compassionate care will never be fully realized until patients are woven into the fabric of healthcare organizations' structures and functions. Planetree has historically deeply listened to and captured the voices of patients and family members discussing their experiences of care and mined these rich insights to inform the model and its components. Seating patients at the conference table to discuss healthcare quality and safety, "routine" processes and procedures changes the tenor of the conversation and adds a compelling perspective to the work of finding compassionate, humane solutions in approaches to care. It is in the co-creation of these solutions by patients and healthcare employees that the best in compassionate care will be fulfilled and compassionate healthcare organizations will be actualized (Taloney and Flores 2013).

In the spirit of continuous quality improvement of our own organizational efforts, Planetree launched a reinvigorated compassion campaign in 2013. This effort began with a focus on our own staff, and included provision of books, discussion groups and webinars on compassion. We then developed compassion tool kits for healthcare providers, adopted the "Compassion in Action" theme for our annual conference and annual Patient-Centered Care Awareness month, developed webinars and educational presentations on "The Business Case for Compassion" for healthcare leaders, and integrated related materials and resources into our "Patient-Centered Nursing" online certification program. The next innovation under development is a motivational tool for healthcare leaders, the "Planetree Compassion Quotient," a composite measure for compassionate, patient-centered culture. The literature suggests that compassion and empathy may be positively impacted: "The exciting news from research is that empathy seems to be a mutable trait. Certain conditions can blunt expressions of empathy and, conversely, certain awareness-building and reflection activities seem to be able to up-regulate empathic behavior" (Malloy and Otto 2012). Integrating coaching and continuing education for healthcare providers that supports compassionate behaviors, and providing a means to measure the impact of such activities over time, may be a catalyst for organizational transformation on a global scale, resulting in healthcare systems that deliver safe, high-quality, *compassionate* care across the continuum.

Introduction to the Point of Care Foundation (Goodrich)

The King's Fund is an independent charitable foundation which aims to improve health and healthcare in England. In 2007 the Point of Care programme was established at The King's Fund, with the twin aims of improving patients' experience in hospital and improving the experience of staff who work in hospitals. In 2008 we published a report "Seeing the person in the patient." The report drew on a literature review, and also drew on our own research with carers and staff in hospitals, and attempted to answer the questions – what do we mean by patient-centered care? How do we know what it is like, and are there any promising interventions to improve care? It was clear that a systematic approach was needed to improve patients' experience in hospital at an individual and at a system level, much in the same way that patient safety has been tackled (Berwick *et al.* 2006). Over the next few years the Point of Care programme has combined research and action, to work with patients and staff together to improve services in hospital, [using an approach called experience-based co-design,]; running a collaborative learning program with hospital teams to improve care [the Patient and Family Centred Care programme] and to pilot an approach to supporting staff to provide compassionate care – Schwartz Center Rounds®. In 2013, The Point of Care Foundation was established as a new and separate charity, to take forward the work of the Point of Care programme, including Schwartz Center Rounds, funded currently by grants from the government's Department of Health, and by Macmillan Cancer Care.

This chapter focuses on the importance of paying attention to staff well-being, We knew that reported stress of health service staff in England is greater than in the general working population and accounts for more than one quarter of staff absence, which itself is higher than in other sectors (Department of Health 2009). Moreover, a workshop held at The King's Fund in 2009 looked at the challenge of providing compassionate care and explored what the barriers might be (Firth-Cozens and Cornwell 2009). A mix of academics and practitioners discussed empathy and compassion and their relationship with stress and burnout. Our work at the Point of Care programme (and now at the Foundation) has built on this, as well as drawing on theoretical and psychological literature. We believe that it is important to understand the context and nature of care in hospitals.

What we know about the nature of the work in hospitals

Context

In recent years hospital activity, especially unplanned work, has been steadily increasing. In England, the number of inpatient hospital admissions, both elective and non-elective has increased to more than 9 million and 5 million respectively per year. There are now about 20 million accident and emergency (A&E) attendances a year, and 20 million outpatient attendances a year (HESOnline (IP) and DH (A&E and OP) 2011).

The number of people working in hospitals over the past 10 years has also increased significantly, with more hospital consultants, nurses and allied health professionals. Non-clinical NHS staff, including managers, porters and administrative staff, traditionally account for about half of all personnel in the NHS, and has also increased (NHS Information Centre 2011). This growth in size and staff numbers, along with the use of new technology and the increased pace of organizational life, have had knock-on effects on relationships between individuals and colleagues and patients. Staff say they miss the personal relationships, face-to-face contact, corridor conversations and informal meetings in the canteen (NHS Confederation and Joint Medical Consultative Council 2007).

In spite of the increase in staff numbers, relationships between staff and patients are more short-term, with less time to get to know patients individually. The increasing specialization in medicine, nursing and the allied health professions, in the context of the continuous striving for greater efficiency, has reduced contact time between individual patients and individual members of staff, and patient care has become more fragmented. The average length of stay has fallen (HES online 2011). Patients over 65 account for 70 percent of hospital bed days and 80 percent of emergency readmissions. More people, in more specialties and departments, are involved in looking after the same patient. The typical inpatient day is increasingly broken up; patients spend less time on their own ward and more time being transported around the hospital to investigations and treatment.

There have been changes in working arrangements – working hours have been affected by the European Working Time Directive, so that junior doctors no longer work very long hours, and patterns of working for nurses has changed so that they often work fewer but longer shifts. This means that both doctors and nurses may not follow a patient's progress as they used to. There have been changes in skill mix, with fewer ward staff being trained nurses, and more health care assistants. There have been changes within and between professions. The boundaries between doctors' and nurses' work have shifted, meaning that nurses now perform more technical tasks, leaving more patient care to health care assistants.

Teamwork and opportunities to reflect can mediate some of the pressures and help individuals to cope. Studies have shown that members of good teams have lower levels of stress. Unfortunately teamwork does not occur spontaneously and has to be worked at. Although staff do work in teams, they are only loosely organized and we know from staff survey data that staff feel isolated, there is a lack of supervision and appraisal (Care Quality Commission 2011).

A large proportion of staff work in "pseudo-teams"– in other words, their teams do not meet the criteria that demonstrate the quality of a team, defined by Carter and West, which include having clearly defined tasks and clear objectives; meeting regularly to review objectives, methods and effectiveness; trusting each other; having a shared commitment to excellent patient care (Carter and West 1999).

With the emphasis on targets, financial efficiency, and throughput, staff are under stress personally, working in big, very busy, pressurized environments with little opportunity to establish good relationships with their patients and colleagues. We also know that stress is caused by a sense of lack of control. The current uncertain environment with job insecurity, the threat of organizational mergers and redundancies, all add to the pressure already there for staff. Reported stress of health service staff in general is greater than in the general working and accounts for more than one quarter of staff absence, which itself is higher than in other sectors (Department of Health 2009).

The work itself

> The job of hospitals is to cope with human bodily and mental vulnerability, death and destruction. In its highly acute form, this is not pretty or easy work . . . As society collectively displaces its discomfort to hospitals and health workers, requiring them emotionally to launder the unspeakable and uncontrollable, it is not surprising that those institutions and workers are under a lot of pressure ...
>
> (Sanders *et al.* 2011).

As shown, the pressurized context in which staff is working makes it challenging to provide high-quality individual care. But theoretical and qualitative research helps us to understand that the very nature of the work staff are doing is incredibly difficult. Continuous contact with patients who are ill, in distress, maybe disfigured or dying means that staff, especially nurses and health care assistants who are with patients continuously, are constantly confronting their own mortality and vulnerability.

Psychologists and others have observed that death and disease, physical and mental degeneration generate a primitive fear in us, particularly in Western cultures. The more serious or terminal the illness, the stronger are the fears and taboos, and one immediate strategy that staff may adopt to deal with this is to distance themselves. Menzies-Lyth has described how people withdraw, perhaps for their own emotional protection, and the uniforms, procedures and targets of modern health care provide organizational barriers to retreat behind (Menzies-Lyth 1988). This natural avoidance, or self-protection strategy, means that compassion and good communication are unlikely to occur unless staff are supported to confront these difficult issues.

The training that doctors, and increasingly nurses receive actually emphasizes the need for detachment, perhaps to the detriment of empathy. It has been shown that junior doctors, for example, feel less empathy as their training progresses (Riess 2010). Again this may be a case of self-defence – becoming "case hardened" to survive, as well as the dominance of the biomedical model that frames their training, which tends to objectify patients.

Consequences for staff

Depression levels in health care staff are high. Depression and high stress affect the ability of staff to provide high-quality care in a variety of ways. With depression in particular, people withdraw, perhaps for their own emotional protection. Burnout is at the extreme end of stress, consisting of three key areas of a lowered sense of personal effectiveness, emotional exhaustion, and depersonalization – which is the area most likely to limit compassion or, worse, to produce cruelty in dealings with patients.

In a busy day, reflective practice is hard to sustain, and our own research with hospital staff revealed that typically they did not talk to colleagues about patients' experience of care or what constitutes "good care."

The consequence for individual members of staff if they are isolated is that they reflect on their own or away from work. They may experience guilt, anxiety and possibly burnout, which itself effects relationships with colleagues and patients

Schwartz Center Rounds®

It was clear that it was a priority for the Point of Care programme to introduce and test an intervention that would provide support for staff – for their sake and for the sake of the patients they cared for. We know that there is a clear relationship between the well-being of staff and patients' well-being, with staff reporting that how they feel affects how they care for patients (Boorman 2009). In the recent Boorman review it was reported that 80 percent of staff felt that their health and well-being impacted on their care for patients, but only 40 percent of staff felt that their employer was proactively trying to do something to improve their health and well-being. An analysis of the national inpatient surveys and national staff surveys has shown a clear relationship between them: to put it crudely, where staff are happy, patients are happy (Raleigh 2011). A recent large study has shown that staff well-being is an antecedent to patient well-being (Maben *et al.* 2012).

Seeing the person in the patient had identified Schwartz Center Rounds as a promising intervention.

The Rounds were developed by the Boston-based Schwartz Center for Compassionate Healthcare (www.theschwartzcenter.org).This is a not-for-profit organization, named after a patient, Kenneth Schwartz, who had written about his experience of being cared for in hospital by caregivers who, he observed, made the "unbearable, bearable" by their acts of kindness (Schwartz 1995). He saw that it cost caregivers to give of themselves in this way and wanted the Schwartz Center to support them, and thus to strengthen the relationship between caregiver and patient. The Rounds are the Schwartz Center's biggest program, now running for 15 years, in over 300 sites in the States. A Round is a multidisciplinary forum, designed for staff from across the hospital to come together once a month to discuss the non-clinical aspect of caring for patients – that is, the emotional and social challenges associated with their jobs. They give staff an opportunity to reflect on their experiences of delivering care, including both its rewards and frustrations – on what the Schwartz Center calls the "human dimension of medicine" (www.theschwartzcenter.org/ViewPage.aspx?pageId=20). Rounds typically take place once a month and are held at lunchtime, with lunch provided. They last one hour: a patient's case or story is presented by the team who cared for him or her, and then the themes that emerge are opened up for discussion, guided by a skilled facilitator, together with a senior doctor, for the rest of the hour.

Very often the Rounds raise issues for discussion which are about caring for difficult or challenging patients and their families – and have included Rounds where the issues of caring for frail elderly patients have been explored. For example, one patient's story recently told in a UK hospital started with this:

> It was hard to care for him, an ongoing battle, because he was delirious. He screamed every time he was moved, but the family were always at the bedside, asking questions, asking him to be moved constantly. Dr A's lasting memory is of seeing him on the Monday and his heart sinking as he realized there was little he could do for him. He did settle down but continued to deteriorate. His last admission was for six weeks. The dilemma was how long to go on treating.

> N [one of the nurses] described how looking after this patient was very challenging - biting, spitting (nurses had to wear masks when caring for him) and kicking. It took four members of staff to lift him or do any interventions. It was distressing for staff. The family were questioning staff day and night – for example they were keen for him to be got out of bed and put into the chair, even though staff disagreed that it was the best thing. Nurses started to avoid the patient because of the pressure from the family and it was hard as ward manager to allocate staff to look after him. Staff felt they had got to the stage where they were treating the family and not the patient. There was almost a sense of relief when he died.

Other Rounds have had titles which illustrate the typical dilemmas staff have to deal with: "Caught between the patient and the family"; "Balancing reality with hope"; "A question of mental capacity," "A patient I will never forget."

Impact of rounds

In 2009 The Point of Care signed an agreement with the Schwartz Center to pilot Rounds in the UK. (The only license held outside the States). The pilot period for the Rounds was one year – between October 2009 and October 2010 – and Rounds were implemented in two hospitals: the Royal Free Hospital and Cheltenham Hospital. Evaluation of the pilot showed that the Rounds had transferred successfully to the UK, and were showing the same positive benefits for staff who attended and for their relationships with colleagues and patients, as they do in the States (Goodrich 2012). Now other hospitals, and some hospices have implemented, or are planning to implement, Rounds. Before they do so they have to meet certain criteria: demonstrable support from the trust's chief executive and board; a skilled facilitator available; a senior clinical person to lead the Rounds; dedicated administrative support; a commitment by the hospital to provide lunch for those who attend; a multidisciplinary steering group to plan ahead the topics and cases to be presented, manage the advance publicity for the Rounds, and evaluate each month. This is the tried and tested way in which the Rounds are organized in the States, and has not been changed for the UK.

The license to run Rounds is now held by the Point of Care Foundation and Rounds are now running at 30 sites, with good attendance, ranging from 40 to 140 attending at any one time. Facilitators at more hospitals, and hospices, are currently being trained and support to start Rounds is being provided by the Point of Care Foundation.

In 2006–7, research was undertaken to evaluate the impact Rounds had on participating staff, on their beliefs about patient care, on teamwork, on staff perceptions of their levels of stress and support in the workplace, and on changes in institutional practices and policies. In their statistical analysis of this research, Lown and Manning (2010) found that following Rounds:

- participants reported better teamwork and perceived themselves as experiencing less stress
- Rounds enhanced participants' "likelihood of attending to psychosocial and emotional aspects of care"
- Rounds "enhanced their beliefs about the importance of empathy"
- the impact of Rounds on these outcomes increased with the number of Rounds participants attended.

The evaluation of the pilot shows that staff attending the Rounds feel supported and that relationships are improving among staff and with their patients. We have seen that Rounds have successfully transferred to England, are firmly established with support from the top of the organizations, have demonstrated a need, and are greatly valued by staff who take part:

> I have really enjoyed them as they have helped me realise I am not alone! We all do a difficult job as well as we can.
>
> (Rounds participant)

> People are taking the concerns of staff seriously - opening ourselves to hear what people are struggling with. And in the context of mid-Staffs staff are expressing things and the Rounds are a sign that it is safe to speak. It is all very well to say we have an open culture, but this demonstrated that value.
>
> (Trust board member)

The Rounds are consciously linked to work on culture change, and will be linked to patient experience work. Also linked to how we look after our staff, who then give better care; there is good evidence for this. There is also good evidence that if staff are very stressed and can't process things, that affects them cognitively and they make mistakes. With the increasing workload, that also makes it a patient safety issue.

(Trust board member and participant)

Schwartz rounds were new to me, but from what I understand about the philosophy, it is reconnecting people with what we are here to do. It is a reminder of how bloody tough it is.

(Rounds participant)

Everyone else has benefited from doctors talking about the emotional impact on them. It is not part of the culture of medicine to talk about the emotional content, and these are senior consultants talking too. It is important for staff to hear it. Having the Round made it happen.

(Steering group member)

I really appreciated the language. You hear words used you don't normally hear such as anger, guilt, shame and frustration. They are obviously there but there is no outlet for them.

(Rounds participant)

Summary

Hospitals are very challenging environments and the nature of the work staff do is very difficult, complex, and requires attention. We believe that Rounds are one way that senior staff and trust boards can signal that care is a priority and show that they recognize the demands on individuals.

Evidence from those attending Rounds is that they find them beneficial and want to attend. Rounds do not replace good teams but they do provide space to reflect on the nature of work.

We are convinced that staff need to be given the means and the support to withstand the pressures of working in a highly pressurized hospital environment, caring for the very sick with the attendant emotional challenges.

Conclusion (Goodrich and Frampton)

It is striking that both Planetree and Schwartz Center Rounds came about through the vision of patients. Both Angelica Thieriot and Kenneth Schwartz recognized, through their own experience, that the best care, while being technically excellent, is provided with kindness – and that requires careful attention.

This attention includes listening – both to patients and staff, whose experience is interconnected. Planetree has listened to and captured the voices of patients and their families talking about their experiences of care, and Schwartz Center Rounds provide a way for organizations to hear the voices of their caregivers, and for caregivers to listen to each other. Building on this, Planetree and the Point of Care have developed practical ways to improve patients' experience – which will be successful, so long as both patients and staff continue to be heard and are meaningfully engaged. Then their experience, and the culture of their organizations, can begin to be truly transformed.

Care Experiences: calling 111

John (UK)

The screams of agony from my partner Linda started at around two o'clock in the morning, it all happened so quickly after what had been an earlier routine visit to the GP. I don't think that I panicked, certainly I was worried sick, but more importantly I didn't really have a clue what to do! I remembered seeing a notice on the GP surgery door that *for out of hours medical help dial 111.* I called to Linda who was doubled up with acute stomach pain *I'll call an ambulance on 999!* For whatever reason, she refused to let me do this, so in desperation I dialed 111. I waited for an indeterminable length of time, for the receiver at the other end to be picked up. The voice when it answered was calm and helpful enough and proceeded to take me through a series of questions about Linda. With Linda's loud screams going on in the background I tried to answer these as carefully as possible, *name, date of birth, problem etc.* "OK" I thought having completed these, "now please get me a doctor or an ambulance." But no! The voice on the other end said *I'll get a nurse to call you back within the hour.* I waited and waited for over an hour but still no call back. So I called 111 again. After what seemed a lengthy wait I explained to the new voice what had happened, expecting to be told that the previous call was recorded. But the voice, much less friendlier than last time said *I'll have to take you through some questions*, to which I timidly replied *I've answered all of these in my previous telephone conversation.* The voice rather sharply said, *you'll still have to answer them.* Linda's screams were getting louder and the voice must have heard, so I hurried through the next same set of questions. I was told after this, *we are extremely busy but I'll get someone to call you back!* Before I could say anything the line went dead. By this time two hours had passed, and by now my anger was boiling over, *how dare I be treated like this, I'm a pensioner, have always worked and paid my taxes, have always supported the NHS etc.* I called again and the

(continued)

(continued)

wait for an answer was even longer, but I was ready. Before, *I'll need to take you . . .* I said *I've answered your questions twice to no effect, no one has called me back, I've been cut off, can you hear the screams? Are you going to be able to help me or should I dial 999.* To this the third voice replied, *you'd better dial 999.* Calling 999 which was answered promptly, *I'll have to take you through some questions,* me now in tears, *please, can you hear the screams, please, please, get me an ambulance.* The ambulance thankfully came quite quickly and the medics were brilliant. But it had taken us almost four hours to get to hospital.

References

Béliveau, J., Corriveau, M.A., Leclerc, L., Giroux, M.C., Audet, M. (2013) *Results of the Inter-case Analysis from the First Loop of Learning History of the CIHR-Planetree Research Project*, presented at the Board of Directors Meeting, Reseau Planetree Quebec, Sherbrooke.

Boorman, S. (2009) *NHS Health and Well-being Review: Interim Report* and *Final Report* London: Department of Health.

Care Quality Commission (2011) *NHS Staff Survey 2010.*

Carter, A.J., West, M. (1999) Sharing the burden: Teamwork in health care settings, in Firth-Cozens, J., Payne, R.L. (eds), *Stress in Health Professionals*, pp. 191–202. Chichester: Wiley.

Department of Health (2009) *NHS Health and Well-being Review* London: Department of Health.

Firth-Cozens, J. and Cornwell, J. (2009) *Enabling Compassionate Care in Acute Hospital Settings.* London: The King's Fund.

Frampton, S.B., Charmel, P. (2009) *Putting Patients First*, 2nd edn. San Francisco, CA: Jossey-Bass.

Frampton, S.B., Charmel, P., Guastello, S. (2013) *The Putting Patients First Field Guide: Global Lessons in Designing and Implementing Patient-Centered Care.* San Francisco, CA: Jossey-Bass.

Goodrich, J. (2012) Supporting hospital staff to deliver compassionate care: Do Schwartz Center Rounds work in English hospitals? *Journal of the Royal Society of Medicine* 105(3), 117–122.

HES Online October 2011. Available at www.hscic.gov.uk/hes (accessed 18 March 2014).

HES Online (IP) and DH (A&E & OP) 2011. Available at www.hscic.gov.uk/hes (accessed 18 March 2014).

Berwick, D.M., Calkins, D.R., McCannon, C.J., Hackbarth, A.D. (2006) The 100,000 lives campaign: Setting a goal and a deadline for improving health care quality. *Journal of the American Medical Association* 295(3), 324–327.

IOM (Institute of Medicine) (2001) *Crossing the Quality Chasm: A New Health System for the 21st Century. Appendix B: Redesigning Health Care with Insights from the Science of Complex Adaptive Systems.* Washington, DC: National Academies Press.

Lown, B.A., Manning, M.A. (2010) The Schwartz Center Rounds: Evaluation of an interdisciplinary approach to enhancing patient-centered communication, teamwork, and provider support *Academic Medicine* 85, 1073–1081.

Maben, J., Peccei, R., Adams, M. (2012) *Exploring the relationship between patients' experiences of care and the influence of staff motivation, affect and wellbeing.* Southampton: NIHR [SDO project 08/1819/213 (November 2012) NIHR Service Delivery and Organisation programme].

McHugh, M.D., Kutney-Lee, A., Cimiotti, J.P., Sloane, D.M., Aiken, L.H. (2011) Nurses' widespread job dissatisfaction, burnout, and frustration with health benefits signal problems for patient care *Health Affairs (Millwood)*, 30(2), 202–210.

Malloy, R., Otto, J. (2012) *A Steady Dose of Empathy.* Hospital & Health Networks. Available at: http://www.hhnmag.com/hhnmag/HHNDaily/HHNDailyDisplay.dhtml?id=7800008222 (accessed 7 June 2012).

Marklein, M.B. (2013) *Higher Education = Lower Joy on Job? USA Today,* July 18, p.2B.

Martin, D.P., Diehr, P., Conrad, D.A., Davis, J.H., Leickly, R., Perrin, E.B. (1998) Randomized trial of a patient-centered hospital unit *Patient Education and Counseling* 34, 125–133.

Menzies-Lyth, I. (1988) *Containing Anxiety in Institutions.* London: Free Association Press.

NHS Confederation and Joint Medical Consultative Council (2007) *A Clinical Vision of a Reformed NHS.* London: NHS Confederation.

NHS Information Centre (2011) *NHS Workforce: Summary of staff in the NHS: Results from September 2010 Census.* London: The Health and Social Care Information Centre.

Planetree (2011) Planetree Contributes to National Priorities Partnership Report Submitted to Secretary Kathleen Sebelius (2011) *PlaneTalk,* November, p. 15.

Raleigh, V.S., Hussey, D, Seccombe, I., Qi, R. (2009) Do associations between staff and inpatient feedback have the potential for improving patient experience?: An analysis of surveys in NHS acute trusts in England. *Quality and Safety in Health Care* 18(5), 347–354.

Riess, H. (2010) Empathy in medicine-a neurobiological perspective *JAMA* 304(14), 1604–1605.

Sanders, K., Pattison, S., Hurwitz, B. (2011) Tracking shame and humiliation in Accident and Emergency *Nursing Philosophy* 12, 83–93.

Schwartz Center for Compassionate Healthcare. Available at: www.theschwartz-center.org.

Schwartz, K.B. (1995) A patient's story *The Boston Globe Magazine,* July 16. Available at www.theschwartzcenter.org/ViewPage.aspx?pageId=50.

www.theschwartzcenter.org/ViewPage.aspx?pageId=20

Spence Laschinger, H.K., Leiter, M., Day, A., Gilin, D. (2009) Workplace empowerment, incivility, and burnout: Impact on staff nurse recruitment and retention outcomes *Journal of Nursing Management* 17(3), 302–311.

Stevenson, A.C. (2002) Compassion and patient centered care *Australian Family Physician* 31(12), 1103–1106.

Stone, S. (2008) A retrospective evaluation of the impact of the Planetree Patient Centered Model of Care Program on inpatient quality outcomes *Health Environments Research and Design Journal* 1(4), 55–69.

Taloney, L., Flores, G. (2013) Building blocks for successful patient and family advisory boards: Collaboration, communication and commitment *Nursing Administration Quarterly* 37(3), 247–253.

Thieriot, A. (2010) Personal communication.

Williams, S.C., Schmaltz, S.P., Morton, D.J., Koss, R.G., Loeb, J.M. (2005) Quality of care in U.S. hospitals as reflected by standardized measures, 2002–2004 *New England Journal of Medicine* 353(3), 255–264.

15 Understanding and protecting against compassion fatigue

Adelais Markaki

Introduction

Compassion fatigue (CF) is a contemporary label for a phenomenon that still lacks consensus among scientists. This euphemistic term describes the condition of gradual lessening of compassion over time, brought on by an exposure to trauma on a regular basis (Boyle 2011). Also known as secondary traumatic stress (STS), it conveys sociological connotations, particularly in regards to media and community responses to natural disasters or human-induced emergencies. Historically, the condition has been studied in diverse professional populations, such as emergency first responders, nurses, physicians, psychologists, counsellors, social workers and lawyers. During the last years, emphasis has been given on both professional and lay caregivers' reactions specific to the helping process, as encountered in hospitals, long-term care and palliative care settings.

Caregivers suffering from CF exhibit an array of symptoms, including constant stress and anxiety, hopelessness, sleeplessness or nightmares, and an overall negative attitude. Decreased productivity, inability to focus, proneness for medical errors, feelings of incompetency and self-doubt are some of the most common professional and personal CF implications:

> The expectation that we can be immersed in suffering and loss daily and not be touched by it is as unrealistic as expecting to be able to walk on water without getting wet. This sort of denial is no small matter.
>
> (Remen 1996, p. 52).

Becoming aware, and understanding the significance of CF is crucial in empowering health professionals, as well as healthcare organizations, to take measures towards self-care promotion, patient outcome improvement, and therapeutic relationship strengthening. Towards that goal, this chapter begins by defining CF, distinguishing it from other occupational stress entities, outlining risk factors and symptoms, and introducing the main theoretical models for its study. Second, significance and implications of CF are discussed at a personal, professional and organizational level. Third, approaches and measures to prevent and counteract CF are presented.

Last, chapter conclusions are followed by two practical appendixes with suggested resources for preventing and counteracting CF as well as screening and diagnostic tools.

Background

Definitions

Since the early 1980s, the 'cost of caring' for people facing emotional pain has been studied by the field of traumatology. Bridging behavioural science and medicine, traumatology refers to the development and application of psychological and counselling services for people who have experienced extreme events. This 'cost of caring' has also been known as 'secondary traumatic stress' (Figley 1989), 'vicarious traumatization' (Pearlman and MacIan 1995), and 'secondary survivor' (Remer and Witten 1988).

The term 'compassion fatigue' was first used by Joinson (1992) in the context of a nurses' burnout study. It was coined to describe the 'loss of the ability to nurture', observed among emergency department nurses. In 1995, Figley used the term in describing secondary traumatic stress disorder (STSD) resulting from helping or desiring to help a person suffering from traumatic events. His groundbreaking observations among mental health workers revealed that:

> Professionals who listen to clients' stories of fear, pain and suffering may feel similar fear, pain and suffering because they care. Sometimes we feel we are losing our own sense of self to the clients we serve.
>
> (p. 1).

Some literature has called compassion fatigue a form of 'burnout'. However, unlike CF, burnout is related to chronic workplace and career distress, rather than exposure to specific kinds of client problems, such as trauma (Beck 2011). Despite somewhat conflicting academic perspectives, there seems to be an across the border agreement that CF exhibits a more sudden and acute onset than burnout, a condition that gradually wears down overwhelmed caregivers (Abendroth 2011).

Another occupational stress condition that needs to be differentiated from CF is 'vicarious traumatization' (VT). The term describes the psychological distress experienced by healthcare professionals in their work with patients who have been traumatized (Pearlman and MacIan 1995). Unlike compassion fatigue, VT is a theory-based construct, specific to trauma workers. Burnout and vicarious trauma can coexist.

Given the ambiguity that exists around the phenomenon of compassion fatigue, as well as the confusion caused by the synonymous use of several terms, every effort has been made to simplify the presentation of what is known, while highlighting areas that deserve further attention.

Risk factors – early signs

Compassion fatigue needs to be addressed in its earliest phases to avoid permanent 'disability'. Thus, it is critical for healthcare providers at all levels and settings to be aware of the risk factors and early signs in order to intervene appropriately. An overview of key triggers, onset chronology, hallmark signs, and outcomes among burnout, compassion fatigue and vicarious traumatization is presented in Table 15.1.

Several personal and professional attributes place a person at risk for developing compassion fatigue or other occupational stress related conditions. Persons who are overly conscientious, perfectionists, and self-giving, have low levels of social support or high levels of stress in their personal life are more likely to develop STS or CF. Also, previous histories of trauma that led to negative coping skills, such as bottling up or avoiding emotions, increase STS risk (Meadors *et al.* 2008).

At the professional level, researchers have suggested that CF is connected to the therapeutic relationship between healthcare provider and patient. Imbalanced, empathic, relationship-based care has been identified as a contributing factor (Sabo 2011; Lombard and Eyre 2011). An individual's capacity for empathy and ability to engage into a therapeutic relationship is considered to be central, with those displaying high levels of empathy being more vulnerable to experiencing CF (Figley 1995; Adams *et al.* 2006).

Organizational stressors, such as heavier workloads and long shifts along with more complex patient needs (i.e. pain, traumatic injury, and emotional distress), are known to result in healthcare professionals feeling tired, depressed, angry, ineffective, apathetic and detached (Boyle 2011). Among hospital and home care nurses who worked 8-hour versus 12-hour shifts, CF scores were found to differ significantly, with nurses who worked the longest shift scoring higher (Yoder 2010). Somatic complaints in nurses (i.e. headaches, insomnia, and gastrointestinal distress) have also been noted. Compassion fatigue escalates gradually over time as a result of cumulative stress, particularly when symptoms are ignored and not timely attended (Bush 2009).

Other organizational attributes in the healthcare field also contribute to employees' compassion fatigue. A 'culture of silence', where stressful events are not discussed after the event is over, as well as poor training in the risks associated with high-stress jobs, are known to contribute to high rates of STSD (Meadors *et al.* 2008).

Compared to post-traumatic stress disorder (PTSD), CF's symptomatology is nearly identical, except that CF applies to caregivers who were affected by the trauma of others (Abendroth 2011). Caregivers with CF may seek to re-live their patients' trauma, while showing symptoms of persistent anxiety and arousal (i.e. difficulty falling or staying asleep, irritability or outbursts of anger, and/or exaggerated startle responses). Ultimately, these caregivers have reduced capacity for, or interest in being empathic toward the suffering of others (Abendroth 2011).

Table 15.1 Overview of compassion fatigue and differentiation from related constructs

Compassion fatigue (or secondary traumatic stress)	Burn-out	Vicarious traumatization
Etiology/key triggers	*Etiology/key triggers*	*Etiology/key triggers*
Relational: consequences of caring for those who are suffering or are dependent on caregivers (i.e. inability to change course of a painful scenario or disease trajectory)	*Reactional:* response to work or environmental stressors, organizational attributes (i.e. staffing, workload, inadequate supplies or resources, managerial style, decision making locus)	*Relational:* long-term consequence of caring for those traumatized
Chronology	*Chronology*	*Chronology*
Sudden, acute onset, can occur from work with a single client	Gradual, over time	Across time – across clients
Hallmark signs	*Hallmark signs*	*Hallmark signs*
Sadness and grief Nightmares Avoidance Addiction Somatic complaints Psychological arousal Changes in beliefs, expectations, assumptions 'witness guilt' Detachment Decreased intimacy	Anger and frustration Fatigue Negative reactions towards others Cynicism Negativity Withdrawal	Signs and symptoms parallel those of direct trauma, although less intense. Anxiety, sadness, confusion, apathy Intrusive imagery Somatic complaints Loss of control, trust and independence Decreased intimacy Relational disturbances (crossover to personal life)
Outcomes	*Outcomes*	*Outcomes*
Imbalance of empathy and objectivity (may ultimately leave position)	Decreased empathic responses Withdrawal (may leave position or transfer)	Changes in spirituality and the sense of meaning and hope

*Adapted from Sabo (2011) and Boyle (2011).

Theoretical models

An established theoretical model for the study of CF has been the 'stress-process model', with key elements the empathic ability, empathic response, and residual compassion stress (Figley 2002; Adams *et al.* 2006). Despite some model limitations, Sabo (2011) has suggested that adding the personal characteristics of resilience and hope, as well as the nature of relationships, could provide better understanding of empathy and engagement as contributors to CF. However, other researchers have argued that there is not enough empirical evidence to support a theoretical framework for CF and vicarious traumatization (Bride *et al.* 2004; Jenkins and Baird 2002; Thomas and Wilson 2004).

On the other hand, the construct of burnout has been studied through a multidimensional model, comprising three elements: emotional exhaustion, depersonalization and reduced personal accomplishment (Demerouti *et al.* 2003; Kitaoka-Higashiguchi *et al.* 2004; Maslach *et al.* 2001). Viewed from that perspective, researchers have suggested that burnout may be a precondition for the other types of occupational stress, namely CF and vicarious traumatization, by creating the fertile ground for these types of stress to develop (Boyle 2011).

Assessing the impact of CF

Significance and prevalence

Caring for dependent people, whose suffering is continuous and unresolved, can be a major trigger of compassion fatigue and burnout. Although a professional might still provide care as mandated by policy, the desire to help and the ability to show empathy can be significantly impacted. This phenomenon mostly occurs among professionals involved in emergency and intensive care services, long-term care, oncology, mental health care, hospice, and child welfare. However, it can also occur among lay caregivers who are primary care providers for chronically or terminally ill patients, showing symptoms of depression, stress and apathy.

Estimates of compassion fatigue prevalence among health care professionals range from 16 per cent to 85 per cent, depending on the setting and the professional category (Wikipedia). According to the latest American Nurses' Association (2011) web-based poll, 62 per cent of all nurses reported suffering from compassion fatigue. An emergency room study found 85 per cent of nurses meeting the criteria for CF (Hooper *et al.* 2010), whereas more than 25 per cent of ambulance paramedics had severe ranges of post-traumatic symptoms (Beck 2011). In two separate studies of hospice nurses, 34 per cent met the criteria for CF (Beck 2011) with hospice nurses in the 'moderate to high risk' category demonstrating 'self-sacrificing behavior' as the major contributing risk factor (Abendroth and Flannery 2006).

In regards to burnout, measured by the Maslach Burnout Inventory tool, a Pulse survey of 1,800 British GPs classified 43 per cent of them at a very high risk (Davies 2013). Similarly, burnout risk among Greek medical residents was found to be 49.5 per cent (Msaouel *et al.* 2010), more than twofold higher compared to data from other European Union countries (Prins *et al.* 2007; Van der Heijden 2008). In another survey of 500 British GPs, 46 per cent were found to be emotionally exhausted, 42 per cent were depersonalized and 34 per cent felt they were not achieving a great deal (Orton *et al.* 2012). This compared with much higher rates of 72 per cent, 41 per cent and 97 per cent, respectively found in the Pulse survey (Davies 2013).

Personal level implications

Caregivers afflicted with CF may develop persistent arousal and anxiety, including difficulty falling or staying asleep, irritability or outbursts of anger, and/or exaggerated startle responses. Other physical symptoms include headaches, digestive problems (diarrhoea, constipation, upset stomach), muscle tension, chest pain/pressure, palpitations or tachycardia. Most importantly, caregivers experience a reduced capacity for, or interest in being empathic towards patients or families (Lombard and Eyre 2011).

Mental health and child welfare professionals are more at risk for CF. Repeated exposure to trauma and violence experienced by clients can create a shift in their perceptions of the world and themselves. Furthermore, it increases their sense of vulnerability by disrupting the counsellor's sense of safety, trust, self-esteem, control and relationships with significant others (Van Hook and Rothenberg 2009).

Professional and organizational level implications

Compassion fatigue is known to impact employees' job satisfaction and performance ability (Lombard and Eyre 2011). Medication errors, decreased documentation accuracy, poor record-keeping, avoidance of intense patient situations, stereotypical/impersonal communications are only some of the reported professional consequences. Organizational negative impacts include reduced productivity, tardiness, absenteeism and frequent use of sick days, having a direct effect on co-workers, managers and ultimately patients (Showalter 2010).

Exploring how CF might affect patient satisfaction and patient safety has lately been the subject of rising interest (Potter *et al.* 2010; Yang and Huang 2005). Recent hikes in health professionals' workloads, such as the newly negotiated GP contract in the UK for 2013/14, assigning GPs responsibility for 24/7 patient care (Davies 2013), are expected to place greater pressure on clinicians as well as researchers to establish the alleged effects of CF and burnout on recipients' quality of care.

Counteracting CF

There are different approaches to address compassion fatigue. All of them entail awareness, balance, and connection.

The role of self-care and self-compassion the need for resilience

Although no clinical treatment options for compassion fatigue exist, there are several recommended preventative measures based on the concepts of self-care and self-compassion. The common premise for both concepts is that we cannot give what we don't have and that both require practice and perseverance.

On a personal self-care level, the use of exercise and attention to diet are central to work/life balance. Focusing attention on pleasurable, non-work-related activities that promote pacing and personal planning, such as journaling and meditation, is an effective self-care strategy (Boyle 2011). Participating in breathing exercises, physical exercise and other recreational activities, taking a break from work, and practicing stress reduction, can all have a shielding effect against CF. A successful strategy for stress reduction is the positive mental training program that has been shown to build resilience and decrease burnout for NHS staff (see Appendix A, entry 5). Setting clear, professional boundaries while accepting the fact that successful outcomes are not always achievable, can also limit the effects of STS (Huggard 2003). Recognizing that work/life balance requires both introspection and ongoing action is the key to ensuring professional longevity (Boyle 2011).

On a professional self-care level, social and peer support have been shown to be crucial for maintaining a balanced perspective. Establishing a diverse network of social support, from colleagues to pets, promotes a positive psychological state and can protect against STS (Huggard 2003). But since many caregivers find it difficult to 'leave problems at home,' professional counselling at work is considered essential. Looking out for danger-signal responses, such as blaming others, utilizing self-medication with alcohol, or other addictive behaviours, can make the difference in receiving, or not, timely help.

All of the above personal and professional self-care strategies need to be integrated in undergraduate health science curricula in order for self-care to become a first-line defence, rather than a therapeutic intervention. Teaching CF prevention strategies and measures could prove an excellent opportunity for interdisciplinary and interprofessional innovative learning initiatives.

The role of research

Investigating the particular needs of distinct professional groups offers valuable guidance for developing targeted intervention programs. Applying supporting evidence in the design of an employee assistance or stress-reduction program allows human resource managers or compassion fatigue training specialists to target the specific needs of that group (Potter *et al.* 2010). Towards that direction, a recent Canadian study explored how compassion satisfaction (CS), CF and burnout among hospice and palliative care workforce interact with key practice characteristics (Slocum-Gori *et al.* 2013).

Another field of inquiry has focused on the correlation between self-compassion and emotional intelligence, attempting to identify nurses who need training in self-compassion and the most appropriate ways to help them (Heffernan *et al.* 2010). In contrast, there have been few, if any studies exploring self-sacrificing behaviour and the possible effects it may have on the psychosocial health of particular groups of healthcare providers, i.e. physicians, nurses, social workers. Further research may also be helpful in explaining whether and how factors, such as (a) duration of the relationship; (b) level of experience; (c) individual characteristics of the caregiver; and (d) patient characteristics may increase the risk for CF and vicarious traumatization (Sabo 2011).

Although numerous models have been developed to guide researchers in comprehending the phenomenon of CF, further construct clarification is still needed. Towards that end, several research questions have been raised by scientists, including the following:

a) What are the relationships between the different types of occupational stress?
b) Does compassion fatigue exist on a continuum of occupational stress? If so, is burnout a precondition for compassion fatigue?
c) How is resiliency related to maintaining the balance between CS and CF?
d) What is the correlation between self-compassion and levels of stress?

Available tools for assessing CF are rather limited in scope and provide minimal help for those who need workplace interventions, such as counselling, support groups, and/or debriefing sessions. A compilation of the most widely used tools for screening/diagnosing compassion satisfaction, compassion fatigue, secondary traumatic stress and burnout is presented in Appendix B.

The role of education

Compassion fatigue is preventable and treatable; yet, it is a phenomenon 'loaded' by cultural beliefs and societal expectations in regards to the caregiving role that extend far beyond the caregiver-patient relationship (Abendroth 2011). Even more, CF problems are often exacerbated by a lack of basic communication skills, since most healthcare professionals are not adequately prepared on how to deal with families under stress, or complex care scenarios (Boyle 2011). This knowledge/skill gap is attempted to be addressed through a variety of venues in the workplace. Continuing education programmes, patient rounds, and interdisciplinary team meetings are all ideal modalities for developing these skills.

Hence, addressing both compassion fatigue and burnout, since they often go hand in hand, is becoming a top educational agenda item for Continuing Education and Human Resource Departments in hospitals and primary care settings. Given that CF can permanently affect a caregiver's ability to provide compassionate care, every effort is made to prevent its onset or ameliorate its consequences.

Certified compassion fatigue training specialists teach workshops to healthcare professionals on how to avoid CF by raising their levels of self-compassion while reducing their levels of stress (Stringer 2010). They help caregivers strengthen their interpersonal and communication skills, gaining insight into stressors that contribute to CF, and helping them develop their own recovery plans (Lombard and Eyre 2011). Interestingly, a 'training-as-treatment' effect of those sessions has been reported among mental health providers (Gentry *et al.* 2004).

Learning and practicing the three components of self-compassion – self-kindness, acknowledging imperfection as part of the shared human experience, and mindfulness – is the first step towards reaching the goal of a healthy work-life balance. To that end, several professional organizations, educational centres and institutes also provide valuable resources and guidance (see Appendix A).

The role of administration/workplace interventions

There is growing research in the clinical workplace on how to prevent or minimize the ramifications of repeated exposure to traumatic events. Problems associated with CF can be counteracted by patient reassignment, formal mentoring programmes, employee training, and a compassionate organizational culture. Performance referrals for behaviours linked to CF, instituted among US health care settings, is one of the less favourable interventions, receiving mixed reviews (Boertje and Ferron 2013). On the other hand, problems associated with burnout can be overcome with radical restructuring and shift of organizational culture. Inspirational leadership, sharing a common vision, empowering employees and adopting a bottoms-up approach are some of the key attributes for a burn-out-free work environment.

Particularly in the mental health field, acknowledging the existence of the 'wounded healers' and encouraging greater openness and support, is essential in breaking away from widespread silence and stigma (Zerubavel and Wright 2012). Mental health managers are urged to become aware of the higher risk for CF and burnout among community-based psychiatrists and social workers (Rossi *et al.* 2012). Similarly, hospice and palliative care administration is called to improve employees' compassion satisfaction through policy and institutional level programs (Slocum-Gori *et al.* 2013). Ignoring CF can prove detrimental not only to the caregiver, but also to the caregiver's employer, and patients.

The role of health policy

Given the economic pressures faced by most of the western hemisphere countries, compassion fatigue can be very costly for caregivers as well as for institutions (Lombard and Eyre 2011). Rising levels of burnout, as a result of unsustainable work levels mandated by tightened national contracts or health coverage providers, are causing a deterioration of professional practice standards. Recent plans of NHS England to cut funding for occupational health services, used by the rising numbers of GPs with symptoms of burnout, indicate that researchers, academicians and clinicians need to publicize their concerns from a cost-benefit point of view (Davies 2013).

Thus, evidence linking CF and burnout with increased risk for medical errors, greater rates of nurse absenteeism and patient avoidance, as well as diminished patient satisfaction should become a banner for a new campaign. Professional organizations and mass media should ring the alarm bells, urging policy makers to demonstrate political will to solve the problem or risk losing seasoned caregivers tired of caring (Landro 2012; Davies 2013). Towards that end, healthcare systems should invest in creating healthy work environments that prevent compassion fatigue and enhance caregiver resilience, productivity and retention even in difficult times.

Conclusions – epilogue

The synonymous use of several terms to describe compassion fatigue, and the absence of consensus on one definition has hindered the study of this important occupational distress phenomenon encountered across clinical care settings. Nevertheless, there is a growing body of evidence in regards to compassion fatigue's risk factors, prevalence, implications and significance.

Professional caregivers need to guard against CF by maintaining optimal health and well-being, balancing work-life demands, practicing self-care and self-compassion, and being aware of CF risk factors and early signs. Building-up the necessary resilience to deal with stressful events, shields caregivers from fatigue, optimizing therapeutic relationships and reinforcing compassionate care. In the midst of sweeping health care system reforms, more targeted attention from managers, educators, researchers, and policy makers will be urgently needed in the next years.

**Care Experiences: compassion conversations 19 –
detachment or non-attachment?**

Written by Dr Robin Youngson (New Zealand)
http://heartsinhealthcare.com

At medical school, a high value is placed on clinical detachment and
objectivity. We are taught that doctors need to be scientists who make
careful observations, sift the evidence, and make objective decisions.
But if we have an emotional connection to our patient it is impossible
to be objective, we are taught.

This cool clinical detachment and objectivity is powerfully reinforced by the language, culture and rituals of healthcare. We dep-
ersonalise patients by stripping away their clothes, their identity and
focusing on the disease, not the person. We talk about 'the hernia on
ward six' and 'the breast lump on ward seven'.

Worse still, the mask of detachment becomes our armour when
we are plunged into the brutalising experiences of early practice. On
my first weekend as a new doctor, I witnessed the deaths of six of my
patients. I was expected to be a robot, to carry on functioning as if
nothing had happened. Over the years, I substituted technical expertise for caring. I became the hero doctor who could treat the sickest
patients using the most complex technology.

But eventually the whole edifice comes crumbling down. Human
beings are incapable of making objective observations. Every perception
is coloured by prior assumptions and expectations. The very idea of being
a separate observer ignores the fact that all beings are intimately connected. We cannot separate the observer from what is being observed.

And as a psychological defence mechanism, clinical detachment
is just a cruel hoax. Every trauma we witness is a wound in our own
heart. If we can share love and compassion, the wounds heal. If we
deny our emotions, the wounds are left to fester.

These are hardly new problems for humanity. More than two thousand years of Buddhist wisdom and practical philosophy offer a guiding light. Thoughts and emotions are inseparable. Every negative
emotion – grief, anger, anxiety, fear, longing, jealousy – distorts our
thinking and our perception. The only mental state that avoids these
distortions is open-hearted compassion.

And what is the source of negative emotions? They arise from
unhealthy attachments – to material possessions, to the better job, to
the perfect outcome. How conditional we made our happiness!

So what does the Dalai Llama counsel? – Open-hearted compassion
with non-attachment. Then we can serve our patients with warmth,
humanity, non-judgement and clarity of perception.

Written by Dr Robin Youngson (http://heartsinhealthcare.com/)

References

Abendroth, M. (2011) Overview and summary: Compassion fatigue: Caregivers at risk *The Online Journal of Issues in Nursing* 16(1).

Abendroth, M., Flannery, J. (2006) Predicting the risk of compassion fatigue: A study of hospice nurses *Journal of Hospice and Palliative Nursing* 8(6), 346–56.

Adams, R., Boscarino, J., Figley, C. (2006) Compassion fatigue and psychological distress among social workers: A validation study *American Journal of Orthopsychiatry* 76(1), 103–8.

American Nurses' Association (2011) Most Online Poll Respondents Reported Suffering from Compassion Fatigue [available at: http://nursingworld.org/EspeciallyForYou/Staff-Nurses/Staff-Nurse-News/Sept-2011-HYS-Poll-Results.html, accessed on 10 April 2011].

Beck, C. (2011) Secondary traumatic stress in nurses: A systematic review *Archives of Psychiatric Nursing* 25(1), 1–10.

Boertje, J., Ferron, L. (2013). Tired of caring? You may have compassion fatigue *American Nurse Today* 8(7), 16–8.

Boyle, D. (2011) Countering compassion fatigue: A requisite nursing agenda *The Online Journal of Issues in Nursing* 16(1), Manuscript 2 [accessed on 31 January 2011].

Bride, B.E., Robinson, M.M., Yegidis, B., Figley, C. (2004) Development and validation of the secondary traumatic stress scale *Research on Social Work Practice* 14(1), 27–35.

Bush, N.J. (2009) Compassion fatigue: Are you at risk? *Oncology Nursing Forum* 36(1), 24–8.

Davies, M. (2013). Revealed: Half of GPs at high risk of burnout [available at: www.pulsetoday.co.uk/home/battling-burnout/revealed-half-of-gps-at-high-risk-of-burnout/20003157.article#.Ud06KaU2UWY, accessed on 4 June 2013].

Demerouti, E., Bakker, A., Vardakou, I., Kantas, A. (2003) The convergent validity of two burnout instruments: A multitrait-multimethod analysis *European Journal of Psychological Assessment* 19(1), 12–23.

Dominguez-Gomez, E. and Rutledge, D.N. (2009). Prevalence of secondary traumatic stress among emergency nurses. *Journal of Emergency Nursing* 35(3), 199–204.

Figley, C. (1995) *Compassion Fatigue: Coping with Secondary Traumatic Stress Disorder in Those who Treat the Traumatized.* New York: Brunner-Routledge.

Figley, C. (2002) Compassion fatigue: Psychotherapists' chronic lack of self care *Psychotherapy in Practice* 58(11), 1433–41.

Figley, C., Nelson, T.S. (1989) Basic family therapy skills, I: Conceptualization and initial findings *Journal of Marital and Family Therapy* 15(4): 349–65.

Gentry, J.E., Baggerly, J., Baranowsky, A. (2004) Training-as-treatment: Effectiveness of the certified compassion fatigue specialist training *International Journal of Emergency Mental Health* 6(3), 147–55.

Heffernan, M., Quinn Griffin, M.T., McNulty, Sister R., Fitzpatrick, J.J. (2010) Self-compassion and emotional intelligence in nurses *International Journal of Nursing Practice* 16(4), 366–73.

Hooper, C., Craig, J., Janvrin, D.R., Wetsel, M.A., Reimels, E. (2010) Compassion satisfaction, burnout, and compassion fatigue among emergency nurses compared with nurses in other selected inpatient specialties *Journal of Emergency Nursing* 36(5), 420–7.

Huggard, P. (2003) Secondary traumatic stress: Doctors at risk *New Ethicals Journal* 6(9), 9–14 [available at: http://home.cogeco.ca/~cmc/Huggard_NewEthJ_2003.pdf].

Jenkins, S.R., Baird, S. (2002) Secondary traumatic stress and vicarious traumatization: A validational study *Journal of Traumatic Stress* 15(5), 423–32.

Joinson, C. (1992) Coping with compassion fatigue *Nursing* 22(4), 116–22.

Kitaoka-Higashiguchi, K., Nakagawa, H., Ishizaki, M., Miura, K., Naruse, Y., Kido, T., *et al.* (2004) Construct validtiy of the maslach burnout inventory-general survey *Stress & Health* 20, 255–60.

Landro, L. (2012) When Nurses Catch Compassion Fatigue, Patients Suffer *Wall Street Journal* [available at: http://online.wsj.com/article/SB1000142405297020 472020457712888210418856.html, accessed on 3 January 2012].

Lombard, B., Eyre, C. (2011). Compassion fatigue: A nurse's primer *The Online Journal of Issues in Nursing* 16(1), Manuscript 3 [accessed on 31 January 2011].

Maslach, C., Schaufeli, W., Leiter, M. (2001) Job burnout *Annual Reviews in Psychology* 52, 397–422.

Meadors, P., Lamson, A. (2008) Compassion fatigue and secondary traumatization: Provider self care on the intensive care units for children *Journal of Pediatric Health Care* (22)1, 24–34.

Msaouel, P., Keramaris, N.C., Tasoulis, A., Kolokythas, D., Syrmos, N., Pararas, N., Thireos, E., Lionis, C. (2010) Burnout and training satisfaction of medical residents in Greece: Will the European Work Time Directive make a difference? *Human Resources for Health* 8(1), 16.

Orton, P., Orton, C., Pereira Gray, D. (2012) Depersonalised doctors: A cross-sectional study of 564 doctors, 760 consultations and 1876 patient reports in UK general practice *BMJ Open* 2: e000274.

Pearlman, L., MacIan, P. (1995) Vicarious traumatization: An empirical study of the effects of trauma work on trauma therapists *Professional Psychology, Research and Practice* 26(6), 558–65.

Potter, P., Deshields, T., Divanbeigi, J., Berger, J., Cipriano, D., Norris, L., Olsen, S. (2010) Compassion fatigue and burnout: Prevalence among oncology nurses *Clinical Journal of Oncology Nursing* 14(5), E56–62.

Prins, J.T., Hoekstra-Weebers, J.E., van de Wiel, H.B., Gazendam-Donofrio, S.M., Sprangers, F., Jaspers, F.C., van der Heijden, F.M. (2007) Burnout among Dutch medical residents *International Journal of Behavioral Medicine* 14, 119–25.

Remen, N.R. (1996) *Kitchen Table Wisdom: Stories That Heal.* New York: Riverhead Books.

Remer, R., Witten, B.J. (1988) Conceptions of rape *Violence and Victims* 3(3), 217–32.

Rossi, A., Cetrano, G., Pertile, R., Rabbi, L., Donisi, V., Grigoletti, L., *et al.* (2012) Burnout, compassion fatigue, and compassion satisfaction among staff in community-based mental health services *Psychiatry Research* 200(2–3), 933–8.

Sabo, B. (2011). Reflecting on the concept of compassion fatigue *The Online Journal of Issues in Nursing* 16(1), Manuscript 1 [accessed on 31 January 2011].

Showalter, S.E. (2010) Compassion fatigue: What is it? Why does it matter? Recognizing the symptoms, acknowledging the impact, developing the tools to prevent compassion fatigue and strengthen the professional already suffering from the effects *American Journal of Hospice & Palliative Medicine* 27(4), 239–42.

Slocum-Gori, S., Hemsworth, D., Chan, W.W., Carson, A., Kazanjian, A. (2013) Understanding compassion satisfaction, compassion fatigue and burnout: A survey of the hospice palliative care workforce *Palliative Medicine* 27(2), 172–8. Epub 2011 Dec16.

Stringer, H. (2010) Your Own Best Friend: Benefits of Self-Compassion [available at: http://news.nurse.com/article/20101122/NATIONAL01/111220028/-1/front page, accessed on 22 November 2010].

Thomas, R., Wilson, J. (2004) Issues and controversies in the understanding and diagnosis of compassion fatigue, vicarious traumatization and secondary traumatic stress disorder *International Journal of Emergency Mental Health* 6(2), 81–92.

Ting, L., Jacobson, J.M., Sanders, S., Bride, B., Harrington, D. (2005). The secondary traumatic stress scale (STSS): Confirmatory factor analyses with a national sample of mental health social workers. *Journal of Human Behavior in the Social Environment: Special Issue on Measurement and Assessment* 11(3), 177–94.

Van der Heijden, F., Dillingh, G., Bakker, A., Prins, J. (2008) Suicidal thoughts among medical residents with burnout *Archives of Suicide Research* 12, 344–6.

Van Hook, M.P., Rothenberg, M. (2009) Quality of life and compassion satisfaction/fatigue and burnout in child welfare workers: A study of the child welfare workers in community based care organizations in central Florida *Social Work & Christianity* 36(1), 36–54.

Wikipedia. Compassion fatigue [available at: https://en.wikipedia.org/wiki/Compassion_fatigue].

Yang, K.P., Huang, C.K. (2005) The effects of nurse morale on patient satisfaction *Journal of Nursing Research* 13(2), 141–51.

Yoder, E.A. (2010) Compassion fatigue in nurses *Applied Nursing Research* 23(4), 191–7.

Zerubavel, N., Wright, M.O. (2012) The dilemma of the wounded healer *Psychotherapy (Chicago Ill)* 49(4), 482–91.

Appendix A

Resources for preventing and protecting against CF*

1   www.theschwartzcenter.org/aboutus/ourstory.aspx
    The Schwartz Center: an autonomous, non-profit organization founded in 1995 by terminally ill patient, Ken Schwartz. The Center's mission is to promote compassionate healthcare so that patients and their caregivers relate to one another in a way that provides hope to the patient, support to caregivers and sustenance to the healing process.

2   www.heartsinhealthcare.com
    Hearts in Healthcare: founded by Dr Robin Youngson, a New Zealand anesthesiologist, is 'an international movement to rehumanize healthcare for both patients and practitioners by restoring compassion as the centre of patient care'.

3   www.nursingworld.org/healthynurse
    American Nurses' Association (ANA) Healthy Nurse initiative: provides resources for nurses to help maintain work-life balance.

4   www.pulsetoday.co.uk/home/battling-burnout
    Battling burnout in GPs: a national UK campaign launched by Pulse Live to raise awareness of the problem both within and outside the profession, lobby for better monitoring of GP workload and more consistent occupational health support.

5   www.foundationforpositivementalhealth.com/what-is-positive-mental-training
    Foundation for Positive Mental Health: runs training workshops, lobbies politicians and medical organizations, and generally seeks to raise the profile of positive thinking and mind body influences on health and well-being. Positive Mental Training has been validated by research as an occupational health programme to treat burnout, depression and stress at work. It is widely used by NHS staff having undergone training for their own benefit. These mental skills can be thought of as an immunization against stress, giving the required resilience to deal with stressful events, thereby promoting good mental health. The Foundation offers training material for practitioners as well as for patients.

6   www.compassionfatigue.org
    Compassion fatigue awareness program (CFAP): founded by Patricia Smith, a U.S. Certified Compassion Fatigue Specialist with more than 20 years of training experience. This site has numerous resources for caregivers working in many professions. Also offers original training materials, workbooks, and texts through its parent organization, Healthy Caregiving LLC [www.healthycaregiving.com].

7   www.proqol.org/Home_Page.php
    Professional quality of life: an international community, led by Dr
    Beth Hudnall Stamm, that has made the ProQOL and advances in the
    Theory of Compassion Satisfaction and Compassion Fatigue possible.
    Presents and offers for use the ProQOL measures and tools, manual,
    bibliography and related presentation aids. The community' philoso-
    phy is that understanding the positive and negative aspects of helping
    those who experience trauma and suffering can improve our ability to
    help them and our ability to keep our own balance.

    Stamm, B.H. (2009). Professional quality of life: Compassion satisfac-
    tion and fatigue. *Version 5 (ProQOL)*.

8   www.dailygood.org/view.php?sid=211
    DailyGood – news that inspires: a resource for self-care and self-com-
    passion. Established in 1998, the DailyGood project promotes positive
    and uplifting news around the world to more than 100,000 subscribers.
    Readers receive a news story, an inspiring quote, and a suggested action
    that each person can take to make a difference in their own lives and
    the world around them. Based on the philosophy 'Be the change that
    you wish to see in the world', the project is run by dedicated volunteers
    who contribute hundreds of hours finding the right stories and quotes.
    All content is distributed and syndicated for free.

* Appendix items are those most frequently used or well-established (not an exhaustive list)

Appendix B

Screening / diagnostic tools*

A   **The Professional Quality of Life Scale (ProQOL):** a screening and research tool that provides information but does not yield a diagnosis. An expression of the positive aspects of caregiving. Developed by Stamm (Stamm 2009; Stamm 2002)
   • includes 30 items (10 each for CF, burnout, and CS)
   • available from www.proqol.org/Home_Page.php

B   **The Compassion Fatigue Scale** (Adams *et al.*, 2006; Adams, Figley, and Boscarino, 2008).

C   **The SCID and CAPS:** clinical diagnostic tools for PTSD or any other psychopathology as a result of work-related trauma exposure.

D   **The Secondary Traumatic Stress Scale (STSS):** developed by Bride *et al.* (2004). Consists of 17 5-point Likert-type scale items, designed to measure the frequency of intrusion, avoidance, and arousal symptoms associated with indirect exposure to traumatic events via one's professional relationships with traumatized patients, over the past 7 days.
   • used by social workers, mental health professionals
   • available from www.cehd.umn.edu/ssw/cascw/events/Secondary Trauma/PDFs/SecondaryTraumaticStressScale.pdf
   • (Bride 2007; Bride et al. 2004; Dominquez-Gomez and Rutledge 2009; Ting, Jacobson, Sanders, Bride, and Harrington, 2005).

E   **The Maslach Burnout Inventory (MBI) tool:** originally created in 1981 by C. Maslach, S.E Jackson, M.P Leiter, W.B Schaufeli and R.L. Schwab. Recognized as the leading measure of burnout, the MBI incorporates the extensive research that has been conducted in the more than 25 years since its initial publication. Its updated edition comprises three separate surveys, each focusing on a distinct work population.

   Purpose: To assess professional burnout in human service, education, business and government professions.

   Administer to: Individuals 13 years and older

   Administration time: 10–15 minutes

   Scoring Options: Hand scorable

   The MBI addresses three general scales:

   o   Emotional Exhaustion: feelings of being emotionally overextended and exhausted by one's work.
   o   Depersonalization: an unfeeling and impersonal response toward recipients of one's service, care treatment or instruction.
   o   Personal Accomplishment: feelings of competence and successful achievement of one's work.

* Appendix items are those most frequently used or well-established (not an exhaustive list)

Care Experiences: personal note from ER doctor written after woman's death goes viral

by Eric Pfeiffer Yahoo! News

An emergency room doctor at New York Presbyterian Hospital has touched the hearts of millions after a personal letter he wrote about the death of a patient went viral on the Internet. The letter was first published on Reddit by the son of the deceased woman, who reportedly died of breast cancer in December 2012. In the letter, the doctor explains that this is the first such note he has written in 20 years of ER work.

The letter has already been viewed by more than 2 million users on Reddit, with thousands leaving comments. The doctor's letter:

Dear Mr (removed),

I am the Emergency Medicine physician who treated your wife Mrs (removed) last Sunday in the Emergency Department at (hospital). I learned only yesterday about her passing away and wanted to write to you to express my sadness. In my twenty years as a doctor in the Emergency Room, I have never written to a patient or a family member, as our encounters are typically hurried and do not always allow for more personal interaction.

However, in your case, I felt a special connection to your wife (removed), who was so engaging and cheerful in spite of her illness and trouble breathing. I was also touched by the fact that you seemed to be a very loving couple. You were highly supportive of her, asking the right questions with calm, care and concern. From my experience as a physician, I find that the love and support of a spouse or a family member is the most soothing gift, bringing peace and serenity to those critically ill.

I am sorry for your loss and I hope you can find comfort in the memory of your wife's great spirit and of your loving bond. My heartfelt condolences go out to you and your family.

The 24-year-old man who posted the letter said in an email interview with the Huffington Post that the outpouring of support from Reddit users has helped him cope with the passing of his mother.

'If my mother were alive to see this, she would want readers to reflect on the power of showing compassion toward a total stranger,' he said in the interview. 'The support I got from Reddit was amazing – doctors, nurses and other Redditors who have lost their mothers to cancer were all shocked and amazed that the doctor took the time to write such a heartfelt, meaningful letter.

Part V

Concluding section

This section is intended to pull together and summarize the previous chapters, drawing on the key points outlined by the contributors. In addition, the section will look at ways of moving further forward on the important topic of compassion, beginning by addressing the question of whether compassion can be taught.

16 Can compassionate care be taught? Experiences from the Leadership in Compassionate Care Programme, Edinburgh Napier University & NHS Lothian: *Liz Adamson and Stephen Smith*
Conclusion: *Sue Shea, Robin Wynyard and Christos Lionis*

16 Can compassionate care be taught? Experiences from the Leadership in Compassionate Care Programme, Edinburgh Napier University and NHS Lothian

Liz Adamson and Stephen Smith

Patients and their families are clear about the value they place on the relational aspects of care. How the nurse or student relates to them as they give the care is as important as the care itself (Firth-Cozens and Cornwell 2009; Pearcey 2010; Smith *et al.* 2010; Edinburgh Napier University and NHS Lothian 2012; Planetree 2012; Dewar 2013; Dewar and Nolan 2013). Compassionate care is not easily defined and measured and there has been much discussion and debate about whether it can be taught (Bradshaw 2009; Shea and Lionis 2010; Adamson and Dewar 2011; Dewar 2011; Curtis 2013). Some people believe that compassion is something that is inherent in a person and cannot be taught (Barker 2013) while others identify that it is a virtue to be cultivated (Bradshaw 2009). Others suggest that we cannot teach compassion but can help students to develop the character and skills that enable them to care compassionately (McLean 2012). The Leadership in Compassionate Care action research programme was developed in response to concerns about the human elements of healthcare practice (Edinburgh Napier University and NHS Lothian 2012). Throughout the programme, health care staff expressed sadness that research such as this was necessary, as they believed that it should be inherent in what they do. This suggests an assumption that the care people experience is compassionate and that those who give that care have the knowledge and skill to provide it. However, we have seen that this is not always the case (*Mid Staffordshire NHS Foundation Public Inquiry* 2013). Similarly the modern context of healthcare is very complex and the expectations of care delivery have changed dramatically; care is increasingly focused on individual needs and preferences; fiscal restrictions and monitoring in healthcare, increasing complexity of treatments and care; waiting time targets and rapid throughput of patients within in-patient care to identify but a few (Youngson 2012; *Mid Staffordshire NHS Foundation Public Inquiry* 2013; Maben *et al.* 2009). It is within this backdrop that we need to consider supporting the development of compassionate caring knowledge and skills within undergraduate nurses.

In order to develop these skills we must first discover what makes care compassionate, or not, and hearing about the experiences of patients, carers and those who provide care can help to inform this.

A good starting place in learning how to provide compassionate care is recognising that we don't always know what patients want and should not make assumptions but consistently check out what is important to them. Listening to the stories of patients and their families, and of those who provide care, can help us to identify the elements of care that make it compassionate and that challenge our assumptions. This heightened awareness and sensitivity to this subject can increase our knowledge and enhance our practice and skills. Stories can help us to reflect on what is important to patients and families (Moon 2010) as listening and reflecting on the stories of others gives us access to the situations, thoughts and experiences of these individuals as they live out their daily lives (McDrury and Alterio 2003). They also support us to reflect on our own practices and experience of caring enabling reflection in action; reflecting in the moment and actively adapting how we do things (Mann *et al.* 2009).

The Leadership in Compassionate Care Programme (LCCP)

In response to concerns about the personalisation and humanity of caring and the experience of compassion within healthcare, the Leadership in Compassionate Care Programme was developed as a joint programme of research between Edinburgh Napier University and NHS Lothian, this programme began in 2007 and research activities continue. The research aims were to embed compassionate nursing within clinical practice and pre-registration nursing education. The focus of inquiry incorporated conducting research within four key areas: first, clinical areas of excellence (28 NHS Lothian in-patient areas including adult, child, mental health and maternity care services); second, with newly qualified staff; third, a Leadership Programme intervention; and the fourth area was embedding learning within the undergraduate nursing and midwifery curriculum. This action research programme adopted theoretical underpinning principles of Appreciative Inquiry and Relationship Centred Care. Appreciative inquiry is an organisational approach based on a premise that within every organisation there are processes that work well. It moves away from a problem-solving approach, focuses attention on success and how this is achieved, and utilises this learning to enhance ways of working (Cooperider *et al.* 2008). Complimentary to this is relationship-centred care which places relationships at the core of every day practice and includes patients, relatives and staff and the inter relationships between and amongst these groups (Nolan *et al.* 2006).

Working with clinical areas of excellence, the research identified and tested key practice development processes that enabled healthcare staff to gather evidence and experiences of care and utilise this evidence through real time feedback, to develop and evaluate compassionate, multidisciplinary healthcare practice. This was gathered from service users, families, staff and students in a variety of ways which included narrative accounts of care, formal and informal observations of practice, beliefs and values focus groups, photo elicitation, interviews with staff and evaluation of action projects. Data were analysed by the LCCP team using a constant comparative method. Evidence and learning from participating clinical areas was shared across NHS Lothian and is currently being disseminated across Scotland. Learning and outcomes from the research conducted within clinical practice has been adapted and implemented within the undergraduate nursing and midwifery curricula through a series of action projects, for example introducing the assessment of compassionate behaviours of students during a simulated clinical assessment scenario and this is described below. An outcome from the LCCP is a model of six key elements of compassionate care; this model is being utilised to further develop practice and education. For example, the model underpins a national education programme for midwifery, infant and maternal health. The model identifies processes related to service users, families and staff and incorporates; caring conversations; feedback; involving, valuing and transparency; person-centred risk taking; knowing you knowing me; creating spaces that work. The final report of the LCCP (Edinburgh Napier University and NHS Lothian 2012) can be found at http://researchrepository.napier.ac.uk/id/eprint/5935.

Within this chapter we will describe and discuss two cases studies where nursing students were given the opportunity to learn and develop skills in compassionate caring.

Case Study 1

This describes a changes implemented in an undergraduate nursing module.

Background to the project

This first case study is set within university where an acute nursing module was modified to make compassionate care more explicit. The module uses simulated practice to teach student nurses how to systematically assess acutely ill patients and how to recognise and respond to signs of deterioration. The underpinning theory is provided online and students are asked to engage with this prior to face to face simulated practice. As the module deals with acutely ill patients the setting was an emergency or acute admissions department. Proving compassionate care in areas of high patients turnover is considered to be challenging as the focus of attention can be the provision of life saving care and minimising deterioration through appropriate and timely interventions. Findings from the LCCP had, however, demonstrated that compassionate care is possible in every care setting and does not necessarily take more time to provide. We therefore set out to encourage the students to focus not only on the technical aspects of care but on the person as an individual and what was important to them at that moment.

Aims of the project

To make compassionate care more explicit within an acute nursing module and to assess it.

To encourage reflective learning and raise awareness of what matters most to patients through listening to the experiences of those involved in giving and receiving care.

Reflection activity

Think of an episode of care that you observed in practice which was compassionate and person centred.
    What were the key elements of this care that made it compassionate?

What we did

We invited students, senior nurses in compassionate care, and lecturers in nursing and clinical staff to participate in an action day where the themes from the LCCP were discussed and how these could be integrated into all aspects of the module and learning experience. One outcome involved briefing the actor patients and encouraging them to use cues that prompt students to think about aspects of compassionate care. For example instructing the actors to say 'You will stay with me won't you nurse?', prompting the students to reassure the patient and sensitively negotiate what is possible.

Actor patients are volunteers who undertake training in role play and working with students. They are given instruction about a specific scenario such as who they are, how they should act and how to respond to the questions students might ask.

Changes to the module

The themes were introduced to the students in the online module materials and excerpts from patients, relatives or staff member's stories were shared to initiate online discussion around aspects of compassionate care. We recorded the stories that had been gathered in clinical practice and released them as podcasts on a dedicated podcast site. The stories helped the students to understand the experience of patients and relatives and how they felt about care. Staff stories helped the students to reflect on what guides the decisions that we make as nurses which can at times involve an element of risk when we do something that is unique and person-centred care.

During practical teaching session when students used jargon such as 'I'll do your obs now' we encouraged actors to question what they meant. The stories gathered within practice demonstrated that making a connection with patients through finding out what they were interested in was an important part of building relationships as demonstrated in the quote below.

Example excerpt from a story:

> It makes a difference if you try to find out something about the person. There is a man in bay 2 and even although it's hard to talk to him – I've managed to have a wee bit of a conversation with him – he likes Hearts (Edinburgh Football Club) – I told him what the Hearts score was yesterday. I look in the notes or speak to the relatives to try to find something– this man had a hearts strip – so I knew. It's good to have common ground to work with. I always try to do this. I've never come across a time when I couldn't make some connection.
>
> Member of staff

We therefore asked the actors to wear something that might provide a clue to the patient's interests such as a badge or a tie with the name of a local golf club or a football scarf.

During the debrief reflective sessions that followed the lecturers fed back to students and encouraged them to identify what they did well, what they might do differently and areas for further development and learning. The actors were also invited to feedback to the students how they felt such as whether they felt safe, listened to and kept informed.

The themes that emerged from the Leadership in Compassionate Care Programme informed the changes that we made such as including elements of compassionate care within the assessment criteria so that students were awarded additional marks when they demonstrated compassionate practice. For example when they ensured that they kept the patient informed of what was happening and what to expect or when they asked the patient if anything was troubling them or what was important to them at that moment this was awarded marks.

What the students said

The students enjoyed listening to the podcasts and discussing the stories. They found that it helped them to understand how patients felt and also helped them to reflect on their own practice and experiences.

The podcasts provide an archive of both the emotional complexities of caring and a reminder of the importance of simple thoughtful actions. The compassion, courage and reflection expressed through Margaret and Elizabeth in their own story is priceless. Thoughtful actions can come from the one's own past experience, and at times these may have been painful. Within nursing it is rare to receive critical feedback from families and the value of sharing these personal stories seems to provide a powerful learning experience.

Student

The students found it helpful to receive feedback from the actors and discuss the scenarios during the debrief reflective sessions.

Listening to the stories injected a new enthusiasm into my work and a belief that I can change things for my patients regardless even in difficult situations.

Student

Case Study 2

This case study describes developments where learning about compassionate care was realised in a clinical practice setting.

What was the background to this development?

The clinical setting for this development was a National Health Service 30-bed in-patient ward for adults who have complex and palliative care needs (Hawthorne Ward), within a small hospital with two wards called Ellens Glen House. Patients are cared for by a comprehensive multidisciplinary team. Undergraduate nursing students from Edinburgh Napier University have the opportunity to experience clinical placements within this setting.

The Senior Charge Nurse (SCN) who leads the team in Hawthorn ward, participated in the 2010 LCCP Leadership Programme; also the other ward (Thistle ward) was one of the first clinical areas of excellence to participate in the programme. These wards have received national and international recognition for their developments in compassionate person-centred care. The UK Patient Experience Network National Award in 2011 for establishing a person-centred caring in-patient environment (Thistle ward) and The International Care Challenge Award 2011 (Hawthorne Ward); this award was for activities that enhance communication between staff and with patients and relatives.

The SCN within Hawthorne Ward was keen to utilise learning from the LCCP Leadership Programme and chose to focus on activities that would influence the student experience. The Leadership Programme utilised theories of relationship-centred care, appreciative inquiry and adopted principles of action research (Cooperrider *et al.* 2008; Nolan *et al.* 2006; Coghlan and Brannick 2010). The programme also supported participants to use a range of tools to listen and respond to feedback in real time, for example rapid feedback forms, emotional touch point process and photo elicitation (Dewar *et al.* 2010; Brand and McMurray 2009; Edinburgh Napier University and NHS Lothian 2012).

The aims of this development?

For undergraduate nursing students to:

*   Further develop an understanding of person-centred compassionate care.
*   To utilise the process of personal reflection to enhance person-centred, compassionate practice.
*   To utilise a creative and fun approach to reflection and learning.
*   To reinforce theoretical approaches in learning (relationship-centred care, appreciative inquiry).

What learning, teaching and assessment strategies were used?

Activity 1

Students were asked to work in pairs or groups and spend approximately one hour away from ward activities participating in a session where they created a collage using flip chart, pens, cuttings from magazines and other creative materials. They were asked the following framing question: think of yourself as a patient in this ward: what would compassionate care look like for you? Students worked collaboratively on the collage and when it was complete the SCN joined them and facilitated a discussion where they talked about the content of their collage, perceptions of individualised compassionate care expressed within it and how this experience might influence how they care for others. The students named their collage and with permission it was put on display in a staff area. This pictorial representation of individual compassion provided an opportunity for the students to share their views and perceptions whilst simultaneously triggering wider discussion amongst staff about person-centred compassionate care. The SCN worked with seven students over a period of 8 months undertaking this learning activity.

Activity 2

At the completion of their clinical placement in Hawthorne Ward, all students were invited to complete a questionnaire based on the Senses framework, which relates to relationship-centred care and achieving the following six senses; security, belonging, continuity, purpose, achievement and significance (Nolan *et al.* 2006; *Smith et al.* 2010) see Figure 16.1. This provided feedback to staff about the student experience of learning and their experiences of care provision while working on the ward. The questionnaire was given to each student commencing their placement as part of a student information pack. The SCN met with each student and discussed their questionnaire responses identifying positive feedback, opportunities for learning and development in regard to the student experience and also the student's individual perceptions of care.

Student nurse Evaluation form for Hawthorn Ward Ellens Glen House

Name   **Date**

Read each statement, indicate on the scale where you feel from 1, totally disagree to 5, fully agree and please expand or explain any aspect you feel necessary.

Factors creating a sense of security	1	2	3	4	5
I felt welcomed to the ward					
The ward environment was supportive					
I was treated as an individual					
I felt safe to participate					
I understand the purpose of the ward					
Comments:					

Factors creating a sense of belonging	1	2	3	4	5
I have/have access to relevant information and materials					
My expectations have been met					
My ideas have been valued and encouraged					
I am encouraged to feel part of the team					
Comments:					

Factors creating a sense of continuity	1	2	3	4	5
I can relate theoretical knowledge to practical experience					
I am receiving adequate information which enhances my learning experience					
Comments:					

Factors creating a sense of purpose	1	2	3	4	5
I understand my role within the ward					
I have identified personal and professional goals to reach for this placement					
I feel there is the potential to make a difference to the quality of care					

Comments:

Factors creating a sense of achievement	1	2	3	4	5
I have actively participated in assessing and planning care					
I have spent time with my mentor					
I have used my own initiative					
I have felt supported/supportive with learning					
I have given/received feedback					

Comments:

Factors creating a sense of achievement	1	2	3	4	5
I have an important contribution to make to patient care					
My contributions have been valued by others					
I have valued others' contributions					
I feel I can make an impact on quality of care					

Comments:

If you could change 3 things about the ward what 3 things would you change:

1.

2.

3.

Figure 16.1 Student nurse evaluation form for Hawthorn Ward Ellens Glen House
Adapted from Nolan *et al.* 2006

What were the findings?

Activity 1 Creating a collage

From a process perspective this was an unfamiliar learning activity, however, all students invited to undertake this learning activity participated in the process despite awareness by the SCN that students felt apprehensive at first about creating a collage. Students indicated that they were proud to have their named collage on display and this generated wider discussions amongst the ward team not only about care, but also how we know what patients and families want, if it is possible to provide and how to action and achieve this. This process identified an overt activity in hearing the students' perspectives, and the SCN perceived that students felt a sense of value which was further investigated in the SENSES questionnaire. The process was quick and easy and cost very little in terms of staff time and materials. This creative and fun activity had a secondary benefit in that it provided stimulating visual images to observe and discuss. The presence of a skilled facilitator and a ward culture where seeking, hearing and responding to feedback was valued and commonplace were vital to the success of this project and therefore important to consider were this activity to be replicated in other settings. Students may feel concerned about participating in this form of learning if they sense an atmosphere of judgement or criticism.

The following feedback from a student identifies some critical reflections regarding doing the right thing in terms of providing care but achieving this whilst incorporating the person's wishes:

> I was asked to prepare a poster on compassionate care taking on the role as a patient in a palliative care setting. As a nurse I believe we all have compassion, at first I did not see the rationale of this project. However, on taking part in this and putting myself in the shoes of the patient, it made me think outside the box, and became apparent how worthwhile it was. I felt this changed my whole outlook of compassionate care and made me focus more on not only what was right but what the patients wishes were. For example if I were a patient in a palliative setting who could no longer manage out of bed to use the toilet, I would prefer to be catheterised rather than being wet in a pad. I would find this demoralising.
>
> (Janet, student nurse, year 3)

Actively hearing and responding to feedback of a person-centred nature has been identified as crucial to the provision of compassionate care (Edinburgh Napier University and NHS Lothian 2012). Janet's views on her wish for catheterisation were she to become bed-bound challenge assumptions about what people would want in this context. The challenge identified by Janet is finding out this person-centred knowledge and working with it in the context of providing care.

The following images and quotes identify similar challenges in hearing and responding to person-centred care and not settling with providing care based on possible assumptions or practice as usual:

'No nappies I'd rather have a catheter'
'Nice food . . . no mush'
'No bad odours'

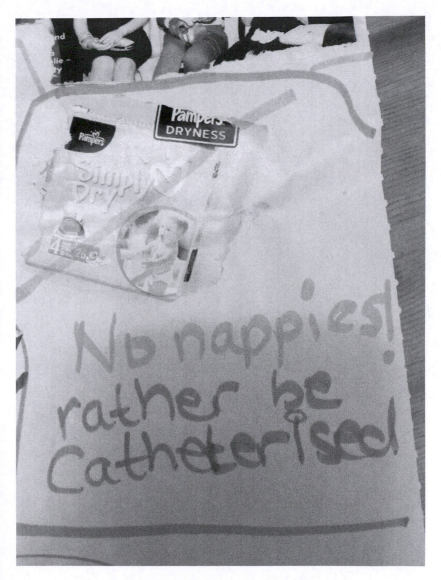

Figure 16.2 Example image 1: No nappies rather be catheterised

'My family, live laugh and love'
Hair done each day . . . Aussie products ☺

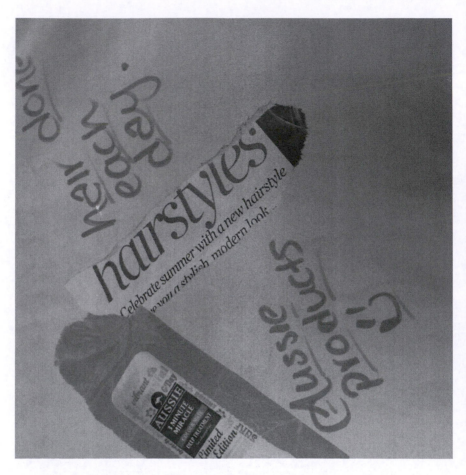

Figure 16.3 Example image 2: Aussie products

'Get outside'

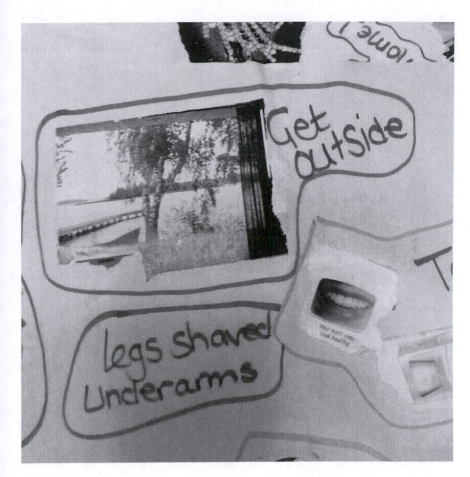

Figure 16.4 Example image 3: Get outside

'Comfy clothes that match'

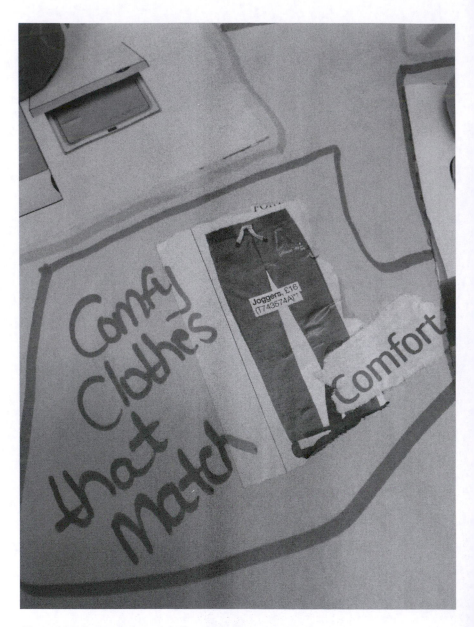

Figure 16.5 Example image 4: Comfy clothes

Activity 2 SENSES evaluation

Feedback from the SCN in regard to using the SENSES evaluation was that it provided a useful and important structure to reflect upon the student's placement. The content of the questionnaire appears highly relevant to students and therefore they are able to complete it with little instruction. The SCN identified the importance of discussing the responses provided by students. Dependent on shift patterns this is not always possible but the students have the questionnaire in their induction pack and they are encouraged to complete it and discuss with their mentor.

The SCN also identified the importance of sharing this feedback with staff, celebrating positive student learning experiences and feedback about care. It is helpful to discuss the feedback where ideas have been expressed and have a think about other opinions and views and debating what we could do differently. Feedback can provide a trigger for staff to consider improvement.

Two examples of feedback that have generated improvement activity included a suggestion that patients and families should be able to access Wi-Fi on the ward and that there could be more use of technology to support patients and relatives. This is currently not available for patients and relatives. With an increasingly diverse age range of patients and the widespread use of social networking, access to the Internet could be a useful way of meeting person-centred needs. Staff have been working with Hospital Facility staff to identify what would make this happen.

A second example related to providing clocks in all the rooms so patients know what time of day it is. At the time of this feedback not all patients had this and staff are looking at and the possibility of purchasing a range of different clocks to ensure patients who have problems with visual acuity can use them.

Examples of feedback relating to the question 'What three things would you change?' can be seen below:

'Have more activities for patients.'

'Wouldn't change anything, enjoyed working on the ward with an excellent team of friendly staff'.

'The amount of time set aside to spend directly with patients, although I appreciate this is difficult everywhere.'

The above examples of improvement are specific; they will not make a difference to all patients but they provide options for staff in caring for someone in a person-centred compassionate way. Hearing and discussing feedback and having caring conversations is an important activity for staff, ensuring that compassionate person-centred care is consistently identified as a core priority within practice.

Can compassionate care be taught? Key aspects to consider

Processes to support learning about compassionate care should incorporate nurturing and building upon existing knowledge, skills and experiences of compassion.

Sharing and hearing individual narratives of what compassionate care looks like, helps to stimulate and challenge how individual practitioners and teams think about and practically deliver this type of care.

Hearing and responding to feedback and having caring conversations can keep the delivery of compassionate care a priority for a healthcare team. Within the LCCP a variety of tools were utilised to elicit evidence of compassionate care and facilitate developments in practice. An example of this was observations of practice. Tools such as this are beneficial; however, they require to be undertaken within a supportive learning culture where compassion is valued and integral to ways of working. Within this environment there also needs ongoing and skilled facilitation supporting practitioners to care compassionately.

There is a growing evidence and awareness identifying that compassionate practice is of central importance to patients, families and multidisciplinary healthcare staff worldwide. The LCCP was undertaken in the United Kingdom; however, it is evident that the activities and findings of the programme are relevant internationally, for example through research collaborations developed in Europe and Australia.

Further research in this area would identify the correlation between the learning activities described in this chapter and a continuing impact on compassionate care practice. This would relate to both individual practitioners and to care teams.

Acknowledgements

The authors would like to acknowledge and thank the following people for their contribution to this article. The acute nursing module team at Edinburgh Napier University; patients, relatives and staff at NHS Lothian who participated in the LCCP; undergraduate nursing students at Edinburgh Napier University who participated in learning activities; the LCCP team; and Senior Charge Nurse Jacqui Brodie, NHS Lothian.

References

Adamson, L., Dewar, B. (2011) Compassion in the nursing curriculum: Making it more explicit *Journal of Holistic Healthcare* 8(3), 42–5.
Barker, K. (2013) Can care and compassion be taught? *British Journal of Midwifery* 21(2), 82.
Bradshaw, A. (2009) Measuring compassion: The McDonaldised nurse? *Journal of Medical Ethics* 35(8), 465–8.
Brand, G., McMurray, A. (2009) Reflection on photographs: Exploring first year nursing students perceptions of older adults *Journal of Gerontological Nursing* 35(11), 30–5.

Firth-Cozens, J., Cornwell, J. (2009) *The Point of Care: Enabling Compassionate Care in Acute Hospital Settings.* London: The Kings Fund.

Coghlan, D., Brannick, T. (2010) *Doing Action Research in Your Organisation*, 2nd edition. London: Sage publications.

Cooperider, D., Whitney, D., Stavros, J. (2008) *Appreciative Inquiry Handbook for Leaders of Change*, 2nd edition. Brunswick, OH: Berret-Koehler.

Curtis, K. (2013) Learning the requirement for compassionate practice: Student vulnerability and courage *Nursing Ethics* http://nej.sagepub.com/content/early/2013/03/15/0969733013478307.full.pdf (accessed 20 March 2013).

Dewar, B. (2011) Caring about caring: An appreciative inquiry about compassionate relationship centred care, PhD, Edinburgh Napier University, Edinburgh [available at: http://researchrepository.napier.ac.uk/id/eprint/4845].

Dewar, B., Nolan, M. (2013) Caring about caring: Developing a model to implement compassionate relationship centred care in an older people care setting *International Journal of Nursing Studies* DOI: 10:1016\j.ijnurstu2013.01.008.

Dewar, B., Mackay, R., Smith, S., Pullin, S., Tocher, R. (2010) Use of emotional touchpoints as a method of tapping into the experience of receiving compassionate care in a hospital setting *Journal of Nursing Research* 15(1), 29–41.

Edinburgh Napier University, NHS Lothian (2012) *Leadership in Compassionate Care Programme, Final Report.* Edinburgh: Edinburgh Napier University.

Maben, J., Cornwell, J., Sweeney, K. (2009) In praise of compassion *Journal of Research in Nursing* 15(1), 9–12.

McDrury, J., Alterio, M. (2003) *Learning through Story Telling in Higher Education: Using Refection and Experience to Improve Learning.* London: Kogan Page.

McLean, C. (2012) The yellow brick road: A values based curriculum model *Nurse Education in Practice* 12, 159–63.

Mann, K., Gordon, J., MacLeod, A. (2009) Reflection and reflective practice in health professions education: A systematic review *Advances in Health Science Education* 14, 595–621.

Mid Staffordshire NHS Foundation Public Inquiry (2013), Report of the Mid Staffordshire NHS Foundation Trust Public Inquiry. London: Stationery Office.

Moon, J. (2010) *Using Story in Higher Education and Professional Development.* London: Routledge.

Nolan, M., Davies, S., Brown, J., Nolan, J., Keady, J. (2006) *The SENSES Framework: Improving Care for Older People through a Relationship Centred Approach.* Getting Research into Practice Series. Sheffield: University of Sheffield.

Shea, S., Lionis, C. (2010) Restoring humanity in health care through the art of compassion: An issue for the teaching and research agenda in rural health care *Rural and Remote Health Journal* 10(4), 1679.

Pearcey, P. (2010) Caring? It's the little things we are not supposed to do anymore *International Journal of Nursing Practice* 16(1), 51–6.

Planetree (2012) Advancing Person Centred Care across the Continuum of Care [available at: www.plantree.org].

Smith, S., Dewar, B., Pullin, S., Tocher, R. (2010) Relationship centred outcomes focused on compassionate care for older people within in-patient settings *International Journal of Older people's Nursing* 5(2), 128–37.

Youngson, R. (2012) *Time to Care.* Raglan, NZ: Rebelheart Publishers.

Conclusion

Sue Shea, Robin Wynyard and Christos Lionis

> When we tell our children about the Great Recession, they will judge us not by growth rates or by deficit reductions. They will judge us by how well we took care of society's most vulnerable, and whether we chose to address our community's most basic health needs . . . The ultimate source of any society's wealth is its people. Investing in their health is a wise choice in the best of times, and an urgent necessity in the worst of times.
>
> (Stuckler and Basu 2013, pp. 145)

The above quote reminds us that in times of austerity, values in health care are of an even greater importance, and the need for compassion is even more visible. However, treating the individual with humanity is crucial at all times.

In the realization of the need and benefits of compassion in health care, and that there is unity in this mission, the aim of this book was to bring together a number of key people, with specific expertise within their chosen fields in order to comprehensively approach elements of compassionate health care. In looking at delivering a broader picture of the concept and implementation of compassion, we have included inspirational contributions from different countries, including England, Scotland, Greece, America and New Zealand.

Both as a word and as a concept, compassion has been brought into sharper focus in health care after events at Mid Staffordshire Hospital UK, and elsewhere. Following the release of the internationally recognized report by Francis (2013), the need for attention to basic health care needs and support for health care staff has become an even more crucial issue at a global level. As Robin Youngson reminds us in the foreword to this book ' . . . personal stories are mirrored by media reports of widespread and scandalous failings of compassionate care . . . '.

However, our intention within this book has been to not only focus on negative experiences, but to also provide examples of positive experiences. In addition to the key chapters of this book, we have also included service-user, carer, and health care professionals' personal experiences, which we feel could provide a valuable learning tool for our readers.

Compassion as a concept may be difficult to quantify, thus there are many varied definitions of compassion provided in the book. Having said this, there is considerable overlap in each of them, and all contributors agree that compassion is a major element in health care both at an organizational level, and in the practical implementation of health care delivery. For example, in Chapter 5, Craig Brown refers to compassion as a 'value' and defines it as ' . . . a soft gentle word that has a deep strength and richness. It is kindness in action. Compassion is a feeling that rises up in response to another's difficulty and urges one to act to alleviate their discomfort . . . '. Thus, compassion can be considered not as a solitary activity, but as a concept containing many features, such as empathy and a genuine need to explore the role of another. Certain approaches lend themselves to this method. Wynyard, in Chapter 1, draws on the work of Irving Goffman and his use of the dramaturgical analogy where in acting out our relationships with others we are either 'front of house' of 'backstage'. In our view, we would argue that health care has to be seen as a holistic practice, with all members of the health care team being attributed equal importance. Everyone working in the health care setting (including administrators, porters, cleaners), ultimately has a responsibility towards the patient, as the patient is the person who is most vulnerable at that moment in time. Thus a patient-centred approach from all individuals involved in the health care system is key.

In addition to the issue of defining compassion, the editors also felt that it was important to explore the nature of the concept. Thus, in Chapter 1, the long historical antecedents of compassion are also drawn upon including reference to the ancient Greeks who thought long and hard about the nature of compassion and the ideas that surround it. They saw that how we act towards others may not always be done in the best or most altruistic way.

The focus of this book was to explore the role of health care practitioners in providing compassionate health care. In Chapter 1, the history of the concept of compassion is addressed at a general level, and following on from the historical context Ann Bradshaw in Chapter 2 focuses on the changing role of nursing over the years, where key figures such as Florence Nightingale are discussed, at a time when nursing was a growing profession imbued with compassion ' . . . witnessed in attentiveness to the practical details of care, in which nothing is too much trouble . . . clearing away vomit, helping the person to the toilet, cleaning faeces off the skin, helping the person to feed and drink . . . willingly with kindness'. With the drive towards a scientific and technological approach in nurse and medical training, perhaps we have lost certain values that traditionally existed in nursing and medicine. However, this may also be partially explained by the nature of financial issues, stress, and the amount of paperwork that health care professionals (HCPs) have to endure.

A further feature of this book, is taking into consideration the conditions under which HCPs are expected to provide compassionate care to their patients. Chapters 3 and 4 deal with the impact of stress on the carers themselves and argue that in keeping compassion alive we have to consider not just the patient, but also the carer. As George Chrousos reminds us:

> not all young physicians, nurses or patient relatives are born with the innate ability to control their emotions and provide care with principled compassion. All of us should be preparing for coping with stress and learn from others, and this is a life-long process . . .

Whilst Martin Seager points to 'a psychologically-minded approach' involving 'looking at the wider system, context and culture of care-giving'. This is a theme also specifically dealt with by Ada Markaki in Chapter 15 where the importance of recognizing early symptoms of compassion fatigue and burn-out is discussed, in order to enable a safe haven for fellow practitioners, so that their patients can always be provided with appropriate care.

In relation to Chapters 3 and 4, Chapter 6 offers a complimentary explanation with regard to the biological effect of compassion. In this chapter Alys Cole-King and Paul Gilbert argue that 'compassion has a very powerful neurophysiological effect and compassion makes our interventions more clinically effective and therefore competent care must also be compassionate care'. The work of both George Chrousos and Alys Cole-King/Paul Gilbert show that by positive techniques, brain chemistry can be altered in oneself and in others giving a more positive outlook on life.

In the introduction to this book, it was noted that compassion is a growing field requiring a multidisciplinary approach. Chapters 6 and 14 mention the importance of the Schwartz Rounds as a way of encouraging multidisciplinary teams to acknowledge and share the emotional impact of working with very distressed patients, and to manage their team dynamics. Again our attention is drawn to the need and importance for HCPs to work together, which could also be a focus of medical and nurse training in terms of training students to work and learn from each other in ways which could benefit both the patient, and the future practitioners' own well-fare. In Chapter 5, Craig Brown looks at the importance of sharing information and discussing the core values of compassion. Drawing on the concept of experiential learning, the benefits of working in small groups is suggested as a useful educational approach to bring about a change in the values, beliefs and behaviour necessary to make compassionate care central in all healthcare settings.

To make more illustrative the provision of compassionate care in chronically ill patients, the book utilized dementia as a clinical entity. Dementia is a condition that is challenging to approach, and where it is important to identify specific practice paradigms that can be presented and discussed. Chapter 10 posits a fascinating and very successful approach into the care of dementia patients. The approach lies in the nature of clowning, in the 'Elderflowers' and 'Clown Doctors' managed by Magdalena Schamberger. Clowning has had a long history of getting people to see both the joy and distress of life in one performance. Sporting old-fashioned clothing and artificial red noses, Schamberger's 'Elderflowers' are able to engage with and compassionately communicate with dementia patients who might otherwise remain inactive. The red nose is a symbol of anonymity, but instantly recognized by the patients and thus distinguishing the Elderflowers from other staff or visitors.

Staying with the issue of chronic illness, and in times of financial crisis, Stathis Papavasiliou, the author of Chapter 11, argues that in the wave of protests in Greece there is the necessity by patients and HCPs alike to 'reevaluate concepts and practices such as compassionate care'. As an endocrinologist, Papavasiliou uses diabetes as a paradigm of chronic illness to show that even in trying circumstances in countries such as Greece, compassion can be exercised if approached in a systematic way. Here he uses a military analogy where a positive outlook always forecasts a victory against odds.

Undoubtedly, an area within which compassionate care is particularly crucial is palliative and end-of-life care. In Chapter 7, Sue Shea discusses the importance of compassionate approaches in palliative and end-of-life care. Shea notes key issues such as patient preferences, the nature of suffering, dignity, and approaches that may reduce suffering and increase the well-being and quality of life for both patients reaching the end of life, and their loved ones.

Economic crisis also features within the book; in particular, this is seen in the work of Alex Kentikelenis *et al.*, who are coming from a Greek perspective on health care. The Greek situation is well known, where Greece – a country close to bankruptcy, has had to endure strict austerity measures, ultimately affecting health care services. The situation in Greece highlights the connection between austerity and healthcare and the impact of financial crisis on the health of people and healthcare systems around the world. In a recently published book Stuckler and Basu (2013) remind us that ' . . . austerity involves the deadliest social policies. Recessions can hurt but austerity kills' (p. xx).

Many chapters of this book have highlighted the importance of compassion in health care but a question that immediately comes to mind is how it can be achieved. Valerie Iles in Chapter 13 demonstrates the importance of recognizing that lack of compassionate care may originate from the organization level, whereby bureaucracy, time management and utilization of scarce resources may take precedence over hands on care of patients. Iles in this chapter shows that renewing the enthusiasm of health care professionals and managerial staff for their role can help them to become more effective and confident in managing people as human beings in their own right. With a similar focus, Susan Frampton and Joanna Goodrich in Chapter 14 put forward current initiatives for improving hospital care and transforming organizational cultures. The authors of this chapter discuss the work of two organizations, one in the UK and one in the USA – both of which emphasize the importance of a patient-centred approach, whilst taking into consideration the organizational structure, thus developing ground breaking programmes aimed at restoring humanity across the organization.

In addition to the organizational changes that health care systems require to successfully implement the provision of compassionate care, it is also important to learn from the analysis of health care providers and patients' experiences. Thus, within Chapter 9, Jill Maben draws on recent research initiatives, discussing patient and health care providers' experiences, and ways in which improving staff well-being can help to improve the patient experience, leading to more compassionate and measurable care delivery.

Although much focus is on hospital care with regard to compassion, the primary health care setting is often the first port of call for illness and disease management. Thus it is a highly suitable setting where compassionate care could be discussed and effective policies could be introduced. In Chapter 8, Christos Lionis and Sue Shea draw attention to the fact that compassionate care is also important within the primary health care setting, pointing out that the concept in its totality appears to currently be missing from the World Organization of Family Doctors (WONCA) current definition of general practice. The authors suggest that the topic of compassion should be included within undergraduate medical teaching, and should also be a focus of family medicine research. Perhaps a major question is whether compassion can be taught, and if so, how. In the concluding section of this book, Liz Adamson and Stephen Smith explore the feasibility of teaching compassion, and the methods which might be instigated in order to achieve this. The chapter draws on some examples of initiatives for teaching compassion that are currently in place, discussing their effectiveness and future relevance to ensuring that compassion is retained as a crucial element of health care.

Service-user and carer contributions

The editors were very grateful to have the valuable input from service-users and carers, which we feel represent a valuable learning tool for our target readership. These contributions have covered treatment of accidents (both in emergency and primary care settings), cancer treatment, clinical depression, amputation, panic attacks, chronic medical conditions, encephalitis, and the importance of hearing and touch in end-of-life care. These contributions not only draw attention to examples of bad care, but also provide examples of very good care, reminding us how good care can be achieved and the sorts of acts of kindness and basic attention to care that are so important to the patient. We are also grateful to the HCPs who provided short accounts of their experiences, poems, and permission to use correspondence, as we feel that these too are valuable learning tools.

Paving the way for enhancing the practice of compassionate health care – summary

A number of issues have been identified in this book, in relation to the provision of compassionate health care and factors that may enhance or prevent it. There are certain key factors that need to be considered to allow for the concept of compassionate to be fully integrated. As we have seen, economic crisis is an obvious influencing factor with regard to the organization of health care services. Within the organization itself, we have been drawn many times to the issue of burn-out and compassion fatigue amongst health care professionals. Thus it is crucial that HCPs themselves are encouraged in the concept of self-care and resilience, and are protected at an organizational level. This book aims to make HCPs more aware about the potential impact of the provision of compassionate care in alleviating the patient's burden, and also to assist in diminishing the risk of burn-out.

The concept of teaching compassion to medical/nurse students and to practising HCPs in all health care settings may crucial, to ensure that the values that they entered the profession with are not lost through the technicalities of training. We have seen that there are a number of initiatives, that can help to promote compassionate health care, and that can introduce new ways of delivering care, and these should be encouraged and developed at all levels. It also seems clear that learning from experiences of patients, carers and HCPs themselves can help us to more fully understand the positives and negatives of health care and factors which can play a major role in the overall patient experience and rate of recovery, disease management and end-of-life acceptance. At this stage, it seems that research into the field of compassionate care, and methods of intervention and evaluation could be enormously helpful. Such research could take place at both a psychosocial, educational and a biological level – designed with a specific focus on the biological effect on both the health care providers and the compassionate care recipient. We hope that this book, will help to pave the way and encourage such research, and that it will offer key theoretical elements to future researchers in this field. We further anticipate that it will be a useful teaching aid, and a helpful reference for both students, and practising HCPs, and for those working in other disciplines with an interest in the importance concept of compassionate care.

We would like to end this book with a poem from the thirteenth-century Persian poet Saadi. This poem is carved in Farsi on the wall just inside the door of the United Nations building in New York. It does not have a title; simply it explores the nature of what it means to be human:

> Human beings come
> From the same source,
> We are one family.
> If a part of the body hurts,
> All parts contract with pain.
> If you are not concerned
> With another's suffering,
> We shall not call you human.
>
> Poem quoted in *Rumi: Bridge to the Soul*
> by Coleman Barks, Harper Collins 2007

Useful links

http://heartsinhealthcare.com

www.jcompassionatehc.com

http://www.jankifoundation.org

http://www.collegeofmedicine.org.uk

http://www.compassionatemind.co.uk

http://www.connectingwithpeople.org

http://researchrepository.napier.ac.uk/id/eprint/4845

http://planetree.org

http://www.heartsminds.org.uk

www.kingsfund.org.uk/joinedupcare

It is never too late to be compassionate and caring!

Throughout this book, we have included real-life experiences from service-users, carers, and accounts from health care professionals. We welcome the opportunity of ending this book with a touching account from Dr David Zigmond, who recalls a fascinating story depicting correspondence from a patient who contacted him 39 years after he had treated her, and his wonderful response to this lady. The story is as follows:

**Physis: healing, growth and the hub
of personal continuity of care**

A 39-year delayed follow-up correspondence with Sally

David Zigmond

Explanatory introduction

Occasionally benign coincidence far exceeds mere serendipity, as if
the cosmos has somehow read and responded to our intent. Receiving
the letter was one of those occasions: its primally evocative and illustrative power far exceeds its apparent brevity and plain speaking. This
needs some explanation.

First the stage

For several years I have been increasingly resolute in pursuing qualitative research into the nature and significance of personal continuity of healthcare. I have been led to this by witnessing and enduring
the consequences of its progressive loss, especially in the latter third
of my professional lifetime. From this has come some understanding. For example, much of this involution derives from the fact that
relationships are more difficult to code, manufacture, manage, quantify and research than, say, drugs or physical procedures. This is a
conundrum. Rather than acknowledging its difficulty we have instead
worsened it by creating something of an academic (then economic
and administrative) oligarchy from the 'safer' confines of more easily
codifiable and quantifiable research and knowledge – the Shibboleths
of 'Evidence Basis', a kind of nouveau riche Ruling Class. This newer
and narrower culture then often wreaks blind damage because subtle, and thus less measurable, aspects of care then become liable to
indifferent neglect or, worse, rationalised hostility and exclusion. In
this arena of collateral damage the loss of personal continuity of care
is one of the most important and egregious examples. When I was a
young practitioner I was encouraged to develop and nurture this earlier longer-term and personal approach. I did not then perceive the
probability of its extinction.

(continued)

(continued)

Now, the events

I am perusing a letter, one of many: there are always more. My eyes scan for the sender, semi-consciously, to decide on priority and degree of attention. The name galvanises my distant memory. I then search for other details, to confirm my guess: it is correct. I have not heard from Sally for thirty-nine years. My visual memory quickly yields her face, its expressions, thence to her mien and spirit; I remember a very sensitive, melancholic and intelligent young woman struggling with her own shadows, intensity and complexity. I cannot remember anything more precise about her symptom-constellation, or her life or family history. I suppose she would be called 'Chronic severe depressive dysthymia': a more adventurous psychiatrist might also risk 'underlying conflicts and struggles with identity formation'.

As I write this I have not refreshed, checked or garnered more details: the account is thus fresh but unrefined. My recollection is that my encounters with Sally spanned about three years and were located in three consecutive Greater London hospitals. I was then a young trainee psychiatrist, very interested in unproceduralised influences of healing. I was certainly receptive to psychotherapeutic ideas but had not (yet) any training. I was only marginally older than Sally and not that differently endowed with resources and problems. I knew this but was able – with care – to sequestrate 'it' but not myself: our roles were then clearly different – our selves and existential predicaments were not. Her letter, after four decades, indicates a further convergence of our common humanity.

Sally's letter is a pithy personal testament of great power and – I believe – importance to all healthcare professionals. Her clear and candid account is suffused with many themes, all of which merit long thought and discussion. I certainly will not attempt to designate these all for the reader, but instead here briefly highlight themes from the *cultures* of care that include yet transcend we two individuals.

For me, most remarkable is the evidence of how, in those previous decades, we were able to create imaginative, sensitive, flexible services. The best of these could, and did, then deliver a much more substantial *person-centred* continuity of care. For several years I worked with such services: they are now very rare. I remember my supervisory consultants being accommodating and encouraging to provide the flexibility of arrangements, space and time for this therapeutic relationship (and others) to run its course and bear its fruit. This was possible because there were, then, far fewer diktats, rules and bureaucratic obelisks stymying autonomous, responsible judgements of wisdom and experience. In those days coded and hegemonic psychiatric diagnosis was far less important than personal connection and understanding; care often proceeded down unmade tracks rather than prescribed tarmacked, generic Care Pathways; care was often a delicate dance improvised between individuals rather than an institutional march decreed by academic or administrative committees.

Sally today would be most unlikely to find such continuity of personal containment and accompaniment in any NHS Psychiatric (not Psychotherapy, remember) Services. What she then received may now seem extraordinary, but it was not uncommon then. I am saddened not just for patients, but also for the working welfare of current doctors: few, if any, will have the licence or latitude for such broad, deep or long contact with individuals, or garner the humanly profound and lasting satisfactions.

Some will say that we cannot now economically afford such bespoke services. I do not agree: such care is much cheaper than the kind of anomic, multidisciplined, multi-teamed approaches that flounder with great expense and poor personal connection in the current NHS. I see this regularly and spend much of my professional time trying to repair the damage. If we do not make good human sense to one another, economic and human costs are much higher.

Sally's letter was a kind of dramatic oxymoron – a shock from the anciently familiar: amidst my current healthcare concerns it rapidly crystallised into a welcome and edifying sense. For the outside reader its private significance for us both is easily imagined. This will produce many individual resonances.

Many may identify *Agape*: non-erotic, unpossessive, unidealised love that is probably essential to *Physis*. The institutional and cultural themes invite opportunities for reflection that should not be missed: hence this invitation to greater readership. After contact and discussion with Sally she agrees. This is thus a documentary presentation, and to anchor authenticity real names are used.

I have attached my reply to her, largely for human interest. The correspondence is unedited, apart from the omission of addresses. Claybury refers to Claybury Hospital, then a large psychiatric hospital in suburban east London. It closed about twenty years ago.

(continued)

(continued)

Letter 1

3 June 2013

Dear David Zigmond

Back in the 1970s I was a patient of yours. At first an outpatient at North Middlesex Hospital and then I became an inpatient in Claybury.

I met John at Claybury and although at the time many people advised against us getting together, we went on to have a happy 30 years. Like everyone we had our ups and downs, had three great kids, Rachel, Paul and Natalie, and now three lovely grandchildren too.

He died 3 days after that anniversary in 2006. I continued my long career in nursing which has changed so much from those early years and in the last decade I focused on palliative care which was more in tune with my own values and beliefs on patient centred care. I retired last year as all the NHS changes finally wore me down!

I'm writing not to just tell you all this information but to let you know what a difference you have made to my life. You really cared, you made me feel like I was important, not just another NHS patient. You listened and believed in me. I don't often talk about that time to many people, but when I do I say how you made me feel safe and I believed that you wouldn't leave me – and you didn't. I left and never told you what a big impact you had on my life and that I knew I would never sink into those dark depths of depression again, I felt healed. That experience influenced every area of my life and work and the person I became.

Radical changes have taken place in mental care over the years but it wasn't just about the system, I was so fortunate to have had you as my Doctor. I don't know how difficult it was in those days to keep me as a patient when you moved hospitals, but you did and it made all the difference. I've never forgotten, it's just taken me a long time and before any more time passes, I just want to say a heartfelt 'Thank you, you saved my life'.

Best wishes
Sally Baynes (Davies)

Letter 2

15 June 2013

Dear Sally

Thank you so much for your candid and unsentimentally heartfelt letter.

I very quickly recalled your face and your spirit though, interestingly, I cannot remember your 'clinical' details, your 'history'. It is instructive, what we retain of one another.

I find your letter remarkable for the span of time you recall and the unaffected clarity and veracity of your account. I am deeply gratified and moved

*that the 'cuttings' I offered you so long ago were cherished, planted and nur-
tured by you and have steadily borne fruit, over a lifetime. In parallel it has
been my conviction, over my working lifetime, that this kind of activity should
often lie at the heart of what we do for one another. In these realms most damage
and most healing is human.*

*It sounds to me as if your 'recovery' has gone far beyond the medically
mapped realms of 'symptom relief' and 'good clinical outcome'. You indicate
that most wondrous and humbling transformation: you have turned your
painful burden into a compassionate and healing gift, for yourself and others.
It seems that this has cascaded through your marriage to two generations of
family, and beyond that to your many recipients of palliative care nursing. All
of this is heartening for me, too: our healing and nourishment of one another
is often unobvious.*

*But there are shadows, too, where I also wish to join you. You refer to your
'patient centred values and beliefs . . . being worn down', leading to your retirement (from the NHS). Likewise, your reference to 'radical changes in mental
healthcare' making your own previous healing experiences most unlikely now. I
resonate with this: such concerns are at the centre of my vocational life.*

*We are here different in our adjustment: you have expediently retired to
your more accessible gratifications of family and grandchildren; I remain
contentiously engaged with heroic obstinacy, possibly because I do not yet have
grandchildren (though the social and biological machinery looks promising).*

*It seems that as we get older we find solace and peace in a few simple and
timeless maxims: 'Counting our Blessings . . . Seeing what is there, not what is
not . . . '. Simple to say, yet often so difficult to live by. It sounds as if you have
managed a great deal.*

*Your letter has particular and intense value for you and I. But I think it
has messages that are universally important, especially for healthcare workers. What you talk of lies before, behind and beyond all trainings, texts, systems, manuals, data and codes which now weary and alienate so many.*

With suitable safeguards, could we publish these letters?

*Whatever your reply I have found it deeply satisfying to have heard from you
in this way: such communications give great difficulties even deeper meaning.*

*With warmest wishes
David Zigmond*

References

Francis, R. QC (2013) *Report of the Mid Staffordshire NHS Foundation Trust Public
Inquiry.* House of Commons: Stationery Office (Vols 1–3).
Stuckler, D. and Basu S. (2013) *The Body Economic: Why Austerity Kills.* London: Allen
Lane.

Glossary

Attachment Theory: Describes the dynamics of long-term relationships between people. It argues that most importantly an infant needs to develop a relationship with at least one primary care giver for normal social and emotional development to occur. It is most associated with the work of psychoanalyst John Bowlby (1907–1990).

Austerity Policy: Is used by governments to reduce the demand for luxuries and consumer goods.

Beveridge Report: Report by Lord Beveridge of 1942 advocating the creation of a NHS.

Care Quality Council (CQC): Is an organization set up by the UK government to check whether hospitals, care homes and care services are meeting national standards.

Compassion Distance: Are structural barriers which prevent compassion taking place.

Concept: An idea especially an abstract idea used by our thought processes to classify the world in some way.

Covenant: Is a binding agreement or contract, usually, but not always, where finance is involved.

Evidence Based Medicine (EBM): Seeks to assess the strength of the evidence of risks and benefits of treatment and diagnostic tests. This helps clinicians predict whether a treatment will do more good than harm.

Experiential Learning: Is the process of making meaning from direct experience i.e. learning by doing. Major theorists include the philosopher and educationalist John Dewey (1859–1952), David A. Kolb educational theorist (1939–) and developmental psychologist Jean Piaget (1896–1980).

Foundation Trust: These are considered mutual structures akin to cooperatives where local people, patients and staff can become members and governors and hold the Trust to account.

Francis Report: The report into the care provided by Mid Staffordshire NHS Foundation Trust published in 2012 under the Inquiry Chairman Robert Frances QC.

Globalisation: The process enabling markets to operate worldwide often providing worldwide and standardized organization, e.g. McDonald's.

Health Care Professional (HCP): A person who by education, training, certification, or licence is qualified to and is engaged in providing health care. This is often extended to health care workers (HCW) those who may not be qualified but who also have a direct input into care e.g. porters, cleaners, hospital cooks etc.

Humanism: Philosophically is the denial of any power or moral value superior to that of humanity. It is often associated with the thought of philosophical or cultural movements e.g. Italian Renaissance

Keogh: Sir Bruce Keogh author of a report a review of 14 NHS 2013 Trusts which proposed a fundamental shift in provision of urgent care, with more extensive services outside hospital and patients with more serious or life threatening conditions receiving treatment in centres with the best clinical teams, expertise and equipment.

The Kings Fund: Is an independent charitable organization that seeks to improve health care in the UK by providing research and health policy analysis and publications. Using the insights from research it helps to shape policy to bring about behavioural change in the health service

Lord Morris of Castle Morris (1930–2001): British poet, critic and professor of literature. He became the Labour Party's deputy chief whip and education spokesman in the House of Lords.

Managerialism: Is the application of managerial techniques to the running of businesses or organizations not necessarily associated with the world of business e.g. the National Health Service.

MeSH: Is an abbreviation derived from *Medical Subject Headings,* the list of medical terms used by the National Library of Medicine (NLM) for its computerized system of storage and retrieval of published medical reports. The system is also used for indexing medical references published in the monthly and annual volumes of *Index Medicus,* published by the NLM.

Mind Blindness: It can be described as a cognitive disorder where an individual is unable to attribute mental states to the self and others. As a result of the disorders the individual is unaware of the mental states of others. The theory asserts that children are unable to exercise empathy with others. This inability hinders normal development in children by not enabling them to experience mental states in others.

National Health Service: UK creation of a comprehensive health and rehabilitation service, from 'the cradle to the grave', for the prevention and care of disease. Implemented across the UK by 1948.

NHS Trust: Is an important part of the UK government's progamme to create a 'patient led' NHS.

Neo-Liberalism: Is an economic philosophy emerging in Europe during the 1930s which attempted to chart a 'Third or Middle Way' between classical liberalism and collectivist central planning. Renewed recently by political parties like the New Labour Party under its then Prime Minister Tony Blair.

Non-Governmental Organisation (NGO) legally constituted organizations worldwide that operate independently from any form of government.

The term is usually applied only to organizations that pursue wider social aims and sometimes political aspects, but are not openly political organization.

Oxymoron. An epigrammatic effect, by which contradictory terms are used in conjunction, e.g. cruel compassion.

Phenomenology: Is a philosophical method of enquiry best associated with Edmund Husserl (1859–1938). As a philosophy it is not an empirical technique but an a priori investigation of meanings.

Planetree Foundation: Was founded in the USA 1978. The major philosophy of the Foundation is based around patient centred care, the basic premise being that health care should be organized first and foremost around the needs of patients. Via this viewpoint it aims to transform the culture of care which it does through a partnering process with health care providers across the USA. The philosophy in bringing about change is always to put the needs of the patients first.

Point of Care Programme: It aims to enable health care staff in hospitals to deliver the quality of care they would want for themselves and their own families. Its premise is to focus on patients' experience and work on methods to intervene and improve current medical practice. 'We define patients' experience as the totality of events and interactions that occur in the course of episodes of care' (Goodrich and Cornwell 2008).

Praxis: Is the process by which a theory, lesson, or skill is enacted, practised, embodied or realized. 'Praxis' may also refer to the act of engaging, applying, exercising, realizing or practising ideas.

Project 2000: A Report by the United Kingdom Central Council for Nursing Midwifery and Health Visiting published in 2000. The Report represented the recommendations of the Council about the best way forward for the development of nursing, midwifery and health visitors. Part of this way forward one of the recommendations was an all degree profession for nurses.

RCGP: Is the Royal College of General Practitioners.

Samaritans: Charity available 24 hours a day to provide confidential emotional support for people who are experiencing feelings of distress, despair or suicidal thoughts.

Schadenfreude. German, meaning delight in another's misfortune.

Schwartz Rounds: The Schwartz Center Rounds brings doctors, nurses and other caregivers together to discuss the human side of healthcare. They provide a monthly one hour service for staff from all health care disciplines to discuss difficult emotional and social issues arising from patient care. The aim of the Rounds is to support health care staff in the provision of compassionate care to their patients.

Stoic: Was a member of the school of philosophy founded in Athens by Zeno of Citrium in the third century BC. Basically stoicism taught that a person needs to behave virtuously and to keep destructive emotions in check. Key words for the Stoic are self-control and fortitude

Symposium: A conference or meeting for discussion especially associated with ancient Greece.

Troika: Is the tripart committee led by the European Commission with the European Central Bank and the International Monetary Fund, that organized loans to the governments of Greece, Ireland, Portugal and Cyprus

WONCA: World Organization of National Colleges, Academies and Academic Associations of General Practitioners. The mission of WONCA is to maintain and improve the quality of life of peoples of the world through defining clear values that help and promote high standards of health care in general practice

Index

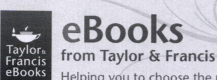

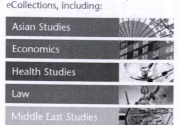